AF801252

International Perspectives on Aging

Volume 47

Series Editors

Jason L. Powell, Department of Social and Political Science, University of Chester Chester, UK

Sheying Chen, Department of Public Administration, Pace University, New York, USA

The study of aging is continuing to increase rapidly across multiple disciplines. This wide-ranging series on International Perspectives on Aging provides readers with much-needed comprehensive texts and critical perspectives on the latest research, policy, and practical developments. Both aging and globalization have become a reality of our times, yet a systematic effort of a global magnitude to address aging is yet to be seen. The series bridges the gaps in the literature and provides cutting-edge debate on new and traditional areas of comparative aging, all from an international perspective. More specifically, this book series on International Perspectives on Aging puts the spotlight on international and comparative studies of aging.

Marja Aartsen • Iuliana Precupetu
Bianca Suanet
Editors

Macro Social Influences on Loneliness in Later Life

Towards a Better Understanding of the Loneliness Paradox in Europe

Springer

Editors
Marja Aartsen
NOVA Norwegian Social Research
OsloMet – Oslo Metropolitan University
Oslo, Norway

Iuliana Precupetu
Research Institute for Quality of Life
Romanian Academy
Bucureşti, Romania

Bianca Suanet
Amstelveen, The Netherlands

ISSN 2197-5841 ISSN 2197-585X (electronic)
International Perspectives on Aging
ISBN 978-3-031-94564-9 ISBN 978-3-031-94565-6 (eBook)
https://doi.org/10.1007/978-3-031-94565-6

This work was supported by Oslo Metropolitan University – OsloMet – NOVA, P.O. Box 4, St. Olavs plass, NO-0130 Oslo, Norway.

© The Editor(s) (if applicable) and The Author(s) 2025. This book is an open access publication.

Open Access This book is licensed under the terms of the Creative Commons Attribution 4.0 International License (http://creativecommons.org/licenses/by/4.0/), which permits use, sharing, adaptation, distribution and reproduction in any medium or format, as long as you give appropriate credit to the original author(s) and the source, provide a link to the Creative Commons license and indicate if changes were made.
The images or other third party material in this book are included in the book's Creative Commons license, unless indicated otherwise in a credit line to the material. If material is not included in the book's Creative Commons license and your intended use is not permitted by statutory regulation or exceeds the permitted use, you will need to obtain permission directly from the copyright holder.
The use of general descriptive names, registered names, trademarks, service marks, etc. in this publication does not imply, even in the absence of a specific statement, that such names are exempt from the relevant protective laws and regulations and therefore free for general use.
The publisher, the authors and the editors are safe to assume that the advice and information in this book are believed to be true and accurate at the date of publication. Neither the publisher nor the authors or the editors give a warranty, expressed or implied, with respect to the material contained herein or for any errors or omissions that may have been made. The publisher remains neutral with regard to jurisdictional claims in published maps and institutional affiliations.

This Springer imprint is published by the registered company Springer Nature Switzerland AG
The registered company address is: Gewerbestrasse 11, 6330 Cham, Switzerland

If disposing of this product, please recycle the paper.

Foreword

When writing a foreword to a book on loneliness, one must surely begin by asking why. Why, over long sweeps of time, does our preoccupation with loneliness endure? Why do we continue to theorize loneliness; to refine our methodological approaches; to search for interventions that will ameliorate its impact? Why would a group of scholars devote the huge amount of effort it takes to write a book that takes such a thorough look at broad societal contexts of loneliness?

There are many reasons for our tenacity. At its core, loneliness reflects our belief in the importance of social connections and the negative consequences of their absence. It follows a tradition of naming social phenomena in a way that underscores how their absence signifies exclusion of some groups of people. Poverty, homelessness, and unemployment are examples. They draw direct attention to the lack of income security, housing and decent work that comprise the material resources that are hallmarks of doing well. Loneliness also draws attention to exclusion from valued resources. In this case, resources are the social connections that many see as fundamental to our humanity.

The alarm about loneliness speaks to its centrality in our thinking about the wellbeing of populations. We see this concern in the language used to describe its rising incidence. We speak of loneliness as an epidemic; as a public health concern; as a crisis. Each reflects a sense of heightened concern that too many people lack the relationships that make life worthwhile. At its darkest, loneliness is seen as an existential threat with people's very survival dependent on their relationships with others who sustain them. In contrast, the metaphor of social capital frames relationships as assets, positing that we draw on our connections to others to live and to thrive in the world. Governments speak of the need to challenge economic measures such as GDP as the indicator of a nation's productivity by shifting the emphasis to wellbeing of nations and positioning social resources as key indicators.

In the introduction to this volume, the editors say that theirs is not the first book on loneliness, nor will it be the last. This statement acknowledges the long journey towards understanding loneliness and reducing its impact. So what's left to do? The longstanding research agenda to understand experiences of loneliness might arguably be seen as successfully completed. We know much about the components of loneliness, its measurement and its outcomes. While we continue to have our conceptual differences about nuances in the definition of loneliness, there is considerable agreement that it reflects a gap between what a person wishes from their social relationships and their evaluation of them. Despite this progress, successful interventions to alleviate loneliness are worryingly elusive. Although loneliness is in the end an individual experience, addressing it through local solutions that are oriented towards lonely individuals has had mixed results at best.

The book reflects the authors' resumption of the narrative. They frame loneliness as an indicator of widening social inequalities in an increasingly divisive world, fuelled by macro-social trends that threaten the formation of valuable social groups. The focus is on older adults. The interrogation is of how community and societal contexts influence patterns of loneliness. The geographic context is Europe. A goal is to unravel the loneliness paradox.

The contextual lens prompts questions about assumptions about settings that are relationship-dense yet have high rates of loneliness. The loneliness paradox was named because of the counter-intuitive finding that the loneliest older people live in countries where there are high rates of co-residence and large, proximate networks. We see in this finding a parallel family paradox worthy of further consideration. Might it be that large proximate family networks or co-residence are not always settings that stave off loneliness among older adults in countries where such living arrangements are common. How might a macro contextual lens be applied to assessing the relationship between familist national policies and loneliness experiences?

Bringing major social trends and disruptions into the loneliness narrative is new to the loneliness narrative. Climate change, political instability, and forced migration all have potential to truncate personal social connections but also to shape the conditions that mitigate or exacerbate loneliness. A critical look at which older people are left behind during these major disruptions will help us track patterns of inequity. It will also help us further clarify the place of loneliness as a metric for exclusion and will add considerably to our knowledge of how older people can be in the world.

University of Stirling, Stirling, United Kingdom Norah Keating
Den Haag, the Netherlands Jenny Gierveld

Acknowledgements

NOVA—Norwegian Social Research at Oslo Metropolitan University has covered the fees associated with open access publishing.

Competing Interests The editors have no conflicts of interest to declare that are relevant to the content of this book.

Contents

Editors and Contributors

About the Editors

Marja Aartsen, PhD, is currently research professor and social gerontologist at NOVA—Norwegian Social Research at OsloMet. She is specialized in longitudinal research on social relations, social exclusion, loneliness, and cognitive functioning in the second half of life. She is interested in social issues related to ageing in place and active or successful ageing. Recent research projects and collaborations include gendered pathways to exclusion from social relations (GENPATH), reducing old-age social exclusion (ROSENET), and a multidimensional approach to social exclusion and its health consequences (AMASE). She was editor of the European Journal of Ageing from 2017 until summer 2022.

Iuliana Precupetu, PhD, is a senior researcher at the Research Institute for Quality of Life, Romanian Academy, and the Research Institute of the University of Bucharest. She is a sociologist specializing in quality of life, health inequalities, and social exclusion in later life. Her current interests include the relationship between social exclusion in older age and mental health, as well as the application of life course methods to quality of life research. Most recently, she coordinated the AMASE research project—A multidimensional approach to social exclusion in later life: health consequences for ageing populations.

Bianca Suanet, PhD, is a sociologist, specializing in loneliness, social relations, and care use among older adults, especially in relation to the impact of societal and policy changes. She was formerly Professor of Ageing and Social Change at the Linköping University in Sweden and Associate Professor in Sociology and Head of the Social Functioning Group of the Longitudinal Aging Study Amsterdam at the Vrije Universiteit Amsterdam in the Netherlands. Currently, her research projects encompass studies on the relationship between macro-level factors and loneliness and optimizing interventions against loneliness based on scientific evidence for older migrants.

Contributors

Marja Aartsen Norwegian Social Research (NOVA), Oslo Metropolitan University, Oslo, Norway

Iuliana Precupetu Research Institute for Quality of Life, Romanian Academy, Bucharest, Romania

Research Institute of the University of Bucharest, Bucharest, Romania

Bianca Suanet Amsterdam, The Netherlands

Fredrica Nyqvist Faculty of Education and Welfare Studies, Social Policy, Åbo Akademi University, Vaasa, Finland

Joanna McHugh Power Department of Psychology, Maynooth University, Kildare, Republic of Ireland

Laura Coll-Planas Research group on Methodology, Methods, Models and Outcomes of Health and Social Sciences (M3O), University of Vic-Central University of Catalonia (UVic-UCC), Vic, Spain

Institute for Research and Innovation, Life Sciences and Health in Central Catalonia (IRIS-CC), Vic, Spain

Theo G. van Tilburg Department of Sociology, Faculty of Social Sciences and Department of Epidemiology & Data Science, Vrije Universiteit Amsterdam and Amsterdam University Medical Centers, Amsterdam, The Netherlands

Sofie Van Regenmortel Society and Ageing Research Lab, Vrije Universiteit Brussel (VUB), Brussels, Belgium

Elisa Tiilikainen Department of Social Sciences, University of Eastern Finland, Kuopio, Finland

Hanna Ristolainen Department of Social Sciences, University of Eastern Finland, Kuopio, Finland

Vanessa Burholt School of Nursing/School of Population Health, University of Auckland, Auckland, New Zealand

Swansea University, Wales, UK

Lena Dahlberg School of Health and Welfare, Dalarna University, Falun, Sweden

Aging Research Center, Karolinska Institutet and Stockholm University, Stockholm, Sweden

Marian Vasile Department of Sociology, Faculty of Sociology and Social Work, University of Bucharest, Bucharest, Romania

Sunwoo Lee Faculty of Physical Culture at Palacký University Olomouc, Olomouc, Czech Republic

Laura Tufă Research Institute for Quality of Life within the Romanian Academy, Bucharest, Romania

Research Institute of the University of Bucharest, Bucharest, Romania

Alexander Seifert University of Applied Sciences Northwestern Switzerland, Olten, Switzerland

Liat Ayalon The Louis and Gabi Weisfeld School of Social Work, Bar Ilan University, Ramat Gan, Israel

Lisa Joanne Klasen German Centre of Gerontology, Berlin, Germany

Department of Psychology, Humboldt-Universität zu Berlin, Berlin, Germany

Mareike Bünning German Centre of Gerontology, Berlin, Germany

Nadiya Kelle German Centre of Gerontology, Berlin, Germany

Clemens Tesch-Römer German Centre of Gerontology, Berlin, Germany

Oliver Huxhold German Centre of Gerontology, Berlin, Germany

Cosmina Pop Research Institute for Quality of Life, Romanian Academy, Bucharest, Romania

George Pavlidis Institute for Social and Psychological Studies, Karlstad University, Karlstad, Sweden

Mihaela Ghenţa National Scientific Institute for Labour and Social Protection (INCSMPS), Bucharest, Romania

Aniela Matei National Scientific Institute for Labour and Social Protection (INCSMPS), Bucharest, Romania

Thomas Hansen Norwegian Institute of Public Health, Oslo, Norway

Part I
Central Theme of the Book

Chapter 1
Introduction. For a Macro-social Perspective on Loneliness

Marja Aartsen, Iuliana Precupetu, and Bianca Suanet

1.1 Introduction

This is a book on loneliness. It is by no means the first, nor will it be the last. Loneliness is a strong negative feeling that arises when there is a mismatch between the number and quality of social relationships one has and those one desires (Perlman & Peplau, 1981). While loneliness often fades over time, it persists for a substantial part of the population with negative consequences for health and mortality (Holt-Lunstad, 2022). Research on loneliness is not new, but the recent spike in cases during the COVID pandemic due to social distancing regulations has put the need for loneliness interventions high on political agendas. Consequently, the volume of research studies on loneliness has increased significantly in recent years. Although there are numerous loneliness interventions, very few can reduce loneliness substantially (Masi et al., 2011; Hickin et al., 2021). Some of the most well-known risk factors for loneliness are not living with a partner, a small social network and social inactivity (e.g., Hawkley & Cacioppo, 2010). One would therefore expect that in countries where many people live alone and families are relatively small, loneliness would be highly prevalent. But this is not what we see. On the contrary! Loneliness is most prevalent in countries where most people live with other people and where opportunities for social interaction are good. This paradoxical result, first observed in 1990 (Jylhä & Jokela, 1990), has been seen repeatedly in the years since (e.g., Yang & Victor, 2011; Hansen & Slagsvold, 2015; Heu et al., 2021). Despite

M. Aartsen (✉)
Norwegian Social Research (NOVA), Oslo Metropolitan University, Oslo, Norway
e-mail: maraar@oslomet.no

I. Precupetu · B. Suanet

Research Institute for Quality of Life, Romanian Academy, Bucharest, Romania

© The Author(s) 2025
M. Aartsen et al. (eds.), *Macro Social Influences on Loneliness in Later Life*, International Perspectives on Aging 47,
https://doi.org/10.1007/978-3-031-94565-6_1

the substantial body of knowledge on loneliness, we have not been able to solve the loneliness paradox.

Much of the research has concentrated on the individual or micro-level, but loneliness, like many other social phenomena, cannot be reduced to an individual problem (Bronfenbrenner, 1995; Cotterell et al., 2018; Kaplan, 2004). The social construction of loneliness has largely been overlooked, and little is known about the potential impact of communities, neighbors, and neighborhoods (the meso-level), as well as the influence of the culture and structure of the society in which people live. Even less attention has been given to the potential impact of recent mega-societal trends on loneliness (e.g., climate change, digitalization, eroding trust). Ignoring the broader social context in loneliness research can be considered a 'mistake' (Chater & Loewenstein, 2022), leading to a biased and incomplete understanding of loneliness. With this book, we argue that without considering the macro-level determinants of loneliness, our understanding of loneliness remains fundamentally incomplete. Future research and interventions must acknowledge and address these broader societal influences to develop more effective and sustainable solutions for loneliness.

The book focuses on older adults (65+), specifically those in their third or fourth age (Laslett, 1989). The third age refers to the post-retirement period marked by relative freedom, few job or caregiving obligations, good health, and an active lifestyle. In contrast, the fourth age is characterized by significant physical and mental decline, increased dependence, and often higher levels of loneliness. The correlates of loneliness are often age-specific, meaning findings from older populations may not necessarily apply to younger individuals. For instance, losing a partner at a young age can have a greater impact on loneliness than in later life, when widowhood is more expected. Additionally, older adults may adopt different strategies to avoid loneliness due to reduced energy for maintaining social relationships (Huxhold & Fiori, 2024), and their motivation to connect with others may shift as their time horizon shortens (Carstensen, 1992). As the population of older adults grows, particularly those reaching very old age, understanding loneliness in later life has become more urgent. Existing knowledge remains limited, especially regarding macro-level factors. By shedding light on how societal structures shape loneliness, this book moves beyond seeing it as purely an individual issue, offering valuable insights for researchers, policymakers, intervention stakeholders, and citizens.

1.2 The History of Loneliness Research

Loneliness has fascinated scientists, writers, and artists for centuries. One of the earliest works addressing loneliness is by the Roman statesman and philosopher Cicero (106-43 BC), who wrote about friendship in his work De Amicitia. While Cicero did not use the term "loneliness" as we understand it today, his writings highlight the importance of friendship as a remedy for the negative feelings that arise from being without significant others. People often have an intuitive understanding of loneliness as a devastating negative feeling that arises when a person feels separated from other people. However, a closer examination of scholarly and artistic works reveals a lack of a unified understanding of loneliness. This likely stems from the various disciplines that have explored the concept, each tapping into different aspects of loneliness. In recent decades, research on loneliness has grown considerably. From 1970 to 1980, a little more than 150 scientific publications written in English included the word "loneliness" in the title, whereas from 2010 to 2020 this number was around 7000, with the majority published in the last four years.

1.2.1 First Generation Loneliness Research

The first systematic scholarly work on loneliness was conducted by Peplau and Perlman in 1982. It was mainly devoted to the classification of explanations for loneliness that were present in the literature at that time. One group of explanations was based on clinical samples. It conceived loneliness generally as a disease that can be attributed to individual factors. The psychodynamic approach sees loneliness rooted in negative childhood experiences (e.g., Fromm-Reichmann, 1959). The phenomenological approach, with Rogers (1970) as prominent representative, perceives loneliness as the consequence of a discrepancy between the true inner self and the self that can be manifested. However, another approach also based on clinical samples did not consider loneliness as a negative state or disease, but as a normal human condition and creative force from which a person can learn (Moustakas, 1972; see also the later work by Mijuskovic, 2012). This approach is referred to as the existential approach by Perlman and Peplau (1982).

The clinical approaches to loneliness were criticized by Bowman (1955) who can be considered an early advocate of the sociological approach to loneliness. Bowman argued that the origins of loneliness lie outside the individual, such as in socialization, life events, and mass media (e.g., Bowman, 1955). Yet another group of explanations considers loneliness as the consequence of both individual and societal factors. For example, the interactionist approach from Weiss (1973) suggests that the origins of loneliness stem from an interaction between both individual attributes and situational factors. Although the role of situational factors, such as role engagements, in shaping the experience of loneliness is acknowledged, these factors are still often viewed primarily in relation to the individual, rather than being considered from a broader societal or contextual perspective. Two other theoretical approaches, the privacy approach (Derlega & Chaikin, 1977) and the general systems approach (Flanders, 1982) claim that the origins of loneliness are at the individual and societal level. The privacy approach assumes that people strive for a balance between the ideal and achieved number of social relations, and that a lack of privacy can also lead to loneliness. The general systems approach perceives loneliness as a feedback mechanism that stimulates the individual and society to maintain an optimal level of contact. Like the existential approach, the general systems approach understands loneliness as something positive and functional.

The cognitive approach developed by Perlman and Peplau (1982) defines loneliness as a negative state of feeling alone that occurs when the number or quality of social relations is lower than expected. Hence, although lonely people are often alone, they can also be surrounded by others (lonely in the crowd) if the quality in the relationships is lower than they wish (Perlman & Peplau, 1982). This approach to loneliness has become the dominant approach to loneliness in western societies. Although it is not so much a theory about the origins of loneliness, it provides a clear conceptualization of loneliness. Since Perlman and Peplau's seminal work on loneliness, more theories on loneliness have emerged. For example, the attachment theory of Bowlby (1982) is in line with the clinical approaches to loneliness and suggests that children who lack secure attachment with a mother or caregiver will be less able to form close relationships in later life and are therefore more prone to loneliness. In line with the general systems approach is the evolutionary theory of loneliness (Cacioppo & Cacioppo, 2018). This approach describes loneliness as a warning system, like hunger, that motivates people to reconnect with other people to enhance survival.

Finally, cultural explanations of loneliness, which emphasize the influence of the wider social context and the role of norms and values, are closely aligned with the sociological approach to loneliness. For example, the collectivistic-individualist explanation suggests that having few social contacts mainly leads to loneliness in collectivistic countries where the norm is to have regular social contact, whereas in individualistic countries being alone is more the norm and therefore less likely to provoke loneliness (Lykes & Kemmelmeier, 2014). Other recent sociological approaches to loneliness refer to loneliness stigma, and how it can reinforce norms for social relations and exclude people who do not adhere to these norms which in turn can induce loneliness (Barreto et al., 2022; Neves & Petersen, 2025). Heu and others (2021) introduced the concept "relational mobility" to explain cultural variations in loneliness prevalence. Relational mobility is the normative freedom to choose the relationships one wants to have as opposed to those one is supposed to have according to the norms in the respective society. In countries with more restrictive or more demanding norms about social relationships, the risk of loneliness may be higher. As loneliness research advances, integrating these perspectives with a clear focus on other macro-level societal influences appears to be a logical next step.

1.2.2 Second Generation of Loneliness Research

A decade ago, a second generation of loneliness theories emerged that further refined the integration of micro- and macro-level influences of loneliness. The first integrated theoretical framework was developed by de Jong Gierveld and Tesch-Römer in 2012. Their model outlines how cultural norms, demographic composition and societal wealth and welfare influence the social expectations of people, thereby modifying the impact of living conditions and social integration on loneliness. Huxhold and Fiori (2024) developed a multi-level model which they labeled the Differential Investment of Resources (DIRe) model (for an application to societal crisis by Klasen et al., 2025: see Chap. 10 of this book). This model is particularly helpful in understanding loneliness as a dynamic element that changes over the course of life. DIRe outlines that maintaining social relations requires time and energy which are known to change with age. Central to their reasoning is that loneliness arises when the individual's expectations about e.g., intimacy, support, fun, and respect, cannot be met by close confidants, broader networks, and/or community involvement. They further argue that contextual factors such as ethnicity, cultural values and the social status of individuals impact the availability of social relations and the individual's ability to maintain social relations.

The HIDECO framework (Historical Changes in Developmental Context), developed by Drewelies et al. (2019), is also noteworthy. While it was not specifically designed to explain the prevalence or emergence of loneliness, it provides valuable insights into how broader social contexts influence individual experiences of loneliness. The framework describes how various aspects of the social context shape individual functioning, including loneliness. Compared to other integrated models, HIDECO offers a more detailed conceptualization of the social environment, considering multiple societal influences. It emphasizes the population distribution of resources for successful aging, such as education, financial security, and access to healthcare, which determine individuals' opportunities for maintaining social relationships. The framework also highlights changes in social and family life, including shifting family structures and evolving intergenerational relationships, which can impact the availability and quality of social connections. Additionally, technological and scientific progress, such as digitalization and medical advancements, plays a crucial role in shaping opportunities for social interaction and support. Lastly, the "Zeitgeist" and societal norms regarding social roles and aging influence expectations about older adults' social engagement, independence, and participation in society. By incorporating these elements, the HIDECO model provides a comprehensive framework for understanding how macro-level changes affect loneliness and other aspects of well-being. Its emphasis on historical and contextual factors makes it a valuable tool for examining how loneliness evolves across generations and societal transformations.

Recently, Suanet and Aartsen developed a sociological life course theory of loneliness (see Chap. 14 of this book; Suanet & Aartsen, 2025), based on a comprehensive review of sociological theories on the construction of loneliness. The model aims to clarify how sociological perspectives can enhance our understanding of the impact of macro-level factors on loneliness. The SOLO model differs from the frameworks proposed by de Jong Gierveld and Tesch-Römer (2012), the DIRe model (Huxhold & Fiori, 2024), and the HIDECO model (Drewelies et al., 2019) in that it provides a more detailed specification of sociological theories relevant to loneliness. It systematically incorporates socio-structural and socio-cultural factors at the meso- and macro-levels, as well as the five principles of life course theory—life span development, agency, time and place, timing of life events, and linked lives

(Elder et al., 2003). Additionally, it integrates the concept of cumulative (dis)advantage (Dannefer, 2003), recognizing how structural inequalities shape loneliness trajectories over the life course and within and between cohorts. By applying these sociological perspectives to loneliness research, the SOLO model introduces a novel and innovative avenue of study, emphasizing the social construction of loneliness. This approach advances our understanding of how macro-level societal structures and cultural norms influence experiences of loneliness across the life course.

1.3 Empirical Approaches to Loneliness

One critical issue in loneliness research is how loneliness is measured. Two main approaches to measure loneliness are a single direct question including the word "lonely" and multiple indirect questions avoiding the word "lonely". Direct questions such as "Do you feel lonely?" are often used due to their efficiency in large-scale surveys. However, direct questions are criticized for underestimating moderate levels of loneliness due to the stigma associated with being lonely (Lau & Gruen, 1992; Schoenmakers, 2020; Barreto et al., 2022). Indeed, a meta-analysis found that loneliness prevalence is lowest when measured with a direct question (Stegen et al., 2024). Indirect questions avoid the word "lonely" but instead use phrases such as "I miss having a really close friend" or "There are plenty of people I can rely on when having problems" (de Jong Gierveld & van Tilburg, 2006). These questions have their roots in the cognitive approach developed by Perlman and Peplau, which defines loneliness as a negative feeling that arises when the quantity or quality of social relationships falls below expectations (Perlman & Peplau, 1981).

These findings highlight the importance of critically evaluating how loneliness is measured in research and policy. A thought-provoking recent study suggested that we could identify loneliness using artificial intelligence by analyzing unstructured speech (Wang et al., 2024). Such technological advancements offer exciting new possibilities for detecting loneliness in natural conversations. As loneliness is a fundamentally subjective experience, shaped both by internal emotions and broader cultural and societal structures, we argue that achieving a more solid conceptualization and measurement of loneliness—through both validated self-report measures and context-sensitive qualitative approaches—remains a top priority for future research, in correspondence with new technologies that will continue to evolve. This also applies to exploring different dimensions of loneliness, such as existential loneliness, as well as understanding how taboos and stigma shape people's willingness to report loneliness.

In empirical research on loneliness, the mechanisms linking micro, meso, and macro conditions to loneliness are often not explicitly specified. However, gaining a deeper understanding of the etiology of later-life loneliness requires examining how these conditions influence both an individual's desired quantity and quality of social relationships, as well as their ability to achieve those relationships. For instance, cultural factors, such as whether a society is collectivistic or individualistic, may strongly shape individuals' expectations regarding their social networks. In contrast, structural factors—including wealth, climate change, and digitalization—play a crucial role in determining the actual opportunities for social connection. These factors also influence how access to social interactions is distributed across different groups within society, potentially reinforcing inequalities. The relevance of this perspective will be revisited in the final chapter, where we reflect on the contributions of the book's chapters and assess whether this approach provides valuable insights for understanding loneliness in later life.

One of the key challenges in studying macro-level influences is that many societal factors overlap, making it difficult to disentangle their individual effects. This has contributed to a lag in empirical research at the macro level. To address this gap, this book introduces Qualitative Comparative Analysis (QCA), a method derived from political science that allows researchers to identify necessary and/or sufficient macro conditions for loneliness. QCA is a set-theoretical approach (Ragin, 2008) that has proven valuable in political science but remains underutilized in loneliness research. By applying this technique in Chap. 11 of this book (Precupetu et al., 2025) this contribution seeks to advance the methodological toolkit for studying macro-social influences on loneliness and provide new insights into the structural and cultural determinants of this growing societal issue.

1.4 Structure of the Book

This book explores the macro-social influences on loneliness in later life, emphasizing how societal structures, cultural contexts, and broader social transformations shape the experience of loneliness. Dedicated to the social construction of loneliness and the notable heterogeneity in its prevalence across European countries, this volume brings together a distinguished selection of experts who share their latest insights on meso- and macro-level influences, cultural and structural theories, and the impact of digitalization, climate change, and societal crises. Divided into five parts, the book addresses key aspects of this complex issue.

The first part introduces the central themes, outlining the relevance of loneliness as a societal concern and discussing the limitations of existing research, which predominantly focuses on individual-level factors. It highlights the need for a multi-level approach that incorporates micro, meso, and macro perspectives to fully understand the contextual influences on loneliness. The second part delves into theoretical perspectives, offering a comprehensive framework for understanding loneliness at different levels. It examines the interplay between individual, relational, and societal factors while also exploring cultural and social exclusion perspectives that shed light on how loneliness manifests across different contexts. The third part presents empirical evidence, focusing on variations in loneliness across different social groups and regions in Europe. It synthesizes research on micro- and meso-level determinants while also providing a review of macro-level influences. This part highlights the role of welfare regimes, demographic trends, and broader societal conditions in shaping the prevalence and experience of loneliness. The fourth part explores recent societal developments that may influence loneliness, including digitalization, migration, climate change, and societal crises. These emerging topics illustrate how macro-level transformations can either alleviate or exacerbate loneliness, depending on how they interact with existing social structures and individual circumstances. The final part discusses methodological advancements and policy implications. It introduces an innovative approach to analyzing macro-social influences on loneliness and revisits the 'loneliness paradox' in light of new findings. The book concludes with policy recommendations and future research directions, emphasizing the need for a holistic approach that integrates individual, relational, and societal dimensions to develop more effective interventions for loneliness.

In sum, by adopting a macro-social lens, this book contributes to a deeper understanding of the societal, cultural, and policy-related determinants of loneliness. It offers a foundation for evidence-based interventions that go beyond individual-level solutions, recognizing loneliness as a socially embedded phenomenon shaped by broader societal forces. It is our hope and expectation that the book and its content will fundamentally change our understanding of loneliness and strategies to combat loneliness.

Competing Interests The authors have no conflicts of interest to declare that are relevant to the content of this chapter.

References

Barreto, M., van Breen, J., Victor, C., Hammond, C., Eccles, A., Richins, M. T., & Qualter, P. (2022). Exploring the nature and variation of the stigma associated with loneliness. *Journal of Social and Personal Relationships, 39*(9), 2658–2679. https://doi.org/10.1177/02654075221087190

Bowlby, J. (1982). Attachment and loss: Retrospect and prospect. *American Journal of Orthopsychiatry, 52*(4), 664–678.

Bowman, C. C. (1955). Loneliness and social change. *American Journal of Psychiatry, 112*(3), 194–198.

Bronfenbrenner, U. (1995). Developmental ecology through space and time: A future perspective. In P. Moen, G. H. Elder Jr., & K. Lüscher (Eds.), *Examining lives in context: Perspectives on the ecology of human development* (pp. 619–647). American Psychological Association. https://doi.org/10.1037/10176-018

Cacioppo, J. T., & Cacioppo, S. (2018). Loneliness in the modern age: An Evolutionary Theory of Loneliness (ETL). *Advances in Experimental Social Psychology, 59*, 127–197. https://doi.org/10.1016/bs.aesp.2018.03.003

Carstensen, L. L. (1992). Social and emotional patterns in adulthood: Support for socioemotional selectivity theory. *Psychology and Aging, 7*(3), 331. https://doi.org/10.1037/0882-7974.7.3.331

Chater, N., & Loewenstein, G. (2022). The i-frame and the s-frame: How focusing on individual-level solutions has led behavioral public policy astray. *Behavioral and Brain Sciences, 46*, e147. https://doi.org/10.1017/S0140525X22002023

Cotterell, N., Buffel, T., & Phillipson, C. (2018). Preventing social isolation in older people. *Maturitas, 113*, 80–84. https://doi.org/10.1016/j.maturitas.2018.04.014

Dannefer, D. (2003). Cumulative advantage/disadvantage and the life course: Cross-fertilizing age and social science theory. *The Journals of Gerontology Series B: Psychological Sciences and Social Sciences, 58*(6), S327–S337. https://doi.org/10.1093/geronb/58.6.S327

de Jong Gierveld, J., & Tesch-Römer, C. (2012). Loneliness in old age in Eastern and Western European societies: Theoretical perspectives. *European Journal of Ageing, 9*(4), 285–295. https://doi.org/10.1007/s10433-012-0248-2

De Jong Gierveld, J., & van Tilburg, T. G. (2006). A 6-item scale for overall, emotional, and social loneliness: Confirmatory tests on survey data. *Research on Aging, 28*(5), 582–598. https://doi.org/10.1177/0164027506289723

Derlega, V. J., & Chaikin, A. L. (1977). Privacy and self-disclosure in social relationships. *Journal of Social Issues, 33*(3), 102–115.

Drewelies, J., Huxhold, O., & Gerstorf, D. (2019). The role of historical change for adult development and aging: Towards a theoretical framework about the how and the why. *Psychology and Aging, 34*(8), 1021–1039. https://doi.org/10.1037/pag0000423

Elder, G. H., Johnson, M. K., & Crosnoe, R. (2003). The emergence and development of life course theory. In J. T. Mortimer & M. J. Shanahan (Eds.), *Handbook of the life course. Handbooks of sociology and social research*. Springer. https://doi.org/10.1007/978-0-306-48247-2_1

Flanders, J. P. (1982). A general systems approach to loneliness. In L. Peplau & D. Perlman (Eds.), *Loneliness: A sourcebook of current theory, research, and therapy*. Wiley.

Fromm-Reichmann, F. (1959). Loneliness. *Psychiatry, 22*, 1–15. https://doi.org/10.1080/00332747.1959.11023153

Hansen, T., & Slagsvold, B. (2015). Late-life loneliness in 11 European countries: Results from the Generations and Gender Survey. *Social Indicators Research, 129*(1), 445–464. https://doi.org/10.1007/s11205-015-1111-6

Hawkley, L. C., & Cacioppo, J. T. (2010). Loneliness matters: A theoretical and empirical review of consequences and mechanisms. *Annals of Behavioral Medicine, 40*(2), 218–227. https://doi.org/10.1007/s12160-010-9210-8

Heu, L. C., Hansen, N., & van Zomeren, M. (2021). Loneliness across cultures with different levels of social embeddedness: A qualitative study. *Personal Relationships, 28*(1), 56–78. https://doi.org/10.1111/pere.12367

Hickin, N., Käll, A., Shafran, R., Sutcliffe, S., Manzotti, G., & Langan, D. (2021). The effectiveness of psychological interventions for loneliness: A systematic review and meta-analysis. *Clinical Psychology Review, 88*, 102066. https://doi.org/10.1016/j.cpr.2021.102066

Holt-Lunstad, J. (2022). Social connection as a public health issue: The evidence and a systemic framework for prioritizing the "social" in social determinants of health. *Annual Review of Public Health, 43*(1), 193–213. https://doi.org/10.1146/annurev-publhealth-052020-110732

Huxhold, O., & Fiori, K. L. (2024). Understanding loneliness in late life. *Current Opinion in Psychology, 57*, 101801. https://doi.org/10.1016/j.copsyc.2024.101801

Jylhä, M., & Jokela, J. (1990). Individual experiences as cultural: A cross-cultural study on loneliness among the elderly. *Ageing and Society, 10*(3), 295–315. https://doi.org/10.1017/S0144686X00008308

Kaplan, G. A. (2004). What's wrong with social epidemiology, and how can we make it better? *Epidemiologic Reviews, 26*, 124–135. https://doi.org/10.1093/epirev/mxh010

Klasen, L. J., Bünning, M., Kelle, N., Tesch-Römer, C., & Huxhold, O. (2025). The influence of societal crises on social integration and loneliness. In M. Aartsen, I. Precupetu, & B. Suanet (Eds.), *Macro social influences on loneliness in later life: Towards a better understanding of the loneliness paradox in later life*. Springer.

Laslett, P. (1989). *A fresh map of life: The emergence of the Third Age*. Harvard University Press.

Lau, S., & Gruen, G. E. (1992). The social stigma of loneliness: Effect of target person's and perceiver's sex. *Personality and Social Psychology Bulletin, 18*(2), 182–189. https://doi.org/10.1177/0146167292182009

Lykes, V. A., & Kemmelmeier, M. (2014). What predicts loneliness? Cultural difference between individualistic and collectivistic societies in Europe. *Journal of Cross-Cultural Psychology, 45*(3), 468–490. https://doi.org/10.1177/0022022113509881

Masi, C. M., Chen, H. Y., Hawkley, L. C., & Cacioppo, J. T. (2011). A meta-analysis of interventions to reduce loneliness. *Personality and Social Psychology Review, 15*(3), 219–266. https://doi.org/10.1177/1088868310377394

Mijuskovic, B. L. (2012). *Loneliness in philosophy, psychology, and literature*. IUniverse.

Moustakas, C. E. (1972). *Loneliness and love*. Prentice Hall.

Neves, B. B., & Petersen, A. (2025). The social stigma of loneliness: A sociological approach to understanding the experiences of older people. *The Sociological Review, 73*(2), 362–383. https://doi.org/10.1177/003802612312121

Perlman, D., & Peplau, L. A. (1981). Toward a social psychology of loneliness. In S. Duck & R. Gilmour (Eds.), *Personal relationships in disorder* (pp. 31–56). London.

Perlman, D., & Peplau, L. A. (1982). Toward a social psychology of loneliness. In L. A. Peplau & D. Perlman (Eds.), *Loneliness, a sourcebook of current theory, research and therapy*. Wiley.

Precupetu, I., Pop, C., & Aartsen, M. (2025). Macro-level influences on loneliness in later life: An fsQCA analysis. In M. Aartsen, I. Precupetu, & B. Suanet (Eds.), *Macro social influences on loneliness in later life: Towards a better understanding of the loneliness paradox in later life*. Springer.

Ragin, C. C. (2008). *Redesigning social inquiry: Fuzzy sets and beyond*. University of Chicago Press. ISBN-13: 978-0-226-70275-9 (paper).

Rogers, C. (1970). *Carl Rogers on Encounter Groups*. HarperCollins.

Schoenmakers, E. (2020). Why and how to talk about loneliness. *Journal of Social Intervention: Theory and Practice, 29*(4), 4–18. https://doi.org/10.18352/jsi.646

Stegen, H., Duppen, D., Savieri, P., Stas, L., Pan, H., Aartsen, M., … & De Donder, L. (2024). Loneliness prevalence of community-dwelling older adults and the impact of the mode of measurement, data collection, and country: A systematic review and meta-analysis. *International Psychogeriatrics*, 1–15. https://doi.org/10.1017/S1041610224000425

Suanet, B., & Aartsen, M. (2025). Linking life course theory to multi-level explanations of loneliness: Towards a Sociology of Loneliness. In M. Aartsen, I. Precupetu, & B. Suanet (Eds.), *Macro social influences on loneliness in later life. Towards of a better understanding of loneliness paradox in later life*. Springer.

Wang, N., Goel, S., Ibrahim, S., Badal, V. D., Depp, C., Bilal, E., Subbalakshmi, K., & Lee, E. (2024). Decoding loneliness: Can explainable AI help in understanding language differences in lonely older adults? *Psychiatry Research, 339*, 116078. https://doi.org/10.1016/j.psychres.2024.116078

Weiss, R. S. (1973). *Loneliness: The experience of emotional and social isolation*. MIT Press.

Yang, K., & Victor, C. R. (2011). Age and loneliness in 25 European nations. *Ageing and Society, 31*(8), 1368–1388. https://doi.org/10.1017/S0144686X1000139X

Marja Aartsen, PhD, is currently research professor and social gerontologist at NOVA—Norwegian Social Research at OsloMet. She is specialized in longitudinal research on social relations, social exclusion, loneliness, and cognitive functioning in the second half of life. She is interested in social issues related to aging in place and active or successful ageing. Resent research projects and collaborations include gendered pathways to exclusion from social relations (GENPATH), reducing old-age social exclusion (ROSENET) and a multidimensional approach to social exclusion and its health consequences (AMASE). She was editor of the European Journal of Ageing from 2017 until summer 2022.

Iuliana Precupetu, PhD, is a senior researcher at the Research Institute for Quality of Life, Romanian Academy, and the Research Institute of the University of Bucharest. She is a sociologist specializing in quality of life, health inequalities and social exclusion in later life. Her current interests include the relationship between social exclusion in older age and mental health, as well as the application of life course methods to quality of life research. Most recently, she coordinated the AMASE research project—A multidimensional approach to social exclusion in later life—health consequences for ageing populations.

Open Access This chapter is licensed under the terms of the Creative Commons Attribution 4.0 International License (http://creativecommons.org/licenses/by/4.0/), which permits use, sharing, adaptation, distribution and reproduction in any medium or format, as long as you give appropriate credit to the original author(s) and the source, provide a link to the Creative Commons license and indicate if changes were made.

The images or other third party material in this chapter are included in the chapter's Creative Commons license, unless indicated otherwise in a credit line to the material. If material is not included in the chapter's Creative Commons license and your intended use is not permitted by statutory regulation or exceeds the permitted use, you will need to obtain permission directly from the copyright holder.

Part II
Theoretical Perspectives

Chapter 2
Theorizing Loneliness in Later Life. Micro, Meso, and Macro Perspectives

Fredrica Nyqvist, Joanna McHugh Power, and Laura Coll-Planas

2.1 Introduction

Loneliness has been addressed theoretically for many years from psychological and social science perspectives and, more recently, by public health. Additionally, loneliness is increasingly recognised as a social justice issue, given that it is caused by structural and social factors which yield unequal distribution (Barreto et al., 2024). The theoretical foundation of loneliness has deep roots. In their highly cited book chapter, *Theoretical Approaches to Loneliness*, Perlman and Peplau (1982) outlined eight different theoretical approaches to loneliness: psychodynamic, phenomenological, existential-humanistic, sociological, interactionist, cognitive, privacy, and systems theory. While some of these approaches emphasize individual psychological traits, the sociological perspective, for example, frames loneliness as a social phenomenon influenced by broader structures, relationships, and cultural norms within society, rather than merely individual or psychological factors. This societal perspective is increasingly valued in the literature, with loneliness even framed as a social justice issue in recent discussion (Barreto et al., 2024).

F. Nyqvist (✉)
Faculty of Education and Welfare Studies, Social Policy, Åbo Akademi University, Vaasa, Finland
e-mail: Fredrica.Nyqvist@abo.fi

J. McHugh Power
Department of Psychology, Maynooth University, Kildare, Republic of Ireland

L. Coll-Planas
Research Group on Methodology, Methods, Models and Outcomes of Health and Social Sciences (M3O), University of Vic-Central University of Catalonia (UVic-UCC), Vic, Spain

Institute for Research and Innovation, Life Sciences and Health in Central Catalonia (IRIS-CC), Vic, Spain

© The Author(s) 2025

M. Aartsen et al. (eds.), *Macro Social Influences on Loneliness in Later Life*, International Perspectives on Aging 47,
https://doi.org/10.1007/978-3-031-94565-6_2

Building on the work of Perlman and Peplau, ecological models such as the Bronfenbrenner ecological model (Bronfenbrenner, 2000) and the socio-ecological model (Dahlberg et al., 2002) offer valuable frameworks which have been borrowed to explain loneliness (McHugh Power et al., 2018; Holt-Lunstad, 2018). Bronfenbrenner's model, which conceptualizes development within multiple layers of environmental influence—ranging from interpersonal processes (termed the "microsystem") to broader societal and cultural contexts ("macrosystem")—provides a useful lens for examining how different levels of influence contribute to human development. Similarly, the socio-ecological model– as it has been applied to loneliness–emphasizes the reciprocal interaction between individual, interpersonal, community, and societal factors, highlighting how micro-level influences can affect meso-level and macro-level outcomes and vice versa (Dahlberg et al., 2002; Victor & Sullivan, 2015).

Relative to the micro-level, the meso- and macro-level perspectives on loneliness have received less attention, both theoretically and empirically. More recent theoretical reviews and models of loneliness such as the synthesized model of loneliness (McHugh Power et al., 2018) and the SOCIAL Framework (Holt-Lunstad, 2022), represent significant advancements by integrating various layers previously described in this introduction. While McHugh Power et al. (2018) address primarily micro- and meso-level factors, the current chapter extends and updates this framework by placing greater focus on the macro-level perspectives. Using the theoretical synthesis by McHugh Power et al. (2018) as a starting point, the aim of this chapter is to chart the main theories of loneliness relevant to older adults within micro-, meso-, and, particularly, the macro-level perspective, which has been hitherto relatively neglected.

2.1.1 Defining Micro-, Meso- and Macro-level

In 2018, McHugh Power and colleagues used the theoretical synthesis approach (Pound & Campbell, 2015) to integrate and combine theories of loneliness across psychology, sociology, public health, and psychiatry. This theoretical synthesis yielded a model of loneliness with five intraindividual factors (developmental, cognitive, existential, personality, and biological), and four interindividual factors (intimate relationships, social networks, situational factors, and cultural determinants of loneliness). Later, an empirical qualitative approach was used to refine and validate this model (Holton et al., 2023).

In planning the current chapter, and in review of Bronfenbrenner's ecological model (2000) and subsequent work, we re-termed intraindividual factors as "micro" level factors determining loneliness. The interindividual level then was divided into the "meso" and the "macro" levels. The three levels are interdependent; macro-level cultural norms about social relationships, filial duty, and familialism, for instance, likely drive micro-level cognitions about others (van Staden & Coetzee, 2010; de Jong Gierveld & Tesch-Römer, 2012; Akhter-Khan et al., 2023). It is also worth noting that the terms micro, meso, and macro are used in different ways across different literatures; within community gerontology, the micro level refers to very proximal relationships, rather than intraindividual processes, and elsewhere, "microsystem" refers to the psychosocial mechanisms through which social relationships impact health (Berkman et al., 2000). As such, it is worth defining the levels as we use them here.

For the purposes of this chapter, *micro-level factors* determining loneliness represent those from within the individual. Essentially, theories operating at this level assume that there are individual characteristics which can determine, to a greater or lesser extent, whether an individual becomes lonely. In our chapter, we define the micro level as constituting intraindividual factors influencing loneliness—in other words, all psychological processes happening within the individual which are theorised to influence loneliness.

We define the *meso level* as the three interindividual levels that correspond to: intimate relationships, social network, and situational factors, encompassing personal context, physical and social environment. Thus, meso-level theories examine loneliness in the context of social relationships, personal situations and community settings. The meso level is the focal construct for community gerontology. This discipline defines community as an overarching level of organization in which ageing is embedded (Greenfield et al., 2019). In other words, the meso level is "beyond the private sphere of home and family but more familiar to us than the wider society" (Crow & Allan, 1994, p. 1). Within the meso-level, the environmental context is defined as the settings in which individuals engage. In some models (e.g. Greenfield et al., 2019), the interpersonal level is considered micro level, but here we classify it as meso level to clearly distinguish psychological mechanisms from those processes involving individuals and networks. This classification approach is consistent with the approach taken by McHugh Power et al. (2018). Moreover, as stated by community gerontologists, the meso level is the continuum of ecological contexts that falls between the micro and the macro levels. It both influences and is influenced by dynamics at these other levels (Greenfield et al., 2019).

Macro-level theories, in contrast, address broader structural and cultural systems, analysing overarching patterns and trends in society, such as economic systems, welfare policies, and cultural norms, often across larger geographical areas like regions, or entire countries (Bronfenbrenner, 2000). While distinct, the micro, meso, and macro levels interact dynamically over time. For example, macro-level cultural norms influence micro-level cognitions (as we describe above) but also evolve based on shifts in individual behaviours and community interactions. In Table 2.1, we provide an overview of the theories on loneliness discussed in this chapter, covering micro-, meso-, and macro-levels, and models that combine these levels.[1]

[1] The theoretical perspectives on loneliness discussed in this chapter were selected based on their ability to provide comprehensive insights into the complexity of loneliness. These theories offer a balanced and nuanced understanding of loneliness from intrapersonal, interpersonal, and societal viewpoints. While we do not attempt an exhaustive review of all theories of loneliness, our perspective is grounded in psychology, public health, and the social sciences, reflecting both our expertise and a broad theoretical approach.

Table 2.1 A summary of the proposed aetiologies of loneliness—both theoretical and evidence-based—across all three levels of analysis (micro, meso, and macro), with special attention to models that integrate multiple levels

Microlevel (intrapersonal aspects)	Mesolevel (interpersonal and environmental aspects)	Macrolevel (societal aspects)	Combination of different levels
Developmental theories, e.g. early childhood experiences, parental relationships)	*Models describing social relationships and social network:* Social network: weak and strong ties Umbrella concepts: social capital and social connection	Structural aspects, e.g. income inequality, welfare institutional arrangement	The integrative model by de Jong Gierveld and Tesch-Römer (2012)
Cognitive theories, e.g. dysfunctional attributions about others, hypervigilance for social threat, social risk avoidance	*Models focusing on the dynamic nature of social relationships:* Convoy model of social relationships Differential Investment of Resources (DIRe) model Dynamic process model of loneliness The Model of relational mobility	Cultural aspects, e.g. individualism and collectivism, religiosity	The synthesized model of loneliness (McHugh Power et al., 2018)
Existential theories—awareness of one's mortality (potentially a subtype of loneliness)		Demographic composition, e.g. marital status, health status, education	The SOCIAL Framework: *The Systemic Framework of Cross-Sector Integration and Action Across the Life Span* (Holt-Lunstad, 2022)
Personality theories, e.g. shyness, affiliation needs, extraversion, the "lonely personality"	*Situational factors:* Personal context: illness and disability; low income and low educational attainment; and stressful situations and transitions Environmental context, e.g. lonelygenic environments conceptual model The virtual context		Conceptual model of exclusion from social relations for older people (Burholt et al., 2020)
Biological theories: evolutionary theory of loneliness; reaffiliation motive			

2.2 The Micro-level Perspective

Following McHugh Power et al. (2018) we consider five domains of micro-level theories of loneliness: developmental, cognitive, existential, personality, and biological. For each domain, we will consider evidence associated with theories of loneliness and highlight what remains unknown before considering their relevance specifically in an older population.

2.2.1 Developmental Theories

In the developmental psychological literature, early attachment experiences are a critical determinant of life-course loneliness (Kumar, 2024; Mikulincer & Shaver, 2014; Fromm Reichmann, 1959; DiTommaso et al., 2003). Attachment theory proposes that early emotional bonds formed with others shape relationships and psychological well-being later in life (Fraley, 2019). By providing a basic framework for understanding and conducting relationships, attachment can be linked to the likelihood of later relationship success and therefore to loneliness (Mikulincer & Shaver, 2014). For instance, having parents who are either lonely themselves or inexpressive (Kupersmidt et al., 1999; Mahon et al., 2006); failure to individuate successfully during childhood (Rosedale, 2007); lack of social support during childhood (Mahon et al., 2006); and difficult parental relationships (Holton et al., 2023) may all yield later-life loneliness, potentially by influencing adult attachment style (Mikulincer & Shaver, 2014). Indeed, attachment insecurity is linked to loneliness among older adults (Spence et al., 2020; Bergman et al., 2024), although it should be noted that attachment insecurity generally decreases with age (Fraley, 2019). Attachment insecurity may cause loneliness by impairing one's ability to enjoy solitude (Mikulincer et al., 2021) which may be particularly problematic in later life when events which cause social isolation are more likely to occur (e.g. retirement, bereavement). More broadly, research into the sequelae of early attachment among older adults is still lacking (Magai et al., 2016), which means that further evidence in relation to the impact of attachment style on older-adult loneliness, particularly, is required.

2.2.2 Cognitive Theories

At the cognitive level, specific beliefs and attitudes are also associated with increased likelihood of loneliness. These include: beliefs about others which do not facilitate social engagement, such as believing that others are hostile (Galanaki & Vassilopoulou, 2007), expectations of others (Akhter-Khan et al., 2023), hypervigilance for social threat (Cacioppo & Hawkley, 2009; Marangoni & Ickes, 1989); a negative self-perception (Heinrich & Gullone, 2006); broader maladaptive social cognition, or errors in the ways we think about and perceive others (Cacioppo & Hawkley, 2009), and social risk avoidance (Heinrich & Gullone, 2006). In one influential definition, loneliness is defined as a perception of social isolation (Cacioppo & Hawkley, 2009). By another influential definition, loneliness is defined as the affective result of a cognitive process—evaluating and comparing one's actual and ideal social relationships (Peplau & Perlman, 1982). Perlman and Peplau have theorised that loneliness is the result of a discrepancy between an individual's actual and desired quality or quantity of social relationships (Peplau & Perlman, 1982). This influential theory positions loneliness as an affective experience which emerges because of cognitive appraisals about one's relationships. Reflecting on the breadth of cognitive processes underlying loneliness, it has been suggested that loneliness arises from a complex interplay of cognitions about the self, relationships, and others (Hawkley & Capitanio, 2015).

While not explicitly about loneliness, the theory of socioemotional selectivity posits that older adults, increasingly aware of their shortening lifespans, make decisions about their social lives which seek to maximise return while minimising effort (Carstensen, 1993)—again ostensibly a cognition-level theory. When applied to loneliness in later life, the socioemotional selectivity theory has been invoked to explain the stability of loneliness in this life stage; older adults may invest more in fewer relationships than younger adults, and jettison less rewarding social ties while maintaining sufficient bonds to avoid loneliness (Mund et al., 2020).

There is an apparent lack of research on the nature in which such cognitive theories may explain loneliness specifically in older age; cognitive theories of loneliness may be applicable at all life stages. One exception is Akhter-Khan's social relationship expectations (SRE) framework (Akhter-Khan et al., 2023). The SRE framework posits that loneliness arises because of unmet expectations in social relationships. Such unmet expectations could arise because of insufficient social provisions (and such a process would belong at the meso-level) or because of high expectation levels. Given the model's focus on expectations, we include it here as a cognitive-level theory of loneliness. With respect to later life in particular, two expectations mentioned by Akhter-Khan are specific to this life-stage: respect and generativity (Akhter-Khan et al., 2023).

There is considerable evidence, then, that cognitions including perceptions and decisions about resources can determine loneliness in later life. This perspective is compatible with attachment theory. For instance, early-life experiences may shape cognitions which determine loneliness in later life. If an individual learns that others are not to be trusted during their early childhood, this belief may persist into adulthood and discourage them from socially engaging with others, leading to loneliness. However, the mechanisms through which this shaping takes place have yet to be elucidated.

2.2.3 *Existential Theories*

Existential theories of loneliness were included in the original theoretical synthesis (McHugh Power et al., 2018). Researchers in this domain characterise loneliness as the inevitable consequence of awareness of one's existence and mortality (Bekhet &

Zauszniewski, 2012; Bolmsjö et al., 2019). Existential loneliness was first described by a generation of psychotherapists and psychiatrists (e.g. Moustakas, 1976) but has since been less evident in the loneliness literature than other subtypes. Alongside social and emotional loneliness, existential loneliness is elsewhere described as a third subtype of loneliness (van Tilburg, 2021) and as such may not overlap substantially with other loneliness subtypes, but it may be particularly pertinent to older adults. Existential loneliness is, because of its association with mortality, most commonly explored in end-of-life populations (Mayers & Svartberg, 2001) and as such, older adults who are at end of life, or whose peers are reaching end of life, would potentially be more likely to experience it (Carr & Fang, 2023). However, when older adults not at end of life were invited to reflect on the existential factors in loneliness, they did not endorse such concerns or feelings, nor did they agree that reflecting on one's existence would cause loneliness (Holton et al., 2023). This led Holton and colleagues to suggest retiring this factor from the theoretical synthesis of loneliness.

Due to the relative neglect of existential loneliness when compared with other subtypes, we yet lack even satisfactory conceptualisation of the topic (Gil Alvarez et al., 2023). Conducting a systematic review of the literature, Gil Alverez and colleagues went on to offer a synthesised definition of existential loneliness—that it is part of human nature, involving an awareness of separateness from others, and of the uniqueness of our experiences, which we can never truly communicate to others. Open issues in the field also remain regarding the cultural variance of the concept, best approaches to measurement (contingent on satisfactory conceptualisation), and whether it is likely to be experienced by those not at end of life (Gil Alvarez et al., 2023; McKenna-Plumley et al., 2024). An interesting point made by McKenna-Plumley and colleagues is that we know little about how existential loneliness may arise from disconnections with spiritual entities or nature more generally; this warrants further exploration particularly in the context of Astell-Burt's lonelygenic environment hypothesis explained in the section on meso-level (Feng & Astell-Burt, 2022).

2.2.4 Personality Theories

Enduring traits such as shyness (Heinrich & Gullone, 2006; Mahon et al., 2006; Marangoni & Ickes, 1989); affiliation needs (Heinrich & Gullone, 2006); sociability (Marangoni & Ickes, 1989), tendency to share information with others (Derlega & Margulis, 1982; Mahon et al., 2006); emotion regulation abilities (Wong et al., 2018; Zysberg, 2015); neuroticism and extraversion (Zysberg, 2015) may drive loneliness. Zysberg proposed a "lonely personality", arising in an individual with a poor sense of self, with deficits in social and emotional skills and information processing, and low extraversion/high neuroticism. Of all personality factors proposed to drive loneliness, the strongest empirical evidence base exists for high neuroticism and low extraversion (Buecker et al., 2020). Interestingly, the genetic basis for loneliness appears to overlap substantially with that of neuroticism (Spithoven et al., 2019), suggesting that there may be overlap between biological and personality theories of loneliness; biology and genetics may provide the basis for individual variation in trait loneliness levels or loneliness proneness. Further evidence for trait loneliness arises in longitudinal studies which demonstrate at a meta-analytic level that loneliness does not change due to age (Mund et al., 2020, 2020).

Reflecting on theories of loneliness arising from specific personality traits, it is perhaps difficult to see how traits (which likely have a genetic basis) can determine loneliness beyond the effects of attachment. Personality traits could of course shape cognitions about loneliness and may act in concert with attachment experiences to determine loneliness levels. Personality traits are also likely to be determined by biology, which makes these theories compatible with biological theories of loneliness. Such interrelations between the domains of the micro-level are underexplored and worth investigating empirically.

2.2.5 Biological Theories

Biological accounts of loneliness can be separated into the evolutionary theory of loneliness and genetic accounts of loneliness. The work of John Cacioppo in particular has been influential. Cacioppo and colleagues (2014a, 2014b) defined loneliness as an adaptive mechanism which serves to redirect the lonely individual towards seeking social connection. This mechanism was further explicated by Qualter et al. (2015) as the "reaffiliation motive"—an unpleasant feeling of loneliness is proposed to trigger reaffiliation behaviours (to withdraw from social situations and make social evaluations), and cognitions to then support reconnection with others. In this manner, loneliness has an adaptive value—it redirects individuals towards social connection. However, according to Qualter and colleagues, the adaptive value of loneliness is attenuated when it becomes chronic. There is indeed evidence to suggest that lonely individuals withdraw socially (Qualter et al., 2015), including lonely older adults (McHugh Power et al., 2019). More broadly the evolutionary account of loneliness developed by Cacioppo and others represented a move away from previous theories which tended to describe loneliness as an unalloyed ill with no redeeming or adaptive benefits.

Genetic accounts of the heritability of loneliness have also been proposed (Boomsma et al., 2005; Goossens et al., 2015) and indeed corroborated (Spithoven et al., 2019), suggesting that loneliness is likely to be partly heritable. Beyond the evolutionary theory of loneliness, which remains dominant as an explanation of the biological underpinnings of loneliness, there is a paucity of theory in this domain. As with cognitive theories of loneliness, there is also a dearth of research into whether such biological theories apply comparably across the lifespan.

2.3 The Meso-level Perspective

In this section, we discuss the meso-level theories framing loneliness by examining different models that have evolved over the decades until now. Without claiming to be exhaustive, theories have been chosen for their complementary approach. Particularly, we will provide an understanding on how interpersonal networks and relationships and their context play a crucial role in shaping the experiences of loneliness in later life. By context we mean situational factors embracing personal context, physical and social environment. Thus, theories presented here are not always specific for loneliness, as was the case in the previous section. Rather, they are existing theories which may be applicable to loneliness.

2.3.1 Models Describing Social Relationships and Social Networks

Research on social networks typically treats the topic as static rather than dynamic over time. In this view, a social network is defined as the structural context in which different types of relationships develop, ranging from strong ties (e.g., intimacy and friendship) to weak ties. The functions and qualities of these relationships create a continuum, with supportive and fulfilling connections on one end, and conflict, withdrawal, and loneliness on the other (Wenger, 1996). Within the sphere of intimate relationships, for instance, emotional loneliness is thought to occur as the result of the loss or absence of a significant intimate figure, such as a partner or spouse (Weiss, 1973). However, it could also happen when there is a primary attachment relationship, but the level of intimacy is perceived as inadequate (Galanaki & Vassilopoulou, 2007; Sullivan, 1953; Weiss, 1973).

In parallel, *umbrella concepts* such as social capital and social connection have been coined to encompass structural and functional aspects of social networks integrating evidence generated by different disciplines. *Social capital*, defined as the value derived from social networks and relationships, has been applied as a concept relevant to the ageing process (Putnam, 2000; Nyqvist, 2009). Accordingly, its structural aspects include social network and social participation, while its cognitive aspects embrace social support, sense of belonging and social trust, to be further discussed in the "macro-level" section of this chapter, below. It is to be highlighted that social capital theory is the only framework distinguishing bonding, bridging and linking social capital, depending on relations between persons belonging to the same social group, to heterogenous groups, or holding unequal levels of power, respectively. Furthermore, social capital is considered both an interpersonal resource and a societal-level characteristic, spanning both meso- and macro-levels (Putnam, 2000). Interestingly, the dark side of social capital has also been described, for instance leading to behavioural contagion and social control (Villalonga-Olives & Kawachi, 2017).

The second umbrella concept worth mentioning is *social connection*, which has emerged as a multifactorial construct on a continuum—from risk, when social connection is low, to protection, when social connection is high (Holt-Lunstad et al., 2017; Holt-Lunstad, 2022). This approach aims to summarize and represent the large body of scientific evidence linking social relationships with health (Holt-Lunstad, 2022). The social connection concept encompasses the structure, function, and quality of social relationships. The structural aspects refer to the existing connections to others in the social network and include the role in those relationships, e.g., social network size and density, marital status, living arrangements, social integration versus social isolation, etc. The functional aspects, comparable to the cognitive aspects of social capital, refer to the sense of connection and result from the social support and inclusion as provided or perceived to be available within those social relationships. Loneliness is framed within the functional items as a perceived lack of support. Each of those social relations might have positive or negative qualities, for example a partnership might be supportive, or pose relationship strain. Positive qualities of social relations will result in social inclusion, while negative qualities will lead to social exclusion.

2.3.2 *Models Focusing on the Dynamic Nature of Social Relationships*

In contrast with the more static theories and constructs explained in the previous section, here we present models with a specific focus on how social ties evolve over time. In 1980, Kahn and Antonucci formulated the *Convoy model of social relationships* (Kahn & Antonucci, 1980). This model explains how individuals are "surrounded by supportive others who move with them throughout the life course", constituting a convoy. These acquaintances, family, and friends can be placed in three concentric rings symbolizing the degree of proximity to the individual, represented at the centre. The convoy model proposes that each individual "has" a social network, but it incorporates both life span and life course perspective. Accordingly, it recognises that over time, the convoy changes due to ageing and life transition. The model provides explanation how relationships change over time, considering determinants such as personal characteristics (micro level) and situational aspects. It also acknowledges macro-level factors such as context, roles, culture and history. Accordingly, within this dynamic process, social ties might become stronger and new social relationships appear, but they might also weaken or even end. Changes leading to a lack or loss of social ties might then be experienced as emotional or social loneliness, depending on the proximity and relevance of that connection.

The *Differential Investment of Resources (DIRe) model* describes how social relationships develop in adulthood, emphasizing that relationships require an investment in time and energy (Huxhold et al., 2022). The DIRe model, in a similar manner to the Convoy model, considers three different layers that constitute the social structure: the first layer includes close confidants providing intimacy and support; in the second layer, we have the broader network and, in the third one, the community. While the first layer would require time to maintain emotional closeness, the second and third layer would require more energy, since they encompass interactions with weak ties involving active self-presentation and situational awareness. Within the DIRe model, the *Dynamic process model of loneliness* has been described (Huxhold & Fiori, 2024). Similarly to the process described in the convoy model, the dynamic nature of investing more or less in different types of social ties might lead to unmet social expectations and thus to loneliness, which would then require new investments to be alleviated. The DIRe model also considers how personal characteristics and context are key to determining the investment made in each layer, and how such investment might change along the ageing process. Specifically, the DIRe model describes the influence of individual characteristics (ostensibly micro-level) in terms of skills, capacity and motivation, as well as societal characteristics (macro-level) i.e. social structure and norms as influencing the investment in terms of energy and time in social relationships (for an application to societal crisis see Chap. 10 of this book; Klasen et al., 2025).

The third and last model explaining how social networks change along the life cycle is the Model *of relational mobility*. Relational mobility is a socio-psychological concept referring to the perceived ease associated with joining or leaving social groups and establish new social contacts (meso-level). Thus, experiencing loneliness but perceiving that there are social opportunities and that there is room for personal choice to generate new social contacts as desired (i.e. high relational mobility), provides a positive outcome (i.e. alleviation of loneliness). Meanwhile, perceiving low relational mobility, i.e. social rigidity, which is also linked to low trust with each other, may result in hopelessness for those feeling lonely. According to this model, level of social flexibility or rigidity is dependent on personal abilities (micro-level) and social norms linked to cultural values (macro-level). An example of cultural values linked to this model would be the Japanese society, which is characterised by a low relational mobility (Badman et al., 2022).

2.3.3 Situational Factors: Personal and Environmental Contexts

Theories mentioned above already refer globally to context as key factor determining social ties. Now, we will refer specifically to *situational factors* at meso-level, distinguishing the personal from the environmental context as mentioned in McHugh Power et al. (2018). The *personal context* comprises different situations that may lead to loneliness, categorised at the meso-level since the micro-level is concerned exclusively with psychological processes happening within the individual. Situational factors, meanwhile, refer to the broader context surrounding the individual, shaping the likelihood of loneliness by influencing more proximal (micro-level) factors. Such situations include illness and disability; socioeconomic status such as low income and low educational attainment; and stressful situations and transitions such as migration, institutionalization or incarceration (McHugh Power et al., 2018). Each of these situational factors has a specific putative pathway to loneliness. For example, acquired disability might interfere in social abilities or hinder participation in social activities, while economic constraints might stress social relationships and result in withdrawal. The intersection of several of these factors may be experienced during the ageing process, leading to potential later-life loneliness.

In terms of *environmental context*, the social environment at meso-level is the community where one lives, which is the context where social relationships are developed, maintained or changed. Cumulative evidence shows which community factors influence loneliness in older people (Meehan et al., 2023). Among them, characteristics of the *neighbourhood* are key influential factors for loneliness and social isolation: safety, density, walkability, availability of green spaces, accessibility to services, transportation and public third places, the socioeconomic status of the area, neighbourhood satisfaction, and level of social cohesion. Moreover, social and physical environments differ in rural and urban areas. While urban environments might offer more social opportunities, they are also fast paced and the individualistic nature of cities can lead to loneliness. On the other hand, in rural areas, close-knit communities may offer stronger personal bonds and higher sense of belonging and place attachment, but loneliness can occur due to geographic and social factors such as lack of diverse social interactions or fewer chances to meet new people (Burholt & Dobbs, 2012). A recent innovative approach worth mentioning is the *Lonelygenic environments conceptual model,* which embraces micro and macro levels while having its strengths at meso level (Feng & Astell-Burt, 2022). This model refers to those complex contextual conditions that can cause or aggravate loneliness, pointing out to the key role of urban planning. Accordingly, stigma towards loneliness and structural discrimination (racism, sexism, ableism, classism) generate social and built environments where particularly people with disadvantages feel lonely. Conversely, public green spaces, which are less typical in lower-income communities, would foster social connections. The lonelygenic environments model emphasises that at personal, relational and collective level, harm can be caused or reduced, and capacities can be built or restored (Feng & Astell-Burt, 2022). This model highlights that loneliness is a social problem requiring community solutions, rather than simply personal-level interventions (see also Chap. 13 of this book; Ghenţa & Matei, 2025). Thus, the lonelygenic environments model challenges individualistic approaches at micro-level that emphasize cognitive or social skills, while contributing a more comprehensive analysis of social structures and environmental factors.

The *virtual context* is also relevant, since online social networking is associated with loneliness. However, current evidence shows contradictory results regarding social media use and whether it might be enhancing or reducing loneliness (Nowland et al., 2018). A model has been proposed to explain this phenomenon whereby there is a bidirectional and dynamic relationship between loneliness and social media use.

On one hand, being connected online may help to alleviate loneliness when it enhances existing relationships and supports the development of new connections. On the other hand, if the digital world is used to displace time spent in offline social activities, it may create or exacerbate loneliness. Nevertheless, when considering specifically older people, evidence on the useful effects of online social networking enhancing the sense of social connection is clear, while the evidence on the harmful effects reinforcing loneliness is low and limited to a problematic use and among people with tendency for upward social comparison (Dwyer, 2024).

2.4 The Macro-level Perspective

Here, we explore the broader structural and cultural elements that might influence an individual's experience of loneliness. This approach is known as the macro-level perspective, a term coined by Bronfenbrenner and exemplified within the socio-ecological model (Holt-Lunstad, 2018; Meehan et al., 2023) which examines how societal and cultural forces play a role in loneliness. We will look at economic conditions, cultural norms, and welfare structures to understand how they might influence and contribute to the occurrence of loneliness in later life.

In terms of socio-economic influences, research conducted by Tapia-Muñoz et al. (2022) in the United States and Europe found that older adults in countries with greater income inequality tend to experience higher levels of loneliness. This correlation persisted even after adjusting for personal attributes and the country's gross domestic product per capita (GDP). The study by Tapia-Muñoz et al. (2022) proposed that the link between national income disparity and loneliness could be attributed to both direct and indirect factors. Direct factors include constrained economic resources and substandard living conditions, while indirect factors involve reduced social capital such as social cohesion and trust. The concept of trust was incorporated into loneliness research to elucidate cross-country variations in loneliness through a social-cultural and historical-political lens (Rapolienė & Aartsen, 2022). Empirical evidence suggests that higher loneliness levels in Easter-European countries transitioning from totalitarian regimes could be in part attributed to lower trust, both interpersonal and institutional. This deficit in trust appears to contribute to increased social disengagement within these populations, which in turn contributes to higher levels of loneliness.

The influence of cultural norms and values on loneliness can be significant. These factors can shape the way individuals interact with one another and perceive their connections within society, which in turn can influence their experiences of loneliness (see McHugh Power et al., 2018). Some studies suggest that people in collectivistic societies, often referred to as traditional societies that put strength on family solidarity and economic interdependence, report higher levels of loneliness compared to those in individualistic societies (Fokkema et al., 2012; Imamoglu et al., 1993; Sundström et al., 2009; Burholt, 2023). Individualistic societies place higher value on personal independence and self-reliance, emphasizing the importance of personal goals and achievements over collectives' ones (Burholt, 2023).

In the European context, it is often posited that countries in the Southern region, along with certain Central and Eastern European countries, tend to exhibit more collectivistic traits (Lykes & Kemmelmeier, 2014; Swader, 2019). Lykes and Kemmelmeier (2014) found that in collectivistic European countries, loneliness was more strongly associated with a lack of family interaction, while in individualistic societies, loneliness correlated more with a lack of friendships and confidants. This suggests that the framework of individualism versus collectivism shapes different expectations and experiences of loneliness. In the literature, living alone has been reported as one of the risk factors for experiencing loneliness. Countries characterized by individualistic values place a strong emphasis on personal autonomy and self-reliance, which often correlates with a higher prevalence of individuals residing alone. However, these countries are reported to have lower incidences of loneliness, a phenomenon that has been termed the "cultural paradox" of loneliness (Heu et al., 2021). Nevertheless, it is important to acknowledge that some studies have indicated an elevated experience of loneliness in individualistic societies (Barreto et al., 2021; Taniguchi & Kaufman, 2022), thereby also challenging the consistency of this pattern, particularly beyond the European region.

Numerous studies have found that regularly attending religious services is linked to reduced feelings of loneliness (e.g. Rote et al., 2013; Upenieks, 2023). In addition to individual religious practices and beliefs, the broader religious context at the macro-level may also shape the experience of loneliness. Countries with higher levels of religiosity might foster social environments where community ties and shared values are strengthened (Schwadel, 2005), indirectly reducing loneliness. In more religious nations, organizations and institutions often reflect religious values, creating a pervasive cultural atmosphere that may shape social interactions and support systems. To our knowledge, little research has focused on macro-level religiosity in relation to loneliness. However, secularism, defined as the state's neutral stance on religion (Kettell, 2019), has been examined in the context of loneliness. It has been theorized that secularism might influence marriage and divorce rates and family formation, potentially reducing the family's role in providing psychosocial support and thereby increasing loneliness. Nevertheless, Das (2022) used data from the Survey of Health, Ageing and Retirement in Europe (SHARE) across ten countries and found that secularism did not lead to increased loneliness or weaker family ties.

2.4.1 Integrative Models: Models Integrating the Micro-, Meso- and Macro-level

To further our understanding, we look at larger structural and cultural factors by using integrative models, which consider influences from multiple levels (Holt-Lunstad, 2018; McHugh Power et al., 2018; Meehan et al., 2023). De Jong Gierveld and Tesch-Römer (2012) introduced such a model that combines individual and societal factors. Their model identifies three main theoretical perspectives on an individual level to explain loneliness. Firstly, it may stem from unmet social contact needs. Secondly, it could be linked to poor living conditions, including low socio-economic status and poor health. Lastly, loneliness may result from discrepancies between desired and achieved social relationships, according to Perlman and Peplau's cognitive model (1982). Additionally, the model indicates that societal factors, such as a country's socio-economic conditions and cultural norms, can shape individuals' social expectations and levels of integration. Demographic variables like age, marital status, health, and education also play a role in the varying degrees of loneliness observed across different countries (Fokkema et al., 2012; Prohaska et al., 2020). Differences in demographic composition have been used to explain why loneliness levels might be higher in Eastern Europe as compared to Western countries (Fokkema et al., 2012; Hansen & Slagsvold, 2016).

Building on de Jong Gierveld and Tesh-Römer's integrative model, Nyqvist et al. (2019) examined the impact of welfare state regimes on loneliness among older adults. Welfare state regimes categorize countries based on how their welfare systems are organized (Esping-Andersen, 1990; Hemerijck, 2013). Nyqvist et al. (2019) analysed five European welfare regimes and found that loneliness levels were lower in the Nordic, Anglo-Saxon, and Continental regimes as compared to Southern and Eastern regimes. This integrative model was also applied to assess loneliness in European welfare regimes before and after the global financial crisis of 2008–2009 (Nyqvist et al., 2021). The theoretical assumption at the macro-level is that in more redistributive welfare regimes such as the Nordic regime, individuals rely less on personal social resources for health and well-being compared to regimes where these outcomes depend more heavily on family ties, the voluntary sector, and the market. It was also hypothesized that the global financial crisis and the resulting recession weakened the role of welfare regimes in mitigating loneliness by pressuring welfare states to adjust their institutional arrangements. The results suggested a somewhat weaker influence of welfare regimes in 2014 than in 2006, possibly reflecting the strain on redistributive policies during economic downturns.

The crowding-in and crowding-out hypotheses provide additional theoretical lenses for understanding the role of welfare regimes in loneliness. The crowding-out hypothesis suggests that generous welfare states might reduce informal social relations by assuming responsibility for those in need. Conversely, the crowding-in argument posits that well-developed welfare states redistribute resources necessary for social contacts to thrive. These hypotheses align with the integrative model's emphasis on societal influences, such as redistributive systems shaping social integration. While evidence generally indicates that comprehensive welfare states do not erode social trust (Rothstein & Stolle, 2008), some support exists for the crowding-out hypothesis regarding social contacts (Reeskens & van Oorschot, 2014).

From the perspective of social isolation, a model worth mentioning is the *Conceptual model of exclusion from social relations for older people* (Burholt et al., 2020; Van Regenmortel et al., 2025). It is framed within the critical human ecological framework, thus integrating the biological aspects with psychological traits and the sociocultural, social-structural, policy, and physical environment as they impact on the human experience, while, at the same time, individuals influence and adapt to their environments (Bronfenbrenner, 1986). Those micro-, meso, and macro-level risk (or protective) factors shape social relations and determine whether the self-evaluation comparing needed or desired social relations with the achieved social relations will result in loneliness. Moreover, this model integrates the micro-level lifespan developmental theory called *Selection, Optimization and Compensation Theory* describing the adaptive mechanisms that individuals undergo throughout their ageing process to maintain functioning in the face of changes (Baltes & Carstensen, 2003).

Finally, from a public health perspective, loneliness has increasingly been viewed through the lens of social connection, with loneliness considered analogous to poor social connection (Holt-Lunstad et al., 2017). In this frame, it has been proposed to be prioritized within the Social Determinants of Health (Holt-Lunstad, 2022). Specifically, the *SOCIAL Framework: The Systemic Framework of Cross-Sector Integration and Action Across the Life Span* has been built on the social connection conceptual model and combined with the socio-ecological model and the cross-sectorial approach of the WHO "Health in All Policies". This is a comprehensive public health framework emphasising intersectionality and considering social factors relevant to health. It is aimed to guide research, intervention, practice and policy by crossing the diverse aspects of social connection with all areas: clinical and population health, transportation, housing, employment, education, leisure and food. Hence, the SOCIAL Framework applies a lifespan approach and embraces diversity to advance in health equity. In summary, this is an integrative framework from a health and health policy perspective, conceptualizing loneliness as opposed to social connection and built on scientific findings linking loneliness to adverse health outcomes.

2.5 Conclusion

Over the past decades, theoretical development in loneliness has shifted from a focus on individual psychological factors (Perlman & Peplau, 1982) to a more comprehensive understanding that includes social, environmental, and structural influences (e.g. de Jong Gierveld & Tesch-Römer, 2012; Victor & Sullivan, 2015; McHugh Power et al., 2018). While the meso-level, especially in community contexts, emphasises social and relational dynamics within neighbourhoods and local environments, the macro-level, encompassing broader societal and cultural structures, highlights the influence of policies, economic conditions, and cultural norms on individual experiences of loneliness.

In this chapter, we defined intraindividual processes as micro-level factors, while recognizing that in other models, the micro level might refer to interindividual processes, such as close personal relationships (e.g. Bronfenbrenner, 2000). This highlights the lack of consensus in how these levels are conceptualized across different disciplines. It is also important to note that the boundaries between these levels are not always clear-cut, and there can be significant overlap and interaction between them. While our overview is not systematic, it provides a broad perspective on the various theories and approaches to understanding loneliness. Building on previous theoretical overviews (e.g. Perlman & Peplau, 1982; McHugh Power et al., 2018), this chapter emphasizes the consideration of theories operating at multiple levels to grasp the complexity of loneliness.

We have looked at micro-, meso-, and macro-levels individually and additionally presented models that propose integrated levels, such as the model by De Jong Gierveld and Tesch-Römer (2012), the SOCIAL Framework: *The Systemic Framework of Cross-Sector Integration and Action Across the Life Span* (Holt-Lunstad, 2022) and *Conceptual model of exclusion from social relations for older people* (Burholt et al., 2020). However, the complexity inherent in these models presents significant challenges that must be acknowledged, such as the multidimensionality of loneliness, including emotional, social, and existential dimensions, as well as temporal changes over time at different levels. Loneliness is not a static experience; it fluctuates and evolves due to various factors, including life transitions, societal changes, and individual development. Such evolution must be taken into account when the goal is to explain the aetiology of loneliness.

With respect to microlevel factors influencing loneliness, which has attracted more attention from researchers in the past decades, there is yet much to be done. Our chapter highlights the lack of systematic evaluation of existing microlevel theories of loneliness, and a valuable contribution to the literature would be such an evaluation. We also need to prioritise our understanding of the manner in which the micro-level factors are influenced and in turn, influence each other, and theories of loneliness at other levels. For instance, biological theories of loneliness are likely to yield insight into personality phenotypes which determine loneliness, but ultimately, the phenotype is also likely to be influenced by cultural and societal factors too. Understanding the complex reciprocal nature of these causal pathways is of necessity to better understand who becomes lonely, and how to intervene.

Theories at meso-level are the most comprehensive in acknowledging the influence of micro- and macro-level factors, which makes them difficult to classify at meso level or consider them as integrative models. However, for the purpose of this paper, when the focus is put in the social relationships, it was considered as meso-level theory. Moreover, theories at meso level are consistently built on the social circles proposed by Kahn and Antonucci (1980), while being complementary on their static or dynamic perspective of social networks. Some theories complement each other by adding specific components such as the role of investments in terms of time and energy in the DIRc. Finally, at meso level, loneliness is seen as the result of unmet social expectations explained by social relationships in the immediate personal context and physical environment.

Based on the theoretical overview from this chapter, one conclusion is that there are fewer theoretical explanations at the macro-level, particularly compared to micro-level theories. Empirical evidence suggests that much of the explanation for loneliness lies in interindividual and interpersonal aspects (Barjaková et al., 2023).

Macro level factors, meanwhile, are shown to explain a smaller portion of the variance in loneliness (e.g., Langenkamp, 2023). This could be one reason why macro-level theories are less explored—they might be perceived as less significant in explaining loneliness. Additionally, as discussed by Swader and Moraru (2023), significant confounding variables complicate the interpretation of the societal impact. Societies reporting lower levels of loneliness, such as those in Northern and Western Europe, frequently share a set of common features, including higher wealth, more developed welfare systems, different population structure, increased social capital, and a higher degree of civic engagement. These factors could collectively influence the experience of loneliness—making it thus challenging to isolate their individual impacts or to evaluate the potential independent effects of nationality on loneliness. Lastly, ageist attitudes in the society, along with structural and cultural changes such as advancement in digital technology and its usage, have also been suggested as potentially affecting loneliness in later life (Fried et al., 2020; Morgan et al., 2021). However, these factors have so far been relatively unexplored from a macro-level theoretical perspective, highlighting the need for further research.

Competing Interests The authors have no conflicts of interest to declare that are relevant to the content of this chapter.

References

Akhter-Khan, S. C., Prina, M., Wong, G. H. Y., Mayston, R., & Li, L. (2023). Understanding and addressing older adults' loneliness: The social relationship expectations framework. *Perspectives on Psychological Science, 18*(4), 762–777. https://doi.org/10.1177/17456916221127218

Badman, R. P., Nordström, R., Ueda, M., & Akaishi, R. (2022). Perceptions of social rigidity predict loneliness across the Japanese population. *Scientific Reports, 12*(1), 16073. https://doi.org/10.1038/s41598-022-20561-5

Baltes, M. M., & Carstensen, L. L. (2003). The process of successful aging: Selection, optimization, and compensation. In P. H. Baltes & O. G. Brim (Eds.), *Understanding human development* (pp. 81–104). Springer US. https://doi.org/10.1007/978-1-4615-0357-6_5

Barjaková, M., Garnero, A., & d'Hombres, B. (2023). Risk factors for loneliness: A literature review. *Social Science & Medicine*, 116163. https://doi.org/10.1016/j.socscimed.2023.116163

Barreto, M., Doyle, D. M., & Qualter, P. (2024). Changing the narrative: Loneliness as a social justice issue. *Advances in Political Psychology, 45*(Suppl. 1), 157–181. https://doi.org/10.1111/pops.12965

Barreto, M., Victor, C., Hammond, C., Eccles, A., Richins, M. T., & Qualter, P. (2021). Loneliness around the world: Age, gender, and cultural differences in loneliness. *Personality and Individual Differences, 169*, 110066. https://doi.org/10.1016/j.paid.2020.110066

Bekhet, A. K., & Zauszniewski, J. A. (2012). Mental health of elders in retirement communities: Is loneliness a key factor? *Archives of Psychiatric Nursing, 26*(3), 214–224. https://doi.org/10.1016/j.apnu.2011.09.007

Bergman, Y. S., Faran, Y., Caspi, E., & Klonover, E. (2024). Subjective age and loneliness in older adults: The moderating role of attachment patterns. *Journal of Applied Gerontology, 43*(7), 970–977. https://doi.org/10.1177/07334648231223357

Berkman, L. F., Glass, T., Brissette, I., & Seeman, T. E. (2000). From social integration to health: Durkheim in the new millennium. *Social Science & Medicine, 51*(6), 843–857. https://doi.org/10.1016/s0277-9536(00)00065-4

Bolmsjö, I., Tengland, P. A., & Rämgård, M. (2019). Existential loneliness: An attempt at an analysis of the concept and the phenomenon. *Nursing Ethics, 26*(5), 1310–1325. https://doi.org/10.1177/0969733017748480

Boomsma, D. I., Willemsen, G., Dolan, C. V., Hawkley, L. C., & Cacioppo, J. T. (2005). Genetic and environmental contributions to loneliness in adults: The Netherlands twin register study. *Behavior Genetics, 35*, 745–752. https://doi.org/10.1007/s10519-005-6040-8

Bronfenbrenner, U. (2000). *Ecological system theory*. Oxford University Press.

Buecker, S., Maes, M., Denissen, J. J. A., & Luhmann, M. (2020). Loneliness and the big five personality traits: A meta–analysis. *European Journal of Personality, 34*(1), 8–28. https://doi.org/10.1002/per.2229

Burholt, V. (2023). Culture, social isolation, and loneliness in later life. In A. Hajek, S. Riedel-Heller, & H. H. König (Eds.), *Loneliness and social isolation in old age* (pp. 51–60). Routledge. https://doi.org/10.4324/9781003289012-8

Burholt, V., & Dobbs, C. (2012). Research on rural ageing: Where have we got to and where are we going in Europe? *Journal of Rural Studies, 28*(4), 432–446. https://doi.org/10.1016/j.jrurstud.2012.01.009

Burholt, V., Winter, B., Aartsen, M., Constantinou, C., Dahlberg, L., Feliciano, V., De Jong Gierveld, J., Van Regenmortel, S., Waldegrave, C., & Working Group on Exclusion from Social Relations, part of the COST-financed Research Network 'Reducing Old-Age Exclusion: Collaborations in Research and Policy' (ROSENet). (2020). A critical review and development of a conceptual model of exclusion from social relations for older people. *European Journal of Ageing, 17*(1), 3–19. https://doi.org/10.1007/s10433-019-00506-0

Cacioppo, J. T., Cacioppo, S., & Boomsma, D. I. (2014a). Evolutionary mechanisms for loneliness. *Cognition and Emotion, 28*, 3–21. https://doi.org/10.1080/02699931.2013.837379

Cacioppo, S., Capitanio, J. P., & Cacioppo, J. T. (2014b). Toward a neurology of loneliness. *Psychological Bulletin, 140*, 1464–1504. https://doi.org/10.1037/a0037618

Cacioppo, J. T., & Hawkley, L. C. (2009). Perceived social isolation and cognition. *Trends in Cognitive Sciences, 13*, 447–454. https://doi.org/10.1016/j.tics.2009.06.005

Carr, S., & Fang, C. (2023). A gradual separation from the world: A qualitative exploration of existential loneliness in old age. *Ageing and Society, 43*(6), 1436–1456. https://doi.org/10.1017/S0144686X21001252

Carstensen, L. L. (1993). Motivation for social contact across the life span: A theory of socioemotional selectivity. In J. E. Jacobs (Ed.), *Nebraska symposium on motivation, 1992: Developmental perspectives on motivation* (pp. 209–254). University of Nebraska Press.

Crow, G., & Allan, G. (1994). *Community life: An introduction to local social relations*. Harvester Wheatsheaf.

Dahlberg, L., Krug, E. G., Mercy, J. A., Zwi, A. B., & Lozano, R. (2002). Chapter 1. Violence: A global public health problem. In *World report on violence and health* (pp. 12–15).

Das, A. (2022). Secularism, family ties and loneliness: A multilevel longitudinal study of ten European societies. *Social Science Research, 101*, 102619. https://doi.org/10.1016/j.ssresearch.2022.102619

De Jong Gierveld, J., & Tesch-Römer, C. (2012). Loneliness in old age in Eastern and Western European societies: Theoretical perspectives. *European Journal of Ageing, 9*, 285–295. https://doi.org/10.1007/s10433-012-0248-2

Derlega, V. J., & Margulis, S. T. (1982). Why loneliness occurs: The interrelationship of social-psychological and privacy concepts. In L. A. Peplau & D. Perlman (Eds.), *Loneliness: A sourcebook of current theory, research and therapy* (pp. 152–164) [13 pages]. Wiley.

DiTommaso, E., Brannen-McNulty, C., Ross, L., & Burgess, M. (2003). Attachment styles, social skills and loneliness in young adults. *Personality and Individual Differences, 35*(2), 303–312. https://doi.org/10.1016/S0191-8869(02)00190-3

Dwyer, L. (2024). Canadian perspectives on loneliness; digital communication as meaningful connection. *Frontiers in Public Health, 12*, 1389099. https://doi.org/10.3389/fpubh.2024.1389099
Feng, X., & Astell-Burt, T. (2022). Lonelygenic environments: A call for research on multilevel determinants of loneliness. *Lancet Planetary Health, 6*(12), e933–e934. https://doi.org/10.1016/S2542-5196(22)00306-0
Fokkema, T., de Jong-Gierveld, J., & Dykstra, P. A. (2012). Cross-national differences in older adult loneliness. *Journal of Psychology, 146*, 201–228. https://doi.org/10.1080/00223980.2011.597012
Fraley, R. C. (2019). Attachment in adulthood: Recent developments, emerging debates, and future directions. *Annual Review of Psychology, 70*(1), 401–422. https://doi.org/10.1146/annurev-psych-010418-102813
Fried, L., Prohaska, T., Burholt, V., Burns, A., Golden, J., Hawkley, L., et al. (2020). A unified approach to loneliness. *The Lancet, 395*(10218). https://doi.org/10.1016/S0140-6736(20)31338-2
Fromm Reichmann, F. (1959). Loneliness. *Psychiatry, 22*(1), 1–15. https://doi.org/10.1080/00332747.1959.11023153
Galanaki, E. P., & Vassilopoulou, H. D. (2007). Teachers and children's loneliness: A review of the literature and educational implications. *European Journal of Psychology of Education, 22*, 455–475.
Ghenţa, M., & Matei, A. (2025). Policy recommendations to address loneliness in later life. In M. Aartsen, I. Precupetu, & B. Suanet (Eds.), *Macro social influences on loneliness in later life: Towards a better understanding of the loneliness paradox in later life*. Springer.
Gil Alvarez, M., Haugan, G., Larsson, H., Sarrelainen, S. M., Duppen, D., & Dezulter, J. (2023). Mapping existential loneliness and isolation: Conceptualisations and operationalisations. *Journal of Humanistic Psychology*. https://doi.org/10.1177/00221678231193780
Goossens, L., Van Roekel, E., Verhagen, M., Cacioppo, J. T., Cacioppo, S., Maes, M., & Boomsma, D. I. (2015). The genetics of loneliness: Linking evolutionary theory to genome-wide genetics, epigenetics, and social science. *Perspectives on Psychological Science, 10*(2), 213–226. https://doi.org/10.1177/1745691614564878
Greenfield EA., Black K., Buffel T. & Yeh J. (2019). Community Gerontology: A Framework for Research, Policy, and Practice on Communities and Aging. *Gerontologist, 59*(5), 803–810. https://doi.org/10.1093/geront/gnx089
Hansen, T., & Slagsvold, B. (2016). Late-life loneliness in 11 European countries: Results from the generations and gender survey. *Social Indicators Research, 129*, 445–464. https://doi.org/10.1007/s11205-015-1180-5
Hawkley, L. C., & Capitanio, J. P. (2015). Perceived social isolation, evolutionary fitness, and health outcomes: A lifespan approach. *Philosophical Transactions of the Royal Society, 370*, 20140114. https://doi.org/10.1098/rstb.2014.0114
Heinrich, L. M., & Gullone, E. (2006). The clinical significance of loneliness: A literature review. *Clinical Psychology Review, 26*, 695–718. https://doi.org/10.1016/j.cpr.2006.04.002
Heu, L. C., van Zomeren, M., & Hansen, N. (2021). Does loneliness thrive in relational freedom or restriction? The culture-loneliness framework. *Review of General Psychology, 25*(1), 60–72. https://doi.org/10.1177/1089268020959033
Holt-Lunstad, J. (2018). Why social relationships are important for physical health: A systems approach to understanding and modifying risk and protection. *Annual Review of Psychology, 69*(1), 437–458. https://doi.org/10.1146/annurev-psych-122216-011902
Holt-Lunstad, J. (2022). Social connection as a public health issue: The evidence and a systemic framework for prioritizing the "social" in social determinants of health. *Annual Review of Public Health, 43*(1), 193–213. https://doi.org/10.1146/annurev-publhealth-052020-110732
Holt-Lunstad, J., Robles, T. F., & Sbarra, D. A. (2017). Advancing social connection as a public health priority in the United States. *The American Psychologist, 72*(6), 517–530. https://doi.org/10.1037/amp0000103

Holton, E., Boyle, N. B., Simons, R., Warters, A., O'Philbin, L., Lawlor, B., et al. (2023). Freedom and loneliness: Dementia caregiver experiences of the nursing home transition. *Age and Ageing, 52*(3), afad033. https://doi.org/10.1093/ageing/afad033

Huxhold, O., & Fiori, K. L. (2024). Understanding loneliness in late life. *Current Opinion in Psychology, 57*, 101801. https://doi.org/10.1016/j.copsyc.2024.101801

Huxhold, O., Fiori, K. L., & Windsor, T. (2022). Rethinking social relationships in adulthood: The differential investment of resources model. *Personality and Social Psychology Review, 26*(1), 57–82. https://doi.org/10.1177/10888683211011525

Imamoglu, E. O., Küller, R., Imamoglu, V., & Küller, M. (1993). The social psychological worlds of Swedes and Turks in and around retirement. *Journal of Cross-Cultural Psychology, 24*(1), 26–41. https://doi.org/10.1177/0022022193241003

Kahn, R. L., & Antonucci, T. C. (1980). Convoys over the life course: Attachment, roles, and social support. In P. B. Baltes & O. G. Brim (Eds.), *Life-span development and behavior* (pp. 253–286). Academic.

Kettell, S. (2019). Secularism and religion. In *Oxford research encyclopedia of politics* (pp. 1–16). Oxford University Press. https://doi.org/10.1093/acrefore/9780190228637.013.378

Klasen, L. J., Bünning, M., Kelle, N., Tesch-Römer, C., & Huxhold, O. (2025). The influence of societal crises on social integration and loneliness. In M. Aartsen, I. Precupetu, & B. Suanet (Eds.), *Macro social influences on loneliness in later life: Towards a better understanding of the loneliness paradox in later life*. Springer.

Kumar, S. (2024). Antecedents of loneliness: A systematic review. *International Journal of Sociology and Social Policy, 44*(1), 1–21. https://doi.org/10.1108/IJSSP-04-2023-0103

Kupersmidt, J. B., Sigda, K. B., Sedikides, C., & Voegler, M. E. (1999). Social self-discrepancy theory and loneliness during childhood and adolescence. *Loneliness in Childhood and Adolescence, 1*, 263–279. https://doi.org/10.1017/CBO9780511551888.013

Langenkamp, A. (2023). The influence of loneliness on perceived connectedness and trust beliefs–longitudinal evidence from The Netherlands. *Journal of Social and Personal Relationships, 40*(7), 2298–2322. https://doi.org/10.1177/02654075221144716

Lykes, V. A., & Kemmelmeier, M. (2014). What predicts loneliness? Cultural difference between individualistic and collectivistic societies in Europe. *Journal of Cross-Cultural Psychology, 45*(3), 468–490. https://doi.org/10.1177/0022022113501205

Magai, C., Frías, M. T., & Shaver, P. R. (2016). Attachment in middle and later life. In J. Cassidy & P. R. Shaver (Eds.), *Handbook of attachment* (3rd ed., pp. 534–552). The Guilford Press.

Mahon, N. E., Yarcheski, A., Yarcheski, T. J., Cannella, B. L., & Hanks, M. M. (2006). A meta-analytic study of predictors for loneliness during adolescence. *Nursing Research, 55*(5), 308–315. https://doi.org/10.1097/00006199-200609000-00003

Marangoni, C., & Ickes, W. (1989). Loneliness: A theoretical review with implications for measurement. *Journal of Social and Personal Relationships, 6*, 93–128. https://doi.org/10.1177/026540758900600107

Mayers, A. M., & Svartberg, M. (2001). Existential loneliness: A review of the concept, its psychosocial precipitants and psychotherapeutic implications for HIV-infected women. *British Journal of Medical Psychology, 74*, 539–553. https://doi.org/10.1348/000711201161082

McHugh Power, J. E., Dolezal, L., Kee, F., & Lawlor, B. A. (2018). Conceptualizing loneliness in health research: Philosophical and psychological ways forward. *Journal of Theoretical and Philosophical Psychology, 38*(4), 219. https://doi.org/10.1037/teo0000099

McHugh Power, J. E., Steptoe, A., Kee, F., & Lawlor, B. A. (2019). Loneliness and social engagement in older adults: A bivariate dual change score analysis. *Psychology and Aging, 34*(1), 152.

McKenna-Plumley, P. E., Turner, R. N., Yang, K., & Groarke, J. M. (2024). The brief scale of existential loneliness: Scale development and psychometric evaluation. *Current Psychology, 43*(42), 32907–32920. https://doi.org/10.1007/s12144-024-06828-2

Meehan, D. E., Grunseit, A., Condie, J., HaGani, N., & Merom, D. (2023). Social-ecological factors influencing loneliness and social isolation in older people: A scoping review. *BMC Geriatrics, 23*(1), 726. https://doi.org/10.1186/s12877-023-04418-8

Mikulincer, M., & Shaver, P. R. (2014). An attachment perspective on loneliness. In R. J. Coplan & J. C. Bowker (Eds.), *The handbook of solitude: Psychological perspectives on social isolation, social withdrawal, and being alone* (pp. 34–50). Wiley Blackwell.

Mikulincer, M., Shaver, P. R., & Gal, I. (2021). An attachment perspective on solitude and loneliness. In R. J. Coplan, J. C. Bowker, & L. J. Nelson (Eds.), *Handbook of solitude* (2nd ed.). Wiley. https://doi.org/10.1002/9781119576457.ch3

Morgan, D., Dahlberg, L., Waldegrave, C., Mikulioniene, S., Rapoliene, G., Lamura, G., & Aartsen, M. (2021). Revisiting loneliness: Individual and country-level changes. In K. Walsh, T. Scharf, A. Wanka, & S. Van Regenmortel (Eds.), *Social exclusion in ageing societies: Interdisciplinary and policy perspectives* (pp. 99–117). Springer. https://doi.org/10.1007/978-3-030-51406-8_8

Moustakas, C. (1976). *Loneliness*. Prentice-Hall.

Mund, M., Freuding, M. M., Möbius, K., Horn, N., & Neyer, F. J. (2020). The stability and change of loneliness across the life span: A meta-analysis of longitudinal studies. *Personality and Social Psychology Review, 24*(1), 24–52. https://doi.org/10.1177/1088868319850738

Mund, M., Lüdtke, O., & Neyer, F. J. (2020). Owner of a lonely heart: The stability of loneliness across the life span. *Journal of Personality and Social Psychology, 119*(2), 497. https://doi.org/10.1037/pspp0000262

Nowland, R., Necka, E. A., & Cacioppo, J. T. (2018). Loneliness and social Internet use: Pathways to reconnection in a digital world? *Perspectives on Psychological Science: A Journal of the Association for Psychological Science, 13*(1), 70–87. https://doi.org/10.1177/1745691617713052

Nyqvist, F. (2009). *Social capital and health: Variations, associations and challenges.* [Dissertation]. Åbo Akademi University.

Nyqvist, F., Nygård, M., & Scharf, T. (2019). Loneliness amongst older people in Europe: A comparative study of welfare regimes. *European Journal of Ageing, 16*, 133–143. https://doi.org/10.1007/s10433-018-0453-y

Nyqvist, F., Nygård, M., & Scharf, T. (2021). Social capital and loneliness in welfare state regimes before and after the global financial crisis: Results based on the European Social Survey. In A. Almakaeva, A. Moreno, & R. Wilkes (Eds.), *Social capital and subjective wellbeing: Insights from cross-cultural studies* (pp. 237–259). Springer.

Peplau, L. A., & Perlman, D. (1982). Perspectives on loneliness. In L. A. Peplau & D. Perlman (Eds.), *Loneliness: A sourcebook of current theory, research and therapy* (pp. 1–20). Wiley.

Perlman, D., & Peplau, L. A. (1982). Theoretical approaches to loneliness. In L. A. Peplau & D. Perlman (Eds.), *Loneliness: A sourcebook of current theory, research and therapy* (pp. 123–134). Wiley.

Pound, P., & Campbell, R. (2015). Exploring the feasibility of theory synthesis: A worked example in the field of health related risk-taking. *Social Science & Medicine, 124*, 57–65. https://doi.org/10.1016/j.socscimed.2014.11.029

Prohaska, T., Burholt, V., Burns, A., Golden, J., Hawkley, L., Lawlor, B., & Fried, L. (2020). Consensus statement: Loneliness in older adults, the 21st century social determinant of health? *BMJ Open, 10*(8), e034967. https://doi.org/10.1136/bmjopen-2019-034967

Putnam, R. D. (2000). Bowling alone: The collapse and revival of American Community: New York: Simon und Schuster, 2001. ISBN. In *Policy analysis* (Vol. 20). https://doi.org/10.2307/3089235

Qualter, P., Vanhalst, J., Harris, R., Van Roekel, E., Lodder, G., Bangee, M., & Verhagen, M. (2015). Loneliness across the life span. *Perspectives on Psychological Science, 10*, 250–264. https://doi.org/10.1177/1745691615568999

Rapolienė, G., & Aartsen, M. (2022). Lonely societies: low trust societies? Further explanations for national variations in loneliness among older Europeans. *European Journal of Ageing, 19*(3), 485–494. https://doi.org/10.1007/s10433-022-00651-5

Reeskens, T., & Van Oorschot, W. (2014). European feelings of deprivation amidst the financial crisis: Effects of welfare state effort and informal social relations. *Acta Sociologica, 57*(3), 191–206. https://doi.org/10.1177/0001699313504231

Rosedale, M. (2007). Loneliness: An exploration of meaning. *Journal of the American Psychiatric Nurses Association, 13*, 201–209. https://doi.org/10.1177/1078390307306617

Rote, S., Hill, T. D., & Ellison, C. G. (2013). Religious attendance and loneliness in later life. *The Gerontologist, 53*(1), 39–50. https://doi.org/10.1093/geront/gns073

Rothstein, B., & Stolle, D. (2008). The state and social capital: An institutional theory of generalized trust. *Comparative Politics, 40*(4), 441–459. https://doi.org/10.5129/001041508X12911362383354

Schwadel, P. (2005). Individual, congregational, and denominational effects on church members' civic participation. *Journal for the Scientific Study of Religion, 44*(2), 159–171. https://doi.org/10.1111/j.1468-5906.2005.00273.x

Spence, R., Jacobs, C., & Bifulco, A. (2020). Attachment style, loneliness and depression in older age women. *Aging & Mental Health, 24*(5), 837–839. https://doi.org/10.1080/13607863.2018.1553141

Spithoven, A. W., Cacioppo, S., Goossens, L., & Cacioppo, J. T. (2019). Genetic contributions to loneliness and their relevance to the evolutionary theory of loneliness. *Perspectives on Psychological Science, 14*(3), 376–396. https://doi.org/10.1177/1745691618812684

Sullivan, H. S. (1953). *The interpersonal theory of psychiatry*. Norton Publishing.

Sundström, G., Fransson, E., Malmberg, B., & Davey, A. (2009). Loneliness among older Europeans. *European Journal of Ageing, 6*, 267–275. https://doi.org/10.1007/s10433-009-0134-8

Swader, C. S. (2019). Loneliness in Europe: Personal and societal individualism-collectivism and their connection to social isolation. *Social Forces, 97*(3), 1307–1336. https://doi.org/10.1093/sf/soy088

Swader, C. S., & Moraru, A. V. (2023). Social infrastructure and the alleviation of loneliness in Europe. *KZfSS Kölner Zeitschrift für Soziologie und Sozialpsychologie, 75*(Suppl 1), 387–414. https://doi.org/10.1007/s11577-023-00827-5

Taniguchi, H., & Kaufman, G. (2022). Family, collectivism, and loneliness from a cross-country perspective. *Applied Research in Quality of Life, 17*(3), 1555–1581. https://doi.org/10.1007/s11482-021-09903-3

Tapia-Muñoz, T., Staudinger, U. M., Allel, K., Steptoe, A., Miranda-Castillo, C., Medina, J. T., & Calvo, E. (2022). Income inequality and its relationship with loneliness prevalence: A cross-sectional study among older adults in the US and 16 European countries. *PLoS One, 17*(12), e0274518. https://doi.org/10.1371/journal.pone.0274518

Upenieks, L. (2023). With you until the end of the age? A longitudinal study of changes in religiosity and loneliness in later life. *Research on Aging, 45*(3–4), 299–319. https://doi.org/10.1177/01640275221109045

Van Regenmortel, S., Tiilikainen, E., Ristolainen, H., Burholt, V., & Dahlberg, L. (2025). Social exclusion perspective on loneliness in later life. In M. Aartsen, I. Precupetu, & B. Suanet (Eds.), *Macro social influences on loneliness in later life: Towards a better understanding of the loneliness paradox in later life*. Springer.

van Staden, W. C., & Coetzee, K. (2010). Conceptual relations between loneliness and culture. *Current Opinion in Psychiatry, 23*(6), 524–529. https://doi.org/10.1097/YCO.0b013e32833f2ff9

van Tilburg, T. G. (2021). Social, emotional, and existential loneliness: A test of the multidimensional concept. *The Gerontologist, 61*(7), e335–e344. https://doi.org/10.1093/geront/gnaa082

Victor, C., & Sullivan, M. P. (2015). Loneliness and isolation. In J. Twigg & W. Martin (Eds.), *Handbook of cultural gerontology* (pp. 252–260). Routledge.

Villalonga-Olives, E., & Kawachi, I. (2017). The dark side of social capital: A systematic review of the negative health effects of social capital. *Social Science & Medicine, 194*, 105–127. https://doi.org/10.1016/j.socscimed.2017.10.020

Weiss, R. S. (1973). *Loneliness: The experience of emotional and social isolation*. The MIT Press.

Wenger, G. C. (1996). Social networks and gerontology. *Reviews in Clinical Gerontology, 6*(3), 285–293.

Wong, N. M., Shao, R., Wu, J., Tao, J., Chen, L., & Lee, T. M. (2019). Cerebellar neural markers of susceptibility to social isolation and positive affective processing. *Brain Structure and Function, 224*, 3339–3351. https://doi.org/10.1007/s00429-019-01965-y

Wong, N. M., Yeung, P. P., & Lee, T. M. (2018). A developmental social neuroscience model for understanding loneliness in adolescence. *Social Neuroscience, 13*(1), 94–103. https://doi.org/10.1080/17470919.2016.1256832

Zysberg, L. (2015). Emotional antecedents of psychological loneliness: A review and an emerging model. In D. L. Rhodes (Ed.), *Loneliness: Psychosocial risk factors, prevalence and impacts on physical and emotional health* (pp. 57–72). Nova Science Publishers.

Fredrica Nyqvist is an Associate Professor of Social Policy at Åbo Akademi University in Finland. Her research focuses on loneliness, civic engagement, social inclusion and exclusion, and active ageing. She currently co-leads the Gerontological Regional Database (GERDA) study in Finland and Sweden, which collects data on loneliness among younger and very old adults, enabling longitudinal and time-trend analyses.

Joanna McHugh Power is Associate Professor in Psychology at Maynooth University, Ireland. She is interested in conceptualising loneliness and in the epidemiology of loneliness—particularly linked to health outcomes—in older adults. She has received funding from the Irish Research Council, Health Research Board, and UK Research and Innovation for her research. Joanna is interested in solutions to loneliness and sits on a national Loneliness Taskforce in Ireland.

Laura Coll-Planas is a medical doctor with a PhD in Public Health. She is Associate Professor in Public Health at Universitat de Vic-Universitat Central de Catalunya, Spain. Her research is focused on loneliness interventions promoting social capital, evaluating their process and impact in adulthood and older adults. She has participated in a leading role on several national and European projects such as Join4joy (ErasmusPlus) and RECETAS (H2020).

Open Access This chapter is licensed under the terms of the Creative Commons Attribution 4.0 International License (http://creativecommons.org/licenses/by/4.0/), which permits use, sharing, adaptation, distribution and reproduction in any medium or format, as long as you give appropriate credit to the original author(s) and the source, provide a link to the Creative Commons license and indicate if changes were made.

The images or other third party material in this chapter are included in the chapter's Creative Commons license, unless indicated otherwise in a credit line to the material. If material is not included in the chapter's Creative Commons license and your intended use is not permitted by statutory regulation or exceeds the permitted use, you will need to obtain permission directly from the copyright holder.

Chapter 3
Unravelling the Socio-cultural Influence on Loneliness

Theo G. van Tilburg

3.1 Introduction

In the common conception of loneliness, it is a characteristic of a person, with individual antecedents. Loneliness is a negative experience of an imbalance (or discrepancy) between realized relationships and the level of desired relationships (Perlman & Peplau, 1981). This includes situations in which the number of existing relationships is smaller than is considered desirable. It also encompasses situations in which the quality or intimacy one desires has not been realized. Although sometimes referred to as a lonely society (Franklin, 2012), by loneliness we refer to the experience of an individual. In addition to individual antecedents of loneliness, however, there are factors in society that increase or decrease the likelihood of loneliness. Therefore, the prevalence of loneliness varies by historical time and geographical space (Luhmann et al., 2023). In this chapter, we discuss socio-cultural influences on loneliness, i.e., related differences in social values and norms.

Values are underlying ideals that are referred to as valuable. They indicate what is considered important. Social values can be adopted by the individual and become personal values and then guide (within any limitations) the individual's behavior. Values describe what is desirable, that is, what is the right choice and better than other choices. For example, values include that it is good to form relationships to receive support, to develop oneself and to be there for others. A satisfying network can be realized, which reduces the chance of loneliness. Social values can be internalized, making the distinction between social values and individual beliefs fluid. In the cognitive approach to loneliness, which underlies Perlman and Peplau's (1981)

T. G. van Tilburg (✉)
Department of Sociology, Faculty of Social Sciences and Department of Epidemiology & Data Science, Vrije Universiteit Amsterdam and Amsterdam University Medical Centers, Amsterdam, The Netherlands
e-mail: theo.van.tilburg@vu.nl

© The Author(s) 2025

M. Aartsen et al. (eds.), *Macro Social Influences on Loneliness in Later Life*, International Perspectives on Aging 47,
https://doi.org/10.1007/978-3-031-94565-6_3

definition, this can be seen in the level of relationship standards. However, social values and individual standards about personal relationships do not always correspond. Thus, to properly understand individual experiences of loneliness, we must consider both social values and individual standards.

Social values have their counterpart in social norms—both influence relationship behavior. Both are part of a moral discourse, but they differ in the way they operate (Hansson, 1991). Values stimulate certain behaviors. Social norms are rules about how groups of individuals are supposed to behave. Norms are prescriptive, prohibitive or permissive. In these different strengths, certain behavior is more or less coercively imposed from the outside. At the same time, norms are often injunctive, meaning that people understand what others expect of them in a social context (Chung & Rimal, 2016). Norms limit the behavior of individuals and indicate, for example, that relationships with people of a different origin, belief or sexual identity are less desirable. Norms are usually unwritten, although for example etiquette, consisting of courtesies and manners, is often described. Behavior that follows the values and does not conflict with the norms is not enforceable. However, deviant behavior can be sanctioned, such as through social disapproval and exclusion, resulting in a restricted personal network and in loneliness.

In this chapter, we elaborate on the relationships between social values and norms and individual relationship standards and behaviors, with the aim of better understanding individual antecedents of loneliness in a socio-cultural context. We start with the introduction and discussion of individualism and collectivism—two social value systems that are usually contrasted. However, these concepts are not unambiguous, and we propose conceptualizing them as two dimensions, which we further explain through the process of modernization. Previous research has modeled socio-cultural influences (Burholt, 2023; de Jong Gierveld & Tesch-Römer, 2012; Luhmann et al., 2023; Tesch-Römer & Huxhold, 2019). We discuss more precisely how social values and norms influence behavior in relationships and loneliness via appraisal and sanctioning, respectively. Inspired by Coleman's (1986) general explanatory model, we introduce a model with paths of socio-cultural influence on the loneliness of an individual. We discuss limitations in the elaboration of the model, including the question of whether, in addition to the loneliness of the individual, there is also a lonely society as a result of social values and norms.

3.2 Individualism and Collectivism

3.2.1 Contrasting Individualistic and Collectivistic Countries

Johnson and Mullins (1987) were among the first to pay attention to loneliness in the context of societies with individualistic values versus societies with collectivistic values. These different value systems reflect themselves in individuals' needs and expectations of social relationships. In individualistic societies, high value is generally given to the individual, and therefore, one gives priority to individual autonomy, achievement, and self-reliance. There are geographically dispersed social ties and families of different generations live independently; the individual puts their own needs before those of the common good (Burholt, 2023). Because relationship needs and expectations are relatively low, it is less likely that there is a discrepancy with the actual emotional bonds. As a result, there is a low likelihood of loneliness. However, in an individualistic society, there can still be loneliness if low needs and expectations are not realized, or if individuals participate in subsystems such as a family or a group of friends within which there are more collectivist values.

In collectivist societies, priority is given to the needs of others (and of the groups to which one belongs) over one's own needs (Schwartz et al., 2010). People belong to a specific group, and this group takes care of them in exchange for loyalty (Hofstede & Bond, 1984). Collectivism includes several other concepts. Familism is a set of values in which family is central as a source of attachment and support, and in which loyalty and obligation to family takes precedence over the fulfillment of one's own needs (Cahill et al., 2021). Familism assumes that family members take care of each other (as a responsibility; it is not required that the family ties be of a high quality), and that few public services are needed (Saraceno, 2016). Communalism—not to be confused with *communism*—emphasizes interdependence of people and conformity to community norms and customs (Jagers & Mock, 1995). In communalism, the interest of the community takes precedence over that of the individual. The citizen is committed to the community formed by tight-knit relationships of family, church, and association. One does not believe in rules imposed by an all-powerful government, and relies on wisdom and the ingrained patterns, customs, and traditions of the community (Etzioni, 2014). Familism and communalism therefore differ somewhat, with the most important difference being that communalism places responsibility on a larger context, which can also be the more abstract form of society as a whole. Both forms of collectivism have in common that the individual does not stand alone. When individuals internalize collectivist values that encourage a high degree of identification with their family or community, but there is insufficient opportunity to maintain the necessary close contacts to realize these values, there is a high probability of loneliness (Heu et al., 2021b).

3.2.2 *Cross-National Differences in Europe: Findings and Measurement*

Various studies have compared the prevalence of loneliness in European countries. Jylhä and Jokela (1990) surveyed older people in six European countries and found that the prevalence of loneliness increases on the linear north-south axis from Finland to Greece. Individuals' ties to family and social community were closer in the south than in the north, but the percentage of people who said they often felt lonely was higher. Similar loneliness differences were observed in studies comparing, for example, Sweden and Turkey (Imamoglu et al., 1993), the Netherlands and Italy (van Tilburg et al., 1998), and a range of northern, western, southern and eastern European countries (Fokkema et al., 2012; Lykes & Kemmelmeier, 2014; Swader, 2019). On the other hand, Barreto et al. (2021) discovered in a worldwide study that the more individualistic a country, the higher the prevalence of loneliness. In another study in five European countries, Heu et al. (2019) found that collectivism was associated with lower loneliness.

The conflicting findings across these studies can stem from differences in the design of the studies and, in particular, the measurement of individualism. One way to measure individualism was to postulate that countries differed in individualism, for example, based on differences in whether the individual was inseparable from family and friends, and whether these ties were the main source of help and care for older adults (Jylhä & Jokela, 1990).

A second way was indirect measurement. For example, de Jong Gierveld and van Tilburg (1999) found that Italians reported less loneliness if they lived with one of their children compared with when they lived alone. Dutch older adults actually reported feeling lonelier when living with one of their children compared to living alone. The researchers linked these findings to a greater emphasis on the importance of family in Italy than in the Netherlands.

A third way was adopted by, for example, Barreto et al. (2021), Lykes and Kemmelmeier (2014) and Stegen et al. (2024). To compare the loneliness prevalence in countries, they used the individualism-collectivism ranking of countries originally developed by Hofstede (1983), with a continuum in which there is appreciation for people who only take care of themselves (and possibly their immediate family), versus in which people are appreciated for belonging to groups in which everyone is taken care of.

Finally, survey participants were asked about their own values. Swader (2019) asked about agreeing with the statement that it is important to make your own decisions about what you do, and be free and not dependent on others. For societal individualism, he took the average score for each country. In the study by Heu et al. (2019), respondents were asked about their internalized collectivism, for example, whether they usually follow the rules of the family. They pooled the data from individuals and did not aggregate it to the national level.

3.2.3 Two Meanings of Individualism: Collectivism

The discussion about operationalizations must be linked to the two different conceptualizations of individualism and collectivism that are recognizable. One conceptualization is the pair that individualism has the meaning that everybody is supposed to look after their own self-interest (and that of their direct family) and thus has an assumed preference for loose and insignificant relationships. In this pair, individualism is contrasted with collectivism, meaning that one should belong to a collectivity or ingroup with tight relationships and that everyone has to look after the interest of their group, with loyalty being rewarded by being looked after (Hofstede, 1983; Luhmann et al., 2023). We label this conceptualization as the solitude-togetherness dimension. A focus on solitude contributes to the social isolation of people, resulting in more loneliness. In contrast, a focus on togetherness protects individuals from loneliness. We indicate that values describe what is desirable, and what is the right choice. In the value pair of togetherness versus solitude, from the perspective of loneliness, it can be said without much debate that togetherness is a positive value because belonging is central here. The fact that some people are more focused on solitude may stem from a situation in which one has noticed that one feels less at home in groups or that one does not have the energy or capabilities to realize a connection in solidarity relationships or groups. People who are more focused on solitude isolate themselves to a greater or lesser extent from other people. In a society based on togetherness, this can be sanctioned by avoidance and neglect.

A second conceptualization is the pair that contrasts individualism, meaning that people can make their own choices, with collectivism, meaning that the opinions, beliefs and behaviors of individuals are subordinate to those in their group (Hofstede, 1983; Lykes & Kemmelmeier, 2014). We label this conceptualization as the dimension of autonomy versus submission to integration in closed groups ('submission' in short). A focus on autonomy contributes to freeing people from unwanted group loyalty and gives them the opportunity to develop satisfying relationships, resulting in less loneliness. A focus on submission, on the other hand, limits the options for individuals to act and increases the chance of loneliness. People can focus on submission to integration in closed groups, for example, because they have organically ended up in such a system (path dependency), because they find it too difficult to make choices independently, because they have not learned to do so or because they do not have the capacity to do so. For these various reasons, a dominant loyalty to one's own group will not increase the risk of loneliness to the same degree for everyone. The value of autonomy emphasizes that appropriate, satisfying relationships can be found outside the closed group. People who are more focused on their autonomy do not necessarily turn away from other people, but they do turn away from the dominant group. This can also be sanctioned by avoidance and neglect from that group.

The dual nature of the collectivist value, namely protective and restrictive, and the dual nature of the individualistic value, namely focused on relationships and on oneself, have now been pulled apart. The distinction between the two dimensions makes it clear that people can enter into meaningful relationships based on the value of togetherness, based on autonomy, or based on both values.

We note here that we are talking about social values. These are systems of ideas that transcend the individual. Much research has focused on comparing (clusters of) countries, but societies also exist on a smaller scale. We have already mentioned the community, the focus of communalism. We can also consider groups of people with a migration background, from a sexual minority, or from a young generation. These groups may have their own culture that differs from the culture within a larger society. Socio-structural differences such as rural-urban and low versus highly educated can also go hand in hand with different subcultures.

Heu et al. (2021a) connected the two conceptualizations in their framework of culture and loneliness. They focused on the restrictiveness of norms regarding social relationships and pointed out that there were different paths to loneliness. In a social environment with more restrictive norms, the risk of physical isolation is lower (with a lower chance of loneliness), but the risk of emotional isolation is higher (with a higher chance of loneliness). The researchers indicate that physical isolation can arise when people want to escape from intrusive and demanding others, and when they are unable to do so, they feel emotionally isolated because the relationship with those others is not of the desired quality. In both cases there is a discrepancy between the desired and the realized relationships. Although their framework is useful, the ambiguity of the concepts of individualism and collectivism has not yet been clarified by introducing a single concept of the restrictiveness of norms regarding social relationships. That is why we propose the value dimensions of solitude-togetherness and autonomy-submission, and will pay separate attention to the restrictiveness of norms. To better understand the need to introduce two dimensions, we will delve deeper into the background of the historical modernization process.

3.3 Togetherness and Autonomy in the Process of Modernization

3.3.1 The Lost Community

Long ago, there was growing concern about the loss of social embeddedness as a result of changes in society that we can summarize as modernization. For example, at the end of the nineteenth century in Germany, Tönnies argued that social connectedness is the result of the human will to live together. This will can take two forms: first, the will to cooperate with others as essential to the social being of humans; second, the deliberate, calculated choice to cooperate with others in order to achieve certain goals. Tönnies described a social development from the first form, which he labelled *Gemeinschaft* (community), to the second form, labelled as *Gesellschaft* (society). You could say that collectivism has been replaced by individualism (for an application of sociological theories to loneliness, see also Chap. 14 of this book; Suanet & Aartsen, 2025). This development meant moving more and more away from a type of society that offered people security and belonging, and in which feelings of togetherness were central, and moving toward a cooler, more calculating relationship style that is anonymous and distant. Examples of such connections are interest groups, business relations and sometimes the social connections formed by residents of a large city. In a groundbreaking study, Wirth (1938) saw that an urban culture and way of life was emerging with superficial, functional encounters characterized by instability and uncertainty. In this process, solidarity was lost. Weakening bonds of local kinship were replaced by impersonal, superficial, transitory, and segmental relationships. In the debate about the development of community under the influence of modernization, this was called the *community lost* position.

With this social change of a lost *Gemeinschaft*, it was assumed that the prevalence of loneliness increased (Schirmer & Michailakis, 2015). Putnam (1995) saw that people were less and less part of organized civic organizations, and more and more on their own. He argued that declining civic engagement and social connectedness threatened the success of society in many areas, including well-being and health. This supposed decline was also reflected in the characterization of loneliness as an epidemic in modern society (Bound Alberti, 2018; Killeen, 1998). At the turn of the twentieth century, the process of digitization began. There was a fear that the rise of social media (use of the Internet and e-mail, and later applications such as Facebook, WhatsApp and TikTok) would lead to meaningful, personal social interaction being blurred by superficial and distant contact in which the individual and not the communal perspective in the contact between people was central. This would lead to an increase in loneliness. The results of an early experimental study by Kraut et al. (1998) confirmed this hypothesis.

In summary, the idea of a lost community has been cited relatively often, perhaps because it is linked to dissatisfaction with the functioning of society. As we will argue in the next paragraph, thorough theoretical and empirical research does show that society has changed, but does not show that cooperation and solidarity have disappeared from our society.

3.3.2 The Saved and Liberated Community

Early empirical studies already provided contrary evidence for the loss of community. For example, Gans (1962) showed that neighborhood and family solidarity continued in the city. This *community saved* position aligned with the continuation of old structures with their associated values and norms in a new environment.

Decades later, Fischer (1982) and Wellman (1979) showed that personal networks had become much more neighborhood-wide, and had taken on a much more diverse composition than just family and neighbors; friends were recognized as a type of relationship that is also important for intimacy, help and support. Close local communities had not disappeared, but primary relationships were organized differently than in the past. People were often part of several networks. Cheap and effective transportation and communication became possible as more and more people had access to cars and telephones, for example. This promoted that people could maintain contacts within spatially dispersed networks, rather than relying solely on neighborhood and family. The community was not *lost*, but *liberated*. This liberation related not only to the previous geographical limitations of social relations, but also to their content. There came a greater scope in access to people and resources, to diverse and differentiated resources not available through local solidarity channels. Much later, there was also early evidence presented indicating that Internet use actually had positive effects on people's social networks (Franzen, 2000) because people had increased opportunities to maintain contact more frequently and over distance.

These insights fit a conceptualization of the modernization process that involved increased autonomy, freedom of choice, and the loss of structural embeddedness in social institutions such as family, church, work, and neighborhood. Giddens (1990) called this process *de-traditionalization*, and Beck (1992) called it *individualization*. Traditional forms of bonding both protected and constrained people. They protected people because social relationships were naturally available from occupying more specific roles such as family member, employee, or neighbor. In a de-traditionalized situation, individuals were able to develop a network fitting with their own preferences, and not be bound to the dominant norms of a traditional community. However, this leaves an individual somewhat alone in the management of their life. The implied liberation from traditional bonds has a downside in the potential shortage of resources to accomplish this task.

In summary, we can state that the liberated community is a combination of what was previously seen as a contradiction, namely the coexistence of collectivism and individualism. The two dimensions of solitude-togetherness and autonomy-submission are therefore more appropriate for describing social changes.

3.3.3 Evidence on Togetherness and Autonomy in Relation to Loneliness

If we continue with the ambiguous terms individualism and the counterpart collectivism, then we cannot properly determine the significance for loneliness. People in a society based on the value of togetherness, i.e., to be socially integrated and to have many social ties (high in togetherness, low in solitude) have a relatively low probability of loneliness when they are able to maintain these social connections. On the other hand, people in a society with a preference for loyalty and conformity to the groups to which they belong over freedom of individual choice (high in submission, low in autonomy) are at high risk of loneliness because realized relationships do not always meet high relationship norms and because prevailing norms limit people's behavior to realizing relationships that fit their personal values.

There is empirical support for distinguishing the autonomy-submission dimension in particular. Santos et al. (2017) operationalized autonomy based on three items from the World Values Survey: a lower emphasis on family over friends, the importance of teaching their children the value of independence, and a preference for self-expression. They found that autonomy values increased from 1960 to 2011. Empirical studies into generational differences in loneliness support the idea that increasing emphasis on autonomy does not mean that social relationships in general are devalued (Luhmann et al., 2023) and therefore does not necessarily increase the risk of loneliness. European studies show no increase in the prevalence of loneliness among older adults in Norway (Nicolaisen et al., 2022), Sweden (Dahlberg et al., 2018; Nyqvist et al., 2017) and Finland (Eloranta et al., 2015), or show a slight decrease in Germany (Hülür et al., 2016) and the Netherlands (Suanet & van Tilburg, 2019; van Tilburg, 2024; van Tilburg et al., 2015).

In addition to this indirect evidence, there is also evidence from research connecting values and loneliness. Interesting for our discourse on the two dimensions, Lykes and Kemmelmeier (2014) showed that in 'collectivist' societies relationships with family were more important for less loneliness, and in 'individualistic' societies relationships with friends and having a confidant were more important. In comparative research among European countries, Swader (2019) used an item on the importance of making one's own decisions to be free and not depending on others to measure autonomy values. He regressed loneliness on individual item scores and country averages. Not living alone, the number of people with whom the respondent can discuss intimate and personal matters and the frequency of social encounters with friends, relatives or co-workers were taken as measures of social integration, which were related to low loneliness. Interestingly, he concluded that there was the least chance of loneliness for people who were highly and variously socially integrated and lived in a society high in autonomy values; what their personal values were, was of less importance. These findings are consistent with the idea that autonomy and an individual choice of social ties are important for less loneliness, and that the underlying values are socially embedded.

3.4 Modelling the Socio-Cultural Influence on Loneliness

Adopting the togetherness-solitude and autonomy-submission dimensions, and acknowledging the importance of social norms results in three paths about the socio-cultural influence on individual's loneliness (Fig. 3.1). For simplicity, we assume for now that the influence effects are one way.

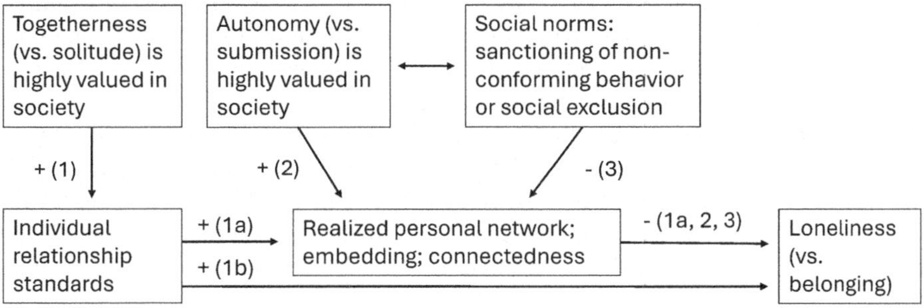

Fig. 3.1 Central concepts and effects on loneliness. Notes. The plus sign indicates a reinforcing effect; a minus sign indicates a weakening effect. Numbers in parentheses refer to the paths

3.4.1 Path 1: Togetherness—Individual Standards—Loneliness

We have already formulated assumptions for the socio-cultural influence on individual's loneliness and are now working out that these effects operate via the individual relationship standards and the realized network of relationships. In the loneliness literature, the value of social relationships at the individual level is labeled relationship standards, i.e., levels against which realized relationships are measured, but other terms are also used. For example, relationship expectations concern characteristics such as support, intimacy, and fun that individuals would like to see in their relationships (Akhter-Khan et al., 2023; Hall, 2012). Filial expectations (or obligations or responsibilities) are a specific form of relationship expectations. It is about mutual expectations that adult children and their parents have regarding the care they are supposed to give (and receive) (Hamon & Blieszner, 1990). It is generally assumed that high togetherness values are reflected in individual relationship standards in which a person wants to affiliate with others. This can lead (path 1a) to less loneliness when people are protected by their embeddedness.

There is some research on relationship standards and loneliness, in which these standards are related to autonomy and have also been measured in individuals. Dykstra (1995) examined the singlehood norm as positive attributes of being single (e.g., "Without a partner one develops a strong personality") and negative attributes of having a partner (e.g., "A partner imposes restrictions on one's life"). The partner standard described the positive aspects of being with a partner (e.g. "A partner enriches oneself") and negative aspects of being single (e.g. "Without a partner one is incomplete as a person"). Older people without partners felt less lonely if they had positive singlehood standards. If their partner standards were high, the likelihood of loneliness was higher. Nowland et al. (2019) conducted a survey of children and found that lower loneliness was associated with higher friendship expectations, measured with the instrument developed by Hall (2012).

However, high togetherness values and corresponding individual relationship standards can also lead (path 1b) to more loneliness when the high ideals about embedding are not fulfilled. High standards can be unrealistic expectations that most likely will not be realized in having a satisfying social network. For example, ten Kate et al. (2021) measured filial expectations in a survey of older Turkish immigrants. A sample item is, "Children should take responsibility for parental care if parents are in need." Filial expectations were only associated with loneliness in interaction with perceived health. Compared to older people in good health, respondents in poor health were more likely to receive care from children, and less likely to have unmet child expectations. Respondents with good health and high filial expectations were relatively high in loneliness; their expectations were not always met and led to conflict with the children. Lowering standards can help to mitigate loneliness (Masi et al., 2011).

3.4.2 Path 2: Autonomy—Personal Network—Loneliness

Path 2 assumes that people in a cultural context in which autonomy values are important are able to form and maintain a good personal network, and thereby reduce their chance of loneliness. There is some evidence for this path. We will first report on an older study that provided a detailed picture of social integration. Emphasizing the importance of togetherness, van Tilburg et al. (1998) found that Italian seniors had smaller personal networks than their peers in the Netherlands, which contributed to the greater loneliness of Italians. They also found that the composition of the household had a different relationship with loneliness in the two countries: older people living without a partner but with one or more children in Italy were less lonely than their peers in the Netherlands, while Dutch people living alone were less lonely than the Italians. Italian older people who had close and frequent contact with their children were less lonely than Italian older people without these kinds of intergenerational ties, but lonelier than Dutch older people who had close and frequent contact with their children. Emphasizing the importance of autonomy, being independent of others but having a good personal network is important to the Dutch. In the cross-national study by Swader (2019), it is found that if an individual finds it important to make their own decisions and be free, the impacts of living alone and relational isolation on increased loneliness are reduced. If there are many respondents in the country who are focused on autonomy, there is less social isolation and less loneliness.

There is also research that finds less social embedding in what they call individualistic countries or among people with individualistic values. Jylhä and Jokela (1990), for example, reports that older people in southern European countries are less likely to live alone and more likely to have good neighborly relationships than older people in northern European countries. However, this does not concern the self-chosen and developed relationship types that focus on autonomy values. In the study by Heu et al. (2019), people who want to be in frequent contact with a close friend, for example, who think that people their age should have a close relationship with their partner, are low on individualistic values and well socially embedded. The values measured here focus more on what we call togetherness and do not focus on the freedom to make one's own choices.

3.4.3 Path 3: Social Norms—Personal Network—Loneliness

Values stimulate individuals to achieve certain relationship goals. We have indicated that the pursuit of the values of solitude and autonomy can be accompanied by social sanctions. Behind these sanctions are social norms that set boundaries within which people are expected to act. Individuals know that they should behave according to accepted norms, and that if they do not, social sanctions may follow. Barreto et al. (2024) argued that the dominant group in society determines what relationship behavior is appropriate. This limits minorities in their choices, preventing them from developing a satisfactory network. Hatzenbuehler and Link (2014) referred to a stigma structurally embedded in society by which circumstances, norms, and policies limit the opportunities, resources, and well-being of specific groups of people.

There is limited research available on the influence of social norms on loneliness. Winter and Burholt (2018) studied cultural exclusion, defined as the extent to which people are able or willing to conform to social norms. They discovered that older adults in rural areas in South Wales felt excluded. During their youth, people were strongly focused on the community, but over time, younger generations and immigrants focused more on their own lives. Their cultural identity was thus at odds with contemporary norms, values, and behaviors. With that, there was a decline in connectedness and sense of community among older residents. From a different perspective, namely that of migrants, Burholt (2023) described their cultural exclusion, which causes them to become socially isolated from society, even though they often create a strongly connected social network within their own group.

In their study of adults belonging to a sexual minority, Elmer et al. (2022) argued that minority stress is a major cause of the difference in loneliness between adults belonging to a sexual majority and minority. Minority stress, i.e., the negative impact of living with a stigmatized identity, takes two forms. In our terminology, there is the sanctioning by others of being sexually deviant through discrimination, harassment, and violence. The individual responds to this through concealment of the sexual orientation from others and through internalized homonegativity, also known as self-stigma, which internalizes the negative social attitudes. The research did not include whether this sanctioning affected the ability to maintain personal relationships, although it showed a correlation with loneliness.

In a study of young-old people who have divorced, van Tilburg et al. (2015) argued that they used to deviate from the social norm and were therefore less integrated socially, which in turn was detrimental to their well-being. They hypothesized that divorced people from later cohorts were less disadvantaged compared to married people and had more opportunities for relationships that suited their individual preferences and social positions than divorced people from earlier cohorts. This idea was based on an assumed increasing normalization of divorce, which was related to the increased divorce rate. Moreover, the married lifestyle was no longer considered the social norm (Gubernskaya, 2010). Marriage seemed to have lost its exclusive right to perform an integrative, protective, and social function, and other life arrangements had become alternatives to marriage. Indeed, van Tilburg et al. (2015) found that the number of personal relationships of divorcees increased between 1992 and 2012 (but that was also the case with the comparison group of married people) and the difference in social loneliness between divorced respondents and those who married for the first time decreased between 1992 and 2012.

3.5 Discussion

We presented a model for the socio-cultural influences on loneliness. Because of our focus on the significance of social values and norms in the process in which loneliness can be a solution, we have not addressed socio-structural and individual-related conditions. For example, what relationship network can be realized depends in part on individual capabilities (such as having financial means to travel so that friendships can be maintained) and limitations (such as being unable to travel for physical or cognitive reasons). Various overviews of risk factors for loneliness are available (Barjaková et al., 2023; de Jong Gierveld et al., 2018). One limitation that results from this is that we did not show the interaction between socio-structural and socio-cultural factors. For example, it is likely that wealth and poor living conditions are related to how important living alone and autonomy are (de Jong Gierveld et al., 2012).

Our model started with social values. As indicated before, value systems do not exist only at the country level and need not be uniform or unambiguous. In complex societies, there is also variation between different parts of society. In a society, dominant groups may determine what values, norms and behaviors are appropriate. But minority groups of people with specific sexual preferences, shared migration backgrounds or deviant demographic behavior such as living alone, for example, may have their own system of values and norms that are guiding in their group (Barreto et al., 2024; Cargan, 1986). Societies in transition may also have fragmented value and norm systems. Values and norms are always fluid, but especially in such a situation. Naming values and norms provides guidance, but also limits our imagination, locking us into specific boxes, and making it difficult for individuals to find their own path to well-being. It sometimes seems that lonely people are trapped in a socio-cultural corset, and that their loneliness is not solvable other than by social upheaval. When we see the socio-cultural context as more layered and more diverse, we also see the possibilities that individual standards can better fit an individual's specific capabilities and desires.

We modelled a path with a unidirectional causal association between individual relationship standards and the realized relationship network: if standards are high, this has a motivating effect on the establishment and maintenance of social relationships, thus counteracting loneliness. We do not exclude the possibility of a reciprocal causal association. A situation of loneliness can motivate the individual to approach others with a positive attitude and try to improve the relationship network. In the study by Bellucci (2020), this was also found, but at the same time, loneliness is also associated with disappointment in how to interact with others, and, on the contrary, negative expectations are developed, along with avoiding others (we have not included this back loop effect in Fig. 3.1). Lonely people are less focused on actively engaging in new contacts, and more focused on avoiding social rejection through psychological coping (Schoenmakers et al., 2015) and engaging in superficial contacts (Tsai & Reis, 2009). As a result, loneliness may be reinforced (Cacioppo & Hawkley, 2009; Qualter et al., 2015; Spithoven et al., 2017).

A related topic is the association between personal and social values. For example, if people are disappointed in their personal relationships, does this also influence social values, i.e., do social values that focus on togetherness become less important as a result? Heu et al. (2019) suggested that the association of sociocultural values and individuals' loneliness may differ between the individual and the country level. The measurement of values and norms in the individual must distinguish between description (the prevalence of behavior as individuals perceive it in their social environment) and injunction (the individual's view of what others in their social environment expect of them in a social context) (Chung & Rimal, 2016). The measurement of values and norms at the level of a society is still underdeveloped, and its association with personal values was not studied. Approaches to this premise do exist. We already pointed to Swader's (2019) study that aggregated respondents' individualism scores into a country characteristic. But this may be too simplistic a representation of the association between personal and social values. It suggests that there are no social values independent of personal values, and that social values are by definition those of the majority of individuals. In our model, we were unable to elaborate on this association. Further research into the interplay of personal and social values is needed. This study must also consider the question of whether (supposed) central social values are widely shared in European societies, or whether there is an increasing presence of fragmented social systems that coexist and sometimes conflict with one another.

We postulated that loneliness is an individual experience. We are not in favor of naming a society as lonely (or not) because using one term with two meanings is confusing. The model we used, depicted in Fig. 3.1, showed a *downstream* influence from social characteristics to an individual experience. Combining the methodological holism and methodological individualism (Coleman, 1986), we can extend this model with a component representing the absence of connectedness and belonging of individuals at the macro level, i.e., a social characteristic. We suggest using the term *alienation* for this characterization. We acknowledge that this term alienation is also used as an individual characteristic: a detachment from yourself, and an alienation from your core and identity, a sense of being cut off from others (estrangement) and a sense of not belonging (Rokach, 1988; Sobirjonovna et al., 2024). In this meaning it is close to the meaning of existential loneliness, the awareness of the fundamental separateness as a human being (Bekhet et al., 2008; Ettema et al., 2010; van Tilburg, 2021). But alienation, human's dissatisfaction in society and the rupture between human individuality and the world of experience, is seen in economic and political philosophy primarily as a characteristic stemming from Karl Marx's social analysis (Musto, 2010). This is not the place to elaborate on the concept of alienation, but instead of a (less or more) lonely society, we feel more comfortable when we speak of a (less or more) alienated society. The methodologically holistic approach calls for an analysis of social causes of an alienated society. The methodological individualist approach, after analyzing the downstream influence from social values to individual standards and experience of loneliness, calls for an analysis of the *upstream* influence from individual loneliness to social alienation. Whereas research on the influence of social characteristics on loneliness is already scarce—we cite in this regard an example of downstream research conducted by Rapolienė and Aartsen (2022) on generalized social trust and loneliness—, the reverse influence (upstream) has not yet been the subject of research to our knowledge. This type of research can contribute to further uncovering the intertwining of social and individual processes around loneliness.

3.6 Conclusion

Previous research identified individualism and collectivism as contrasting socio-cultural value systems that influence the individual experience of loneliness. To clarify the conceptual ambiguity, we proposed distinguishing two dimensions, namely togetherness versus solitude and autonomy versus submission. Both togetherness and autonomy can contribute to less loneliness. We have described the effect of social values on loneliness along three paths. For each of the paths, there is (often still limited) supporting evidence from research. Further research into the interaction between social value systems and the individual experience of loneliness may enhance our understanding of loneliness in today's society.

Competing Interests The author has no conflict of interest to declare that are relevant to the content of this chapter.

References

Akhter-Khan, S. C., Prina, M., Wong, G. H.-Y., Mayston, R., & Li, L. (2023). Understanding and addressing older adults' loneliness: The Social Relationship Expectations Framework. *Perspectives on Psychological Science, 18*(4), 762–777. https://doi.org/10.1177/17456916221127218

Barjaková, M., Garnero, A., & d'Hombres, B. (2023). Risk factors for loneliness: A literature review. *Social Science & Medicine, 334*, 116163. https://doi.org/10.1016/j.socscimed.2023.116163

Barreto, M., Victor, C., Hammond, C., Eccles, A., Richins, M. T., & Qualter, P. (2021). Loneliness around the world: Age, gender, and cultural differences in loneliness. *Personality and Individual Differences, 169*, 110066. https://doi.org/10.1016/j.paid.2020.110066

Barreto, M., Doyle, D. M., & Qualter, P. (2024). Changing the narrative: Loneliness as a social justice issue. *Political Psychology, 45*(S1), 157–181. https://doi.org/10.1111/pops.12965

Beck, U. (1992). *Risk society: Towards a new modernity*. Sage.

Bekhet, A. K., Zauszniewski, J. A., & Nakhla, W. E. (2008). Loneliness: A concept analysis. *Nursing Forum, 43*(4), 207–213. https://doi.org/10.1111/j.1744-6198.2008.00114.x

Bellucci, G. (2020). Positive attitudes and negative expectations in lonely individuals. *Scientific Reports, 10*(1), 18595. https://doi.org/10.1038/s41598-020-75712-3

Bound Alberti, F. (2018). This "modern epidemic": Loneliness as an emotion cluster and a neglected subject in the history of emotions. *Emotion Review, 10*(3), 242–254. https://doi.org/10.1177/1754073918768876

Burholt, V. (2023). Culture, social isolation and loneliness in later life. In A. Hajek, S. G. Riedel-Heller, & H.-H. König (Eds.), *Loneliness and social isolation in old age: Correlates and implications* (pp. 50–60). Routledge. https://doi.org/10.4324/9781003289012-8

Cacioppo, J. T., & Hawkley, L. C. (2009). Perceived social isolation and cognition. *Trends in Cognitive Sciences, 13*(10), 447–454. https://doi.org/10.1016/j.tics.2009.06.005

Cahill, K. M., Updegraff, K. A., Causadias, J. M., & Korous, K. M. (2021). Familism values and adjustment among Hispanic/Latino individuals: A systematic review and meta-analysis. *Psychological Bulletin, 147*(9), 947–985. https://doi.org/10.1037/bul0000336

Cargan, L. (1986). Stereotypes of singles: A cross-cultural comparison. *International Journal of Comparative Sociology, 27*(3–4), 200–208. https://www.proquest.com/scholarly-journals/stereotypes-singles-cross-cultural-comparison/docview/1299975853/se-2?accountid=10978

Chung, A., & Rimal, R. N. (2016). Social norms: A review. *Review of Communication Research, 4*, 1–28. https://doi.org/10.12840/issn.2255-4165.2016.04.01.008

Coleman, J. S. (1986). Social theory, social research, and a theory of action. *American Journal of Sociology, 91*, 1309–1335. https://doi.org/10.1086/228423

Dahlberg, L., Agahi, N., & Lennartsson, C. (2018). Lonelier than ever? Loneliness of older people over two decades. *Archives of Gerontology and Geriatrics, 75*, 96–103. https://doi.org/10.1016/j.archger.2017.11.004

Dykstra, P. A. (1995). Loneliness among the never and formerly married: The importance of supportive friendships and a desire for independence. *Journal of Gerontology, 50B*, S321–S329. https://doi.org/10.1093/geronb/50B.5.S321

Elmer, E. M., van Tilburg, T. G., & Fokkema, T. (2022). Minority stress and loneliness in a global sample of sexual minority adults: The roles of social anxiety, social inhibition, and community involvement. *Archives of Sexual Behavior, 51*, 2269–2298. https://doi.org/10.1007/s10508-021-02132-3

Eloranta, S., Arve, S., Isoaho, H., Lehtonen, A., & Viitanen, M. (2015). Loneliness of older people aged 70: A comparison of two Finnish cohorts born 20 years apart. *Archives of Gerontology and Geriatrics, 61*(2), 254–260. https://doi.org/10.1016/j.archger.2015.06.004

Ettema, E., Derksen, L., & van Leeuwen, E. (2010). Existential loneliness and end-of-life care: A systematic review. *Theoretical Medicine and Bioethics, 31*(2), 141–169. https://doi.org/10.1007/s11017-010-9141-1

Etzioni, A. (2014). Communitarianism revisited. *Journal of Political Ideologies, 19*(3), 241–260. https://doi.org/10.1080/13569317.2014.951142

Fischer, C. S. (1982). The dispersion of kinship ties in modern society: Contemporary data and historical speculation. *Journal of Family History, 7*, 353–375. https://doi.org/10.1177/036319908200700404

Fokkema, T., de Jong Gierveld, J., & Dykstra, P. A. (2012). Cross-national differences in older adult loneliness. *The Journal of Psychology, 146*(1-2), 201–228. https://doi.org/10.1080/00223980.2011.631612

Franklin, A. (2012). A lonely society? Loneliness and liquid modernity in Australia. *Australian Journal of Social Issues, 47*(1), 11–28. https://doi.org/10.1002/j.1839-4655.2012.tb00232.x

Franzen, A. (2000). Does the Internet make us lonely? *European Sociological Review, 16*(4), 427–438. https://doi.org/10.1093/esr/16.4.427

Gans, H. J. (1962). *The urban villagers: Group and class in the life of Italian-Americans*. The Free Press.

Giddens, A. (1990). *The consequences of modernity*. Polity Press.

Gubernskaya, Z. (2010). Changing attitudes toward marriage and children in six countries. *Sociological Perspectives, 53*(2), 179–200. https://doi.org/10.1525/sop.2010.53.2.179

Hall, J. A. (2012). Friendship standards: The dimensions of ideal expectations. *Journal of Social and Personal Relationships, 29*(7), 884–907. https://doi.org/10.1177/0265407512448274

Hamon, R. R., & Blieszner, R. (1990). Filial responsibility expectations among adult child-older parent pairs. *Journal of Gerontology, 45*(3), P110–P112. https://doi.org/10.1093/geronj/45.3.P110

Hansson, S. O. (1991). Norms and values. *Crítica: Revista Hispanoamericana de Filosofía, 23*(67), 3–13. https://www.jstor.org/stable/40104644

Hatzenbuehler, M. L., & Link, B. G. (2014). Introduction to the special issue on structural stigma and health. *Social Science & Medicine, 103*, 1–6. https://doi.org/10.1016/j.socscimed.2013.12.017

Heu, L. C., van Zomeren, M., & Hansen, N. (2019). Lonely alone or lonely together? A cultural-psychological examination of individualism-collectivism and loneliness in five European countries. *Personality and Social Psychology Bulletin, 45*(5), 780–793. https://doi.org/10.1177/0146167218796793

Heu, L. C., Hansen, N., & van Zomeren, M. (2021a). Resolving the cultural loneliness paradox of choice: The role of cultural norms about individual choice regarding relationships in explaining loneliness in four European countries. *Journal of Social and Personal Relationships, 38*(7), 2053–2072. https://doi.org/10.1177/02654075211002663

Heu, L. C., van Zomeren, M., & Hansen, N. (2021b). Does loneliness thrive in relational freedom or restriction? The culture-loneliness framework. *Review of General Psychology, 25*(1), 60–72. https://doi.org/10.1177/1089268020959033

Hofstede, G. (1983). The cultural relativity of organizational practices and theories. *Journal of International Business Studies, 14*(2), 75–89. https://doi.org/10.1057/palgrave.jibs.8490867

Hofstede, G., & Bond, M. H. (1984). Hofstede's culture dimensions. *Journal of Cross-Cultural Psychology, 15*(4), 417–433. https://doi.org/10.1177/0022002184015004003

Hülür, G., Drewelies, J., Eibich, P., Düzel, S., Demuth, I., Ghisletta, P., Steinhagen-Thiessen, E., Wagner, G. G., Lindenberger, U., & Gerstorf, D. (2016). Cohort differences in psychosocial function over 20 years: Current older adults feel less lonely and less dependent on external circumstances. *Gerontology, 62*, 354–361. https://doi.org/10.1159/000438991

Imamoglu, E. O., Kuller, R., Imamoglu, V., & Kuller, M. (1993). The social psychological worlds of Swedes and Turks in and around retirement. *Journal of Cross-Cultural Psychology, 24*, 26–41. https://doi.org/10.1177/0022022193241002

Jagers, R. J., & Mock, L. O. (1995). The Communalism Scale and collectivistic-individualistic tendencies: Some preliminary indings. *Journal of Black Psychology, 21*(2), 153–167. https://doi.org/10.1177/00957984950212004

Johnson, D. P., & Mullins, L. C. (1987). Growing old and lonely in different societies: Toward a comparative perspective. *Journal of Cross-Cultural Gerontology, 2*, 257–275. https://doi.org/10.1007/BF00160684

de Jong Gierveld, J., & Tesch-Römer, C. (2012). Loneliness in old age in Eastern and Western European societies: Theoretical perspectives. *European Journal of Ageing, 9*(4), 285–295. https://doi.org/10.1007/s10433-012-0248-2

de Jong Gierveld, J., & van Tilburg, T. G. (1999). Living arrangements of older adults in the Netherlands and Italy: Coresidence values and behaviour and their consequences for loneliness. *Journal of Cross-Cultural Gerontology, 14*, 1–24. https://doi.org/10.1023/A:1006600082

de Jong Gierveld, J., Dykstra, P. A., & Schenk, N. (2012). Living arrangements, intergenerational support types and older adult loneliness in Eastern and Western Europe. *Demographic Research, 27*(7), 167–200. (In File).

de Jong Gierveld, J., van Tilburg, T. G., & Dykstra, P. A. (2018). New ways of theorizing and conducting research in the field of loneliness and social isolation. In A. L. Vangelisti & D. Perlman (Eds.), *The Cambridge handbook of personal relationships* (pp. 391–404). Cambridge University Press. https://doi.org/10.1017/9781316417867.031

Jylhä, M., & Jokela, J. (1990). Individual experiences as cultural: A cross-cultural study on loneliness among the elderly. *Ageing & Society, 10*(3), 295–315. https://doi.org/10.1017/S0144686X00008308

ten Kate, R. L. F., Bilecen, B., & Steverink, N. (2021). The role of parent-child relationships and filial expectations in loneliness among older Turkish migrants. *Social Inclusion, 9*(4), 291–303. https://doi.org/10.17645/si.v9i4.4508

Killeen, C. (1998). Loneliness: An epidemic in modern society. *Journal of Advanced Nursing, 28*(4), 762–770. https://doi.org/10.1046/j.1365-2648.1998.00703.x

Kraut, R., Patterson, M., Lundmark, V., Kiesler, S., Mukopadhyay, T., & Scherlis, W. (1998). Internet paradox: A social technology that reduces social involvement and psychological well-being? *American Psychologist, 53*(9), 1017–1031. https://doi.org/10.1037/0003-066X.53.9.1017

Luhmann, M., Buecker, S., & Rüsberg, M. (2023). Loneliness across time and space. *Nature Reviews Psychology, 2*(1), 9–23. https://doi.org/10.1038/s44159-022-00124-1

Lykes, V. A., & Kemmelmeier, M. (2014). What predicts loneliness? Cultural difference between individualistic and collectivistic societies in Europe. *Journal of Cross-Cultural Psychology, 45*(3), 468–490. https://doi.org/10.1177/0022022113509881

Masi, C. M., Chen, H. Y., Hawkley, L. C., & Cacioppo, J. T. (2011). A meta-analysis of interventions to reduce loneliness. *Personality and Social Psychology Review, 15*(3), 219–266. https://doi.org/10.1177/1088868310377394

Musto, M. (2010). Revisiting Marx's concept of alienation. *Socialism and Democracy, 24*(3), 79–101. https://doi.org/10.1080/08854300.2010.544075

Nicolaisen, M., Pripp, A. H., & Thorsen, K. (2022). Why not lonely? A longitudinal study of factors related to loneliness and non-loneliness in different age groups among people in the second part of life. *The International Journal of Aging and Human Development, 97*(2), 157–187. https://doi.org/10.1177/00914150221112292

Nowland, R. A., Balmer, D., & Qualter, P. (2019). When friends behave badly: Loneliness and children's expectations of friends and responses to transgressions. *British Journal of Developmental Psychology, 37*(4), 551–570. https://doi.org/10.1111/bjdp.12296

Nyqvist, F., Cattan, M., Conradsson, M., Näsman, M., & Gustafsson, Y. (2017). Prevalence of loneliness over ten years among the oldest old. *Scandinavian Journal of Public Health*, 1403494817697511. https://doi.org/10.1177/1403494817697511

Perlman, D., & Peplau, L. A. (1981). Toward a social psychology of loneliness. In R. Gilmour & S. W. Duck (Eds.), *Personal relationships in disorder* (pp. 31–56). Academic. https://peplau.psych.ucla.edu/wp-content/uploads/sites/141/2017/07/perlman-peplau-81.pdf

Putnam, R. D. (1995). Bowling alone: America's declining social capital. *Journal of Democracy, 6*(1), 65–78. https://doi.org/10.1353/jod.1995.0002

Qualter, P., Vanhalst, J., Harris, R., van Roekel, E., Lodder, G., Bangee, M., Maes, M., & Verhagen, M. (2015). Loneliness across the life span. *Perspectives on Psychological Science, 10*(2), 250–264. https://doi.org/10.1177/1745691615568999

Rapolienė, G., & Aartsen, M. (2022). Lonely societies: Low trust societies? Further explanations for national variations in loneliness among older Europeans. *European Journal of Ageing, 19*, 485–494. https://doi.org/10.1007/s10433-021-00649-z

Rokach, A. (1988). The experience of loneliness: A tri-level model. *The Journal of Psychology, 122*(6), 531–544. https://doi.org/10.1080/00223980.1988.9915528

Santos, H. C., Varnum, M. E. W., & Grossmann, I. (2017). Global increases in individualism. *Psychological Science, 28*(9), 1228–1239. https://doi.org/10.1177/0956797617700622

Saraceno, C. (2016). Varieties of familialism: Comparing four southern European and East Asian welfare regimes. *Journal of European Social Policy, 26*(4), 314–326. https://doi.org/10.1177/0958928716657275

Schirmer, W., & Michailakis, D. (2015). The lost Gemeinschaft: How people working with the elderly explain loneliness. *Journal of Aging Studies, 33*, 1–10. https://doi.org/10.1016/j.jaging.2015.02.001

Schoenmakers, E. C., van Tilburg, T. G., & Fokkema, T. (2015). Problem-focused and emotion-focused coping options and loneliness: How are they related? *European Journal of Ageing, 12*(2), 153–161. https://doi.org/10.1007/s10433-015-0336-1

Schwartz, S. J., Weisskirch, R. S., Hurley, E. A., Zamboanga, B. L., Park, I. J., Kim, S. Y., Umaña-Taylor, A., Castillo, L. G., Brown, E., & Greene, A. D. (2010). Communalism, familism, and filial piety: Are they birds of a collectivist feather? *Cultural Diversity and Ethnic Minority Psychology, 16*(4), 548. https://doi.org/10.1037/a0021370

Sobirjonovna, S. M., Xoliqulovna, B. M., Odiljon, S. D., & Ahror, H. G. (2024). The concept of "loneliness" and "alienation" in the English language. *Excellencia: International Multi-disciplinary Journal of Education, 2*(6), 400–403. https://multijournals.org/index.php/excellencia-imje/article/view/1365/1349

Spithoven, A. W. M., Bijttebier, P., & Goossens, L. (2017). It is all in their mind: A review on information processing bias in lonely individuals. *Clinical Psychology Review, 58*, 97–114. https://doi.org/10.1016/j.cpr.2017.10.003

Stegen, H., Duppen, D., Savieri, P., Stas, L., Pan, H., Aartsen, M., Callewaert, H., Dierckx, E., & de Donder, L. (2024). Loneliness prevalence of community-dwelling older adults and the impact of the mode of measurement, data collection, and country: A systematic review and meta-analysis. *International Psychogeriatrics*. https://doi.org/10.1017/S1041610224000425

Suanet, B., & Aartsen, M. (2025). Linking life course theory to multi-level explanations of loneliness: Towards a sociology of loneliness. In M. Aartsen, I. Precupetu, & B. Suanet (Eds.), *Macro social influences on loneliness in later life: Towards a better understanding of the loneliness paradox in later life*. Springer.

Suanet, B., & van Tilburg, T. G. (2019). Loneliness declines across birth cohorts: The impact of mastery and self-efficacy. *Psychology and Aging, 34*(8), 1134–1143. https://doi.org/10.1037/pag0000357

Swader, C. S. (2019). Loneliness in Europe: Personal and societal individualism-collectivism and their connection to social isolation. *Social Forces, 97*(3), 1307–1336. https://doi.org/10.1093/sf/soy088

Tesch-Römer, C., & Huxhold, O. (2019). Social isolation and loneliness in old age. In *Oxford research encyclopedia of psychology*. Oxford University Press. https://doi.org/10.1093/acrefore/9780190236557.013.393

van Tilburg, T. G. (2021). Social, emotional, and existential loneliness: A test of the multidimensional concept. *The Gerontologist, 61*(7), e335–e344. https://doi.org/10.1093/geront/gnaa082

van Tilburg, T. G. (2024). Residual loneliness in the Netherlands after the COVID-19 pandemic: An application of the single interrupted time series design with pre, peri and post-pandemic observations. *Public Health, 237*, 238–244. https://doi.org/10.1016/j.puhe.2024.10.023

van Tilburg, T. G., de Jong Gierveld, J., Lecchini, L., & Marsiglia, D. (1998). Social integration and loneliness: A comparative study among older adults in the Netherlands and Tuscany, Italy. *Journal of Social and Personal Relationships, 15*, 740–754. https://doi.org/10.1177/0265407598156002

van Tilburg, T. G., Aartsen, M. J., & van der Pas, S. (2015). Loneliness after divorce: A cohort comparison among Dutch young-old adults. *European Sociological Review, 31*(3), 243–252. https://doi.org/10.1093/esr/jcu086

Tsai, F. F., & Reis, H. T. (2009). Perceptions by and of lonely people in social networks. *Personal Relationships, 16*(2), 221–238. https://doi.org/10.1111/j.1475-6811.2009.01220.x

Wellman, B. (1979). The community question: The intimate networks of East Yorkers. *American Journal of Sociology, 84*(5), 1201–1231. https://doi.org/10.1086/226906

Winter, B., & Burholt, V. (2018). The welsh Welsh-Y Cymry cymreig: A study of cultural exclusion among rural-dwelling older people using a critical human ecological framework. *International Journal of Ageing and Later Life, 12*(2), 119–151. https://doi.org/10.3384/ijal.1652-8670.18399

Wirth, L. (1938). Urbanism as a way of life. *American Journal of Sociology, 44*(1), 1–24. https://doi.org/10.1086/217913

Theo G. van Tilburg (PhD in Social Sciences in 1988) is trained in sociology and research methodology. He conducts longitudinal and cohort-comparative research on the prevalence, antecedents and health consequences of loneliness, particularly among older adults, and on interventions that address the problem.

Open Access This chapter is licensed under the terms of the Creative Commons Attribution 4.0 International License (http://creativecommons.org/licenses/by/4.0/), which permits use, sharing, adaptation, distribution and reproduction in any medium or format, as long as you give appropriate credit to the original author(s) and the source, provide a link to the Creative Commons license and indicate if changes were made.

The images or other third party material in this chapter are included in the chapter's Creative Commons license, unless indicated otherwise in a credit line to the material. If material is not included in the chapter's Creative Commons license and your intended use is not permitted by statutory regulation or exceeds the permitted use, you will need to obtain permission directly from the copyright holder.

Chapter 4
Social Exclusion Perspective on Loneliness in Later Life

Sofie Van Regenmortel, Elisa Tiilikainen, Hanna Ristolainen, Vanessa Burholt, and Lena Dahlberg

4.1 Introduction

Loneliness is not evenly distributed across older populations (Beller, 2024). Certain groups are more affected, for example, older adults with a migration background, those with low socio-economic status, and/or with chronic illnesses (Barreto et al., 2023). These disparities reflect broader inequalities in access to opportunities and resources, often linked to discrimination and exclusion from society. However, compared to loneliness, social exclusion of older adults has received less attention in research, policies, and public discourse.

Loneliness and social exclusion in later life are distinct yet related concepts. Whereas loneliness is a subjective experience reflecting the individuals' unfulfilled expectations towards social relations (Perlman & Peplau, 1981; Burholt, 2026), social exclusion stretches beyond (feeling) excluded from social relations and incorporates different domains of life, such as the living environment, communities, services, and civic engagement (Scharf et al., 2005; Walsh et al., 2017). In some studies

---

S. Van Regenmortel (✉)
Society and Ageing Research Lab, Vrije Universiteit Brussel (VUB), Brussels, Belgium
e-mail: Sofie.van.regenmortel@vub.be

E. Tiilikainen · H. Ristolainen
Department of Social Sciences, University of Eastern Finland, Kuopio, Finland

V. Burholt
School of Nursing/School of Population Health, University of Auckland, Auckland, New Zealand

Swansea University, Wales, UK

L. Dahlberg
School of Health and Welfare, Dalarna University, Falun, Sweden

Aging Research Center, Karolinska Institutet and Stockholm University, Stockholm, Sweden

© The Author(s) 2025

M. Aartsen et al. (eds.), *Macro Social Influences on Loneliness in Later Life*, International Perspectives on Aging 47,
https://doi.org/10.1007/978-3-031-94565-6_4

loneliness is an indicator of social exclusion (e.g., Ristolainen et al., 2024b), while in others it has been perceived as an outcome of social exclusion (Burholt & Aartsen, 2021; Dahlberg et al., 2022b). In this chapter, we aim to increase the understanding of the interrelatedness of these concepts and phenomena and examine later life loneliness through the multidimensional framework of old-age social exclusion.

Increasingly, researchers are theorizing integrated and sociological perspectives on loneliness, with some viewing loneliness from socio-ecological perspectives (e.g. Meehan et al., 2023). Sociological theories examine how the individual experience of loneliness is influenced by economic status (recognition), access to resources, sociocultural norms, and social justice (social and political representation, participation, and access to justice) (Burholt, 2026) and attempt to integrate the various levels in one model. We contend that a social-exclusion perspective on loneliness in later life may also be usefully incorporated into integrated models and may help fulfil the aspirations of sociological theories of loneliness. It may address or remind researchers of the potential of meso- and macro-level influences, and the structural and unequal forces at play in fostering loneliness.

In this chapter, we aim to advance current understanding by presenting a social exclusion framework for later life loneliness. This framework incorporates both individual and structural factors influencing the risk of loneliness and provides means to understand the dynamic and multilevel construction and diversity of old-age disadvantage (e.g., Walsh et al., 2017; Van Regenmortel et al., 2018). We begin the chapter by introducing the concept and framework of social exclusion in the context of later life. After this, we present and discuss how loneliness is connected to social exclusion from a multidimensional perspective. In the concluding section, we discuss the frameworks' implications for future research, policies, and interventions highlighting the need to address loneliness as an issue of social justice.

4.2 Social Exclusion in Later Life

The concept of social exclusion stems from the French *les exclus* (Silver, 1994). Renée Lenoir (1974), who is considered the founder of the concept, used the term to group those dependent on social insurance such as the mentally ill, young drug addicts, delinquents, and disabled people (Frétigné, 1999). Social exclusion became a core policy concept in France during the economic crisis of the 1980s. From a focus on various categories of people, the concept narrowed its focus to unemployment. Simultaneously, the term also referred to the increasing instability of social bonds and social disintegration (Silver, 1994). In addition to only describing situations of those who were excluded, the processes leading to exclusion became increasingly highlighted (Martin & Leaper 1996). Besides France, other countries incorporated social exclusion into their policy discourse, such as British social policy in the 1990s (Burchardt et al., 2009). Later, fighting poverty, reducing the number of people at risk of social exclusion and combatting discrimination have been one of the main aims of the Europe 2020 strategy (European Commission, 2014).

Concurrently, more focus has been placed on the social exclusion of older adults across countries (Van Regenmortel et al., 2016; Walsh et al., 2017).

In its simplest form, social exclusion refers to separation from mainstream society and its central arenas, for example, due to low income (Moffatt & Glasgow, 2009). In more detailed—and often used—definitions, social exclusion has been understood as a complex and multi-dimensional process involving a lack of resources, rights, goods, services, relationships, and activities, impacting both the quality of life of individuals and the cohesion of society (Levitas et al., 2007). Social exclusion can occur at any age and is neither specific nor unique to old age. However, it is often experienced and operationalised differently according to life stage (Ibid.)

In later life, several processes increase vulnerability to social exclusion. These include accumulated disadvantages over the course of life and the impacts of ageing processes, for example, decline in functional capabilities and changes in social and support networks. Later life involves critical transitions such as retirement, widowhood, and changes in income opportunities. Older adults' lives are also affected by macro-level developments, such as digitalization and changing family and care patterns, which may increase the risk of social exclusion. Moreover, ageist views and discourses in society lead to discrimination against older adults and consequently foster old-age social exclusion (see Van Regenmortel et al., 2018).

Later life social exclusion has been defined as a multi-dimensional concept influenced by specific features of ageing, such as cumulating life course factors and exclusionary mechanisms occurring over time (Van Regenmortel et al., 2016; Walsh et al., 2017). In a scoping review by Walsh et al. (2017, p. 93), the following definition is provided:

> "Old-age exclusion involves interchanges between multi-level risk factors, processes, and outcomes. Varying in form and degree across the older adult life course, its complexity, impact, and prevalence are amplified by old-age vulnerabilities, accumulated disadvantage for some groups, and constrained opportunities to ameliorate exclusion."

Research on later life social exclusion has often acknowledged social exclusion as a multidimensional phenomenon encompassing different domains of life. A conceptualisation of the following five interconnected domains has been proposed: economic exclusion, exclusion from social relations, exclusion from services, community and spatial exclusion, and civic exclusion (Scharf et al., 2005; Walsh et al., 2021). Within this framework, *economic exclusion* refers to insufficient material conditions and financial resources (Ogg & Myck, 2021), and *exclusion from social relations* refers to insufficient quality and/or quantity of intimate relationships, social networks, social support, and/or social participation (Burholt & Aartsen, 2021). *Exclusion from services* concerns insufficient and/or inadequate availability, access, and use of a variety of services, such as social and health care services or transportation (Draulans & Lamura, 2021). The fourth domain, *community and spatial exclusion,* includes low levels of engagement in local life and of mobility outside and inside a person's home. These relate to both physical and social aspects of place, that is, the built environment as well as attachment, safety, and trust (Tournier & Vidovićová, 2021). Finally, *civic exclusion* comprises exclusion from political and civic participation and violations of rights and it also includes sociocultural and symbolic aspects of old-age exclusion, such as public discourses and ageism (Torres et al., 2020).

Following diverse operationalisations of old-age exclusion as a multidimensional concept, such as those from Scharf et al. (2005) and Walsh et al. (2017), different social exclusion domains have been used in empirical research. These include studies focusing on the well-being of older adults living in rural and urban settings (Dahlberg & McKee, 2018), financially excluded older adults (Van Regenmortel et al., 2021), and older adults receiving formal home care services (Ristolainen et al., 2024a, 2024b). Studies have shown that the domains are highly interrelated, with many older adults experiencing exclusion within multiple domains (Barnes et al., 2006; Becker et al., 2009; Miranti & Yu, 2015; Scharf et al., 2005). Exclusion from one domain can trigger or contribute to other forms of exclusion (Kneale, 2012; MacLeod et al., 2019; Van Regenmortel et al., 2018) potentially stemming from lifelong accumulated disadvantages or from life events and transitions in older age, such as ill health and increased care needs (Barrett et al., 2012; Walsh et al., 2021).

4.3 Social Exclusion and Loneliness in Later Life

As mentioned in the introduction, social exclusion and loneliness in later life are distinct concepts but related to each other in diverse ways. Loneliness can be an outcome of social exclusion (Burholt & Aartsen, 2021), with different dimensions of social exclusion (Dahlberg et al., 2022b) acting as risk factors for loneliness. Conversely, loneliness itself can contribute to social exclusion if a person becomes excluded from social relations and other domains of life due to feelings of loneliness. Interestingly, Huxhold et al. (2022) found that loneliness may, over time, reinforce feelings of social exclusion, but not vice versa. Next, we examine the associations of social exclusion and loneliness by adopting the five-domain framework presented in the previous section and illustrating them with empirical examples.

4.3.1 Economic Exclusion

Economic exclusion involves insufficient material conditions and financial resources. Unlike younger age groups, older adults primarily rely on pensions, although other factors also contribute to economic exclusion in later life (Ogg & Myck, 2021). Given the rising inequality of economic resources in later life (Crystal et al., 2017), adopting a life course perspective is crucial (Ogg & Myck, 2021). Low lifetime earnings, long-term unemployment, and precarious jobs limit pension and asset accumulation, not assuring financial security in retirement. Additionally, health issues and disability throughout life can hinder financial security (Myck et al., 2017). Beyond compounding disadvantage, sudden life events, such as divorce, bankruptcy, widowhood, and illness, can also increase current and future economic vulnerability (Myck et al., 2017; Van Regenmortel et al., 2021). Moreover, significant expenses related to home care (Fret et al., 2020; Myck et al., 2017) or residential accommodation fees, worsen financial insecurity, especially as responsibility for financing old-age care increasingly shifts to individuals (Myck et al., 2017). Economic exclusion thus extends beyond poverty and income and also covers material deprivation (Ogg & Myck, 2021), defined as the inability to afford goods, services, or engage in activities which are perceived as necessities in mainstream society (Fusco et al., 2010).

Various studies link economic exclusion to loneliness in later life. Material deprivation is strongly associated with loneliness levels and the likelihood of becoming lonely in older adulthood, with materially deprived older adults facing higher risks (Gibney et al., 2019; Myck et al., 2021; Tang & Chou, 2024). A review by Ruan and Cheung (2024) found that high economic status correlates with lower levels of loneliness among older adult migrants, although subjective financial status was the primary significant predictor. Subjective aspects of income, such as income discomfort (Dahlberg & McKee, 2014) and having income concerns (Dahlberg et al., 2022b), also increase the risk of loneliness in later life. Furthermore, financial distress, socioeconomic status, and material deprivation in childhood can also influence loneliness later in life (Guthmuller, 2022; Kamiya et al., 2014).

Several theories explain the link between economic exclusion and loneliness. The social relationship expectations model posits that poverty constrains the fulfilment of social relationship expectations (Akhter-Khan et al., 2024). The stress process theory suggests that limited financial resources prevent older adults from coping with stressors, increasing loneliness risk (Tang & Chou, 2024). Additionally, financial hardship reduces participation in social activities, further contributing to loneliness in later life (Guthmuller, 2022; Van Regenmortel et al., 2021). From a life course perspective, childhood experiences are seen as shaping how people see themselves and their social roles. Struggles in childhood, like poverty, poor health, or parental (substance) abuse can harm self-esteem and confidence, leading to feelings of powerlessness and rejection. These effects can last for years, increasing the risk of loneliness in later life (de Jong-Gierveld, 1998; Kamiya et al., 2014).

Other domains of social exclusion may mediate or moderate the relationship between economic exclusion and loneliness. Frequent social participation—such as volunteering, taking courses, playing sports, or joining clubs and community organisations—helps reduce the risk of loneliness. Additionally, it influences the relationship between household wealth and loneliness, meaning that especially for men, social participation can lessen the impact of lower wealth on feelings of loneliness (Niedzwiedz et al., 2016). Tang and Chou (2024) found that engagement in cultural activities fosters social connections and support, which potentially mitigates loneliness. Additionally, neighbourhood collective efficacy moderates the relationship between economic exclusion and loneliness, as strong social bonds and networks in supportive communities can alleviate loneliness among economically excluded older adults (Tang & Chou, 2024).

The influence of financial and material resources goes beyond the individual resources available, as living in countries with low risks of poverty and low risks of material deprivation (a macro-level factor) is associated with lower levels of loneliness in later life (Morgan et al., 2021). According to Wu et al. (2022), there is a micro-macro interplay within the economic domain of exclusion on loneliness, as individual socioeconomic status more strongly affects late-life loneliness in societies with greater income inequality. Conversely, the influence of individual socioeconomic status on late-life loneliness is weaker in societies with more extensive welfare provisions.

4.3.2 Exclusion from Social Relations

Exclusion from social relations reflects the importance of engagement in meaningful relationships with others (Scharf et al., 2005), where exclusion means that there is a lack of or only superficial contacts with other people. Exclusion from social relations has been defined as "*a situation in which people are disconnected from adequate levels and quality of intimate relationships, social networks, social support and/or social opportunities to participate in the wider society*" (Burholt & Aartsen, 2021, p. 78). This dimension of social exclusion is often discussed in terms of social isolation, which refers to the separation of individuals from others and the community (van Tilburg & de Jong Gierveld, 2024). Unlike loneliness, social isolation is an objective state rather than a subjective feeling (Weiss, 1973). Indicators of social isolation are, e.g., living alone, having a small social network, and infrequent social contacts (Holt-Lunstad et al., 2015). Social isolation may also include qualitative aspects of social relations, such as the lack of supporting relations (van Tilburg & de Jong Gierveld, 2024). Similarly, the social exclusion framework acknowledges that social relations can be dysfunctional, for example, when characterised by conflict or abuse (Waldegrave et al., 2021). While loneliness has sometimes been seen as an indicator of social exclusion (Ristolainen et al., 2024b; Van Regenmortel et al., 2018; Walsh et al., 2017), it has been argued that it is an outcome of exclusion from social relations (Burholt et al., 2020).

Social resources play a significant role as risk factors for loneliness in later life. Partners are an important social resource, serving as a protective factor against increasing loneliness over time (Morgan et al., 2021), while widowhood increases the risk of loneliness (Dahlberg et al., 2022a). Additionally, household size plays a role, with those living alone experiencing higher levels of loneliness (Dahlberg et al., 2022b; Gibney et al., 2019). Regarding the quantity of social relations, research indicates that a smaller social network (Dahlberg et al., 2022a, 2022b) and lower frequency of contact with family, friends or colleagues are associated with a greater risk of feeling lonely in later life (Dahlberg et al., 2022b; Gibney et al., 2019). Pan et al. (2023) furthermore found that for non-migrants, cultural migrants and similar-culture migrants, higher social capital was significantly related to lower loneliness in later life. However, the importance of social contacts varies between type of loneliness, with low contact with family and friends significantly predicting social but not emotional loneliness in later life (Dahlberg & McKee, 2014).

On the other hand, not all studies support 'the more the merrier' idiomatic expression. For example, Morgan et al. (2021) found that a greater frequency of contact with children and an increase in the number of grandchildren was significantly related to an increase in loneliness. While these findings may seem surprising, a greater frequency in contact with children may be a result of a worsening personal situation, for example, in terms of health declines, while a greater number of grandchildren may raise the expectation of social interaction at the same time as the children are more engaged in their own children than in their parent (Morgan et al., 2021). Social relations may also include involvement in informal care. A review has shown that older adults who provide informal care to a spouse have an increased risk of loneliness, while caring for grandchildren decreases this risk (Akhter-Kahn et al., 2023).

Besides the quantity of social relationships, the quality of social relations plays a role in loneliness. People who are unsatisfied with their social networks have a higher chance of feeling very lonely (Kemperman et al., 2019), and the quality of social relations is of greater importance for loneliness than the quantity of social relations (Norlin et al., 2025). Similarly, not only high quantity, but also high quality of non-kin ties seems to significantly protect against loneliness among older migrants (Ruan & Cheung, 2024). Being unsatisfied with one's social relations relates to cognitive discrepancy theory, where loneliness is defined as being the result of a discrepancy between one's desired and actual social relations (Perlman & Peplau, 1981; Burholt, 2026).

A lack of emotional support from one's network is also significantly related with loneliness in Denmark, Finland, and Sweden, but not in Norway (Dahlberg et al., 2022b). A lack of (and need for) emotional support might point towards the social needs perspective on loneliness (Burholt, 2026). According to this perspective, sometimes called the 'deficit approach,' loneliness is the result of unfulfilled social needs such as an intimate partner, family member, friends, or acquaintances (de Jong-Gierveld & Tesch-Römer, 2012).

Social relations can have a significant role in loneliness also at the country level. Those living in countries with a higher average level of social contact are, for instance, more likely to feel lonely (Morgan et al., 2021). While this is counter-intuitive, several explanations have been proposed. Living in a society with collectivistic norms means that the expectation of social contact and support is likely to be higher than in individualistic societies, and loneliness is more likely to arise if these high expectations are not fulfilled (Dykstra, 2009). Another explanation is provided by the resource perspective on loneliness, which argues that resources such as health and socioeconomic status help individuals to maintain social activities and decrease the risk of social isolation and, in turn, loneliness (Tesch-Roemer & Huxhold, 2019).

4.3.3 Exclusion from Services

Exclusion from services includes inequities in relation to the access, usage, or appropriateness of services for older adults and the exclusion of older adults from decision-making regarding the design and implementation of services related to their needs and preferences (Barbarella et al., 2020). In the context of later life, it has been defined as the condition (and the processes leading to it) involving the lack or denial of services to a larger extent than what might be considered as 'normal' for most people (Draulans & Lamura, 2021). Within the framework of old-age social exclusion, a large body of research has focused on the accessibility and availability of public services, particularly social and health care (ibid.). Exclusion from care services is connected to the concept of 'care poverty,' referring to lack of adequate coverage of care needs resulting from interplay between individual and societal factors (Kröger et al., 2019; Kröger, 2022). However, exclusion from services is often viewed more broadly, acknowledging also services related to transportation, mobility, and communication technologies (Barbarella et al., 2020; Draulans & Lamura, 2021).

The availability, adequacy, and accessibility of services play a key role in later life loneliness. Older adults experiencing difficulties with transport have a greater risk of loneliness (Gibney et al., 2019). Transportation offers a means to reach and meet other people but also plays a role as a place for social contacts, for example, on public buses and at bus stops (Green et al., 2019). According to a systematic review by Williams et al. (2024), transport behaviours can be a cause of loneliness when opportunities for mobility are reduced due to functional limitations and lack of social networks. Meanwhile, transport behaviours can also be a consequence of loneliness if feelings of loneliness reduce likelihood to travel (ibid.). Older adults who are mobile and use a variety of transportation modes (bicycle, car, and public transport) experience less loneliness as it provides a means to sustain social contacts and relation beyond one's vicinity (van den Berg et al., 2016).

Besides transport and mobility, studies have shown that satisfaction with local amenities and services, such as public spaces, parks, and community centres, is indirectly associated with loneliness via social network satisfaction (Kemperman et al., 2019). These services play a vital role as a social infrastructure, as discussed further within the community and spatial domain. From the perspective of exclusion from services, studies have often focused on the accessibility of health and social care services, in particular. Accessibility of health and social care services includes several dimensions, such as availability, awareness, and affordability, which all have an impact on older adults' ability to reach adequate services in difficult life situations (Peiponen et al., 2024). Being excluded from services may be triggered by economic exclusion if the older person is not able to financially cover the costs of services (ibid.; Fret et al., 2019, 2020). Lower levels of loneliness have been found in welfare regimes that promote social integration and make older adults less dependent on individual social resources (Nyqvist et al., 2019).

Across Europe, challenges in accessing services are increasingly impacted by the decrease of state's responsibility to provide public services and restrictions on who is eligible for care services aimed at older adults (e.g., Kröger, 2022). Studies have shown that older adults with unmet healthcare needs or challenges accessing social services are more likely to be lonely (Chamberlain et al., 2023; Gibney et al., 2019). Furthermore, inadequate help and support have been associated with loneliness among older adults receiving formal home care services on a regular basis (Ristolainen et al., 2024a; Kadowaki et al., 2015). These findings indicate that even though services exist, they may not always be adequate in addressing older adults' social needs in situations where everyday life is challenged by health problems and functional decline. Loneliness may be an emotional outcome of the inadequacy of help and support in daily life (Ristolainen et al., 2024a).

In contrast, some studies have found higher levels of loneliness among older adults who use the most social and health care services (Smith & Victor, 2022; Chamberlain et al., 2022), which may refer to cumulative consequences of multimorbidity or a mismatch between the care given and sought. Conversely, other studies have not found an association between loneliness and the use of social and health services (see Smith & Victor, 2022). In an analysis of individual and country-level changes in loneliness, Morgan et al. (2021) found that better access to health care services at the country-level was associated with increased levels of loneliness among older adults. This finding is surprising and at odds with what could be expected from the perspective of exclusion from services. Hence, Morgan et al. (2021) suggest that the awareness of health care services may increase expectations towards services, leading to feelings of loneliness if health care needs are not met. In contrast, Wagner and Brandt (2018) found that the availability of formal long-term care services was associated with lower loneliness among spousal caregivers. Based on this, it may be argued that inadequate care services have negative consequences for older families and contribute to loneliness through increased caring responsibilities. It is also noteworthy that unpaid caregiving crosscuts several domains of exclusion, and in addition to social and services domain, may be considered from the perspective of civic exclusion, as presented in Sect. 4.3.5.

4.3.4 Community and Spatial Exclusion

Home, place, and environment have been influential and evolving themes in ageing studies (Yarker et al., 2023) and ageing is increasingly understood as spatial (Decker, 2023). Two decades ago, Scharf et al. (2005) underscored the particular importance of the neighbourhood domain in social exclusion in later life compared to other age groups. Today, this is no less the case, as older adults still tend to and prefer to age in place (Burholt, 2024a). Additionally, many older people have spent a considerable period of their lives in the same neighbourhood (Social Exclusion Unit, 2006), which may lead to a stronger investment in the surrounding community and increased place attachment (Burholt, 2024a). The fourth domain, *community and spatial exclusion,* therefore, refers to the unintended, yet decreased engagement in local life and the unintended decreased mobility outside and inside of a person's home. Community and spatial exclusion relate to social and relational aspects of a place, including local amenities, the built environment, and place-based policies. They also encompass feelings of belonging, safety, and trust (Tournier & Vidovićová, 2021). These forms of exclusion partly overlap with exclusion from services, as not only the local availability of resources such as shops, facilities, parks, and social organizations matters, but also the ability of older adults to access and use these resources (Decker, 2023).

A review by Lyu and Forsyth (2022) underlines the importance of structural factors in the community such as walkability, overall environment quality, housing options and a range of proximal transport in combating loneliness in later life. Additionally, living in compact neighbourhoods with higher population and housing density, more access to green space (Lam & Wang, 2022) and living closer to a highway (van den Berg et al., 2016) is related with lower levels of loneliness compared to living in neighbourhoods with lower population and housing density, less access to green spaces and longer distances from transit routes. Local infrastructure, such as public spaces, parks, and cafes, fosters encounters, interaction, and connection (Fried, 2020; Smith et al., 2023), promotes mobility, strengthens individuals' sense of belonging (Smith et al., 2023), and enhances connections to society and social life (Fried, 2020), all of which may prevent or reduce feelings of loneliness.

Beyond the service domain, accessibility is also essential from the perspective of community and spatial exclusion. Accessible community spaces encourage physical activity, such as walking, and they provide a medium for social interaction and community building. They are, thus, key places in fighting loneliness in later life (Jing et al., 2024). Research emphasises that the design, development, and implementation of social and community infrastructure should involve community members, particularly marginalised groups, such as older adults with impairments (Smith et al., 2023). However, despite the potential benefits of accessible community infrastructure in reducing loneliness in later life, not all older adults benefit from it equally (Rhubart et al., 2022). For example, austerity measures influence the availability and accessibility of social infrastructure, but also impacts mental health and well-being directly, including loneliness (Mcgrath et al., 2016; MacLeavy, 2023).

Besides the availability and accessibility of neighbourhood places and services, how residents relate to their neighbourhood also plays a key role. Low perceived community integration is, for instance, a significant predictor of social loneliness (Dahlberg & McKee, 2014), and stronger neighbourhood attachment is related to lower levels of loneliness (Kemperman et al., 2019). Length of residence is a crucial factor, as older adults who have lived in the neighbourhood for longer than others, tend to feel less lonely (van den Berg et al., 2016). Furthermore, perceived neighbourhood safety is indirectly related to loneliness (Dahlberg et al., 2022b; Kemperman et al., 2019; Meehan et al., 2023), and this effect has also been observed at the country (macro) level (Morgan et al., 2021). In general, older adults who are satisfied with their neighbourhood and its facilities are less likely to feel lonely (van den Berg et al., 2016).

4.3.5 Civic Exclusion

As the fifth and final domain, *civic exclusion,* comprises two aspects: civic participation and socio-cultural elements influencing older adults' ability to exercise their citizenship. The first includes engagement in civic activities, such as volunteering, community involvement, voting, and political participation, while socio-cultural aspects include the symbolic and discursive spheres of society, such as discrimination and ageism (Torres et al., 2020; Torres, 2021). Both elements are related. Negative stereotypes and discriminatory practices limit older adults' opportunities to contribute meaningfully to society, resulting in reduced civic engagement (von Humboldt et al., 2024). Within the social exclusion framework, the domain of civic exclusion has received the least attention and therefore lacks established operationalisation: some studies make the distinction between civic participation and socio-cultural elements (Walsh et al., 2017), and others consider both aspects under the domain of civic exclusion (e.g., Ristolainen et al., 2024a). Here, we take the latter approach and acknowledge civic exclusion as a multi-level driver of later life loneliness.

Several studies have shown that older adults who are infrequently engaged in formal social activities, such as educational courses or training, sports/social/other clubs (Nissanholtz-Gannot & Peretz-Dayan, 2023), and political or community organisations (Gibney et al., 2019; Pikhartova et al., 2016), have a higher risk of loneliness in later life than those frequently engaged in these activities. Older people who are volunteers in organisations (Akhter-Khan et al., 2023; Nissanholtz-Gannot & Peretz-Dayan, 2023), especially youth or charity organisations (Lee, 2022), are less lonely than those who do not engage in volunteer activities. If community participation in later life is impeded by barriers, such as cost, inaccessibility or lack of interest, the risk of loneliness increases (Gibney et al., 2019). A study focusing on the general adult population found that loneliness is associated with lower voting intention and a lower sense of duty to vote (Langenkamp, 2021).

As noted earlier, unpaid caregiving is often regarded as a form of civic engagement, which unlike other forms may increase the risk of feeling lonely. Spousal caregivers and caregivers who are still employed in work tend to experience more loneliness compared to non-carers (Akhter-Khan et al., 2023; Zeng et al., 2023). Due to the vigilance and demands on caregivers, this type of civic participation may impede opportunities for unpaid caregivers to fully engage in other types of civic activity, thereby impacting on loneliness (Vercauteren et al., 2024). Grandparental caregiving in turn, is associated with less loneliness (Akhter-Khan et al., 2023). This may indicate differences in caregiver roles, with grandparenting as a source of social well-being rather than mandatory responsibility. Being a caregiver may negatively impact the interpersonal relationships between the caregiver and care receiver, influencing not only civic participation but also exclusion from social relations due to conflicts in family relations or lack of social support (Waldegrave et al., 2021), for example.

According to the review of Walsh et al. (2017), socio-cultural aspects of exclusion consist of three dimensions, namely, identity exclusion, symbolic and discourse exclusion, and ageism and age discrimination. Regarding identity exclusion (i.e. reduction to one-dimensional identities (Walsh et al., 2017)), Ruan and Cheung (2024) found that a low sense of belonging towards one's ethnic group or that of the host area tends to be related to higher levels of loneliness among older adult migrants (Ruan & Cheung, 2024). At the macro level, dominant cultural norms provide a framework of societal expectations of needed or desired relations, which influences one's individual evaluation of the quantity and/or quality of one's social network. Cultural identity (self-categorised) but also cultural position (ascribed) status might be in line with or differ from dominant cultural norms. Both influence one's likelihood of being socially isolated and feeling lonely (Burholt, 2023).

Recently, the association between loneliness and ageism has received more attention in gerontological research, and studies have found that stereotypes, prejudices, and discrimination towards older adults increase the risk of loneliness in later life (Gibney et al., 2019; Pan et al., 2023; Shiovitz-Ezra et al., 2023). Shiovitz-Ezra et al. (2018) propose three mechanisms through which ageism contributes to loneliness: chronic social rejection leading to older adults' avoidance and withdrawal from social participation; self-embodied stereotypes of lonely old-age, and, thirdly, age-based discriminatory practices increasing social exclusion of older adults. In a similar vein, Barreto et al. (2022) found that feelings of loneliness are interrelated with stigma: the lonelier people felt, the more they perceived loneliness as stigmatised in their community. Negative stereotypes towards and expectations about loneliness itself have also been found to increase the risk of reporting loneliness in later life (Pikhartova et al., 2016).

Socio-cultural aspects of civic exclusion also include other forms of discrimination, not only ageism. Studies have indicated that discrimination based on physical disability, appearance, race, ancestry, sex, and sexual orientation is related to higher levels of loneliness in later adulthood (Sutin et al., 2015). To date, studies linking theories of intersectionality and social exclusion have been scarce, but recent efforts have been made to acknowledge the impacts of diverse social positions and locations on civic engagement in later life (Serrat et al., 2021). As shown in Chap. 2 in this book (Nyqvist et al., 2025), intersectional factors such as gender, race, socioeconomic status, and disability play a significant role in shaping why and how older adults with different, often overlapping identities are affected by loneliness during their life course.

4.4 Implications for Future Research and Practice

The review of evidence above shows how different dimensions of social exclusion are key indicators of loneliness in later life, with economic exclusion, exclusion from social relations, exclusion from services, community/spatial exclusion, and civic exclusion all potentially fostering feelings of loneliness. In other words, not only do one's attachment, social needs, personality, and sociodemographic and health characteristics influence loneliness in later life, but opportunities to meet, to belong, to participate in the community and to be engaged in wider society also matter.

Additionally, there are indications that the more domains of social exclusion from which an older adult is excluded, the lonelier they are (Aartsen et al., 2023). Social exclusion is a multidimensional concept composed of different dimensions of disadvantage, in which exclusion in one dimension can affect those in other dimensions, and dimensions of disadvantage tend to co-occur (Van Regenmortel et al., 2018), while disadvantages are often accumulated over the course of older people's lives (Dannefer, 2003). These interrelations between domains of exclusion, might impact the relation with loneliness differently. Related to economic exclusion for instance, we described how participation in civic or social activities mediated or moderated the association between low income and loneliness (Niedzwiedz et al., 2016; Tang & Chou, 2024). Conversely, a study by Nissanholtz-Gannot and Peretz-Dayan (2023, p.1982) found that income (economic domain) acted as a moderator for the relation between participation (civic domain) and loneliness: "Infrequently participating older adults with low-to-moderate income were more vulnerable to loneliness than higher income older adults, for whom infrequent participation did not increase loneliness." Also, one's perception of being excluded from society may prevent individuals from using opportunities for social participation that are available to them (Hommerich, 2015; Huxhold et al., 2022), leading to loneliness.

Based on what is known about loneliness and its associated factors, there is a need for a multidimensional and multilevel understanding of loneliness in later life, integrating individual factors (micro), community factors (meso) and societal factors (macro) (Meehan et al., 2023). A social exclusion perspective is useful as it is multidimensional and combines individual, community, and societal factors. Social exclusion is a process outside the control of the individual, which can be linked to structures. The advantage of a social exclusion perspective on loneliness is that it opens a broad view on the importance of a variety of resources in different life domains beyond social and economic resources and the role that they have in enabling sufficient and meaningful relationships to match one's needs and expectations. Social exclusion, with its multiple dimensions, covers financial and social resources, but also accessible and adequate services, resources in the community, representation (civic participation) and recognition (ageism and discrimination).

Viewing later life loneliness from the perspective of social exclusion highlights the importance of recognising loneliness as a matter of social justice (see also Barreto et al., 2024). The different domains of social exclusion align well with Fraser's tripartite theory of social justice-redistribution, recognition, and representation/participation (Dahl et al., 2004; Fraser, 1998) yet bring in the complex interplay between the different domains. The social exclusion framework captures multilevel barriers and exclusionary mechanisms affecting people's resources and opportunities for social connectedness. From the perspective of social justice, social exclusion and experiences of loneliness shed light on the (in)ability to use societal resources to participate and consequently reveal injustices at distinct levels of society.

To move towards a multilevel, multidimensional integrated understanding of loneliness, there are some recommendations for research. Existing research on the role of social exclusion in loneliness in later life tend to overemphasisze individual and personal indicators of social exclusion domains and does not fully incorporate some of the structural influences at the community and societal level, that are inherent to social exclusion in later life (see also Chap. 12 of this book; Suanet & Pavlidis, 2025). Furthermore, we must be wary of generalising results from large-scale studies, which is only meaningful if socio-structural and cultural characteristics are the same. Consequently, further attention should be given to the contextualisation of research to gain further insights into loneliness across different cultures and societies. There are methodological implications of incorporating a social exclusion perspective into an integrated model. Large-scale epidemiological studies are tied to specific countries or regions and look at cross-sectional associations with loneliness, longitudinal trajectories of loneliness, or cohort differences in loneliness. However, they rarely contextualise findings. As such, we do not have sufficient evidence of the impact of social changes, geographical differences and policies on loneliness for older people, which means there are blind spots in the multilevel understanding of loneliness in later life (Burholt, 2024b). Without considering the broader context, such as community dynamics, societal norms and the organisation of welfare services, research may overlook critical elements that contribute to loneliness in different settings. Contextualizing helps to capture the complexities of loneliness and provides a more comprehensive understanding of how it is experienced across diverse populations and environments. Taking a social exclusion perspective, and contextualising research can help us understand the relationships between the factors on all levels.

In a multilevel and multidimensional perspective on loneliness, the chronosystem should not be overlooked, as life course mechanisms contribute to loneliness in later life. The chronosystem captures changes over time, and it is known that loneliness is dynamic and can also develop gradually (Burholt, 2024b). The cumulative advantage/disadvantage model (Dannefer, 2003), for instance, shows how early life conditions can shape future opportunities: individual choice and circumstances, alongside long-standing institutional structures, favour some people over others. Consequently, inequities influence resources and opportunities across the life course and may increase the likelihood of loneliness in later life. Those experiencing loneliness earlier in life are indeed more likely to experience loneliness in later life (Victor et al., 2022). Stability and continuity of relationships tend to be key factors in preventing loneliness (Lam et al., 2022) and later life loneliness is often affected by life course inequalities (Hagan et al., 2020; Tiilikainen et al., 2024). Consideration of domains of social exclusion across the life course may provide a more comprehensive, integrated model for understanding loneliness, as it highlights how exclusions in areas such as economic resources, social relationships, services, community, and civic engagement accumulate over time. This approach captures the complex interplay of life course inequalities and systemic factors that shape the risk of loneliness, underscoring the need to address multiple exclusion domains to mitigate loneliness in later life.

In this chapter, we have demonstrated that loneliness itself is not just personal; it also has structural causes (Barreto et al., 2024; Wilkinson, 2022). These are often left unaddressed in favour of solutions that individualise and blame lonely citizens for their own position (Jentoft et al., 2024, p.1). From the perspective of social exclusion, there is a need for a whole-system approach to address loneliness in later life. This requires a focus on the macro- and meso-level factors influencing loneliness across the social exclusion domains. Successful intervention strategies are likely to require a combination of initiatives that target the general population-level, and programs aimed at older adults who have an increased risk of loneliness.

Research evidence shows that many older adults have difficulties in leaving their home and participating in their local communities due to environmental barriers. Therefore, it is important to consider intervention strategies addressing these environmental barriers. This could be done by developing and implementing neighbourhood-level or community-based interventions. Despite the existing evidence on the role of age-friendly and inclusive environments in loneliness in later life (Gibney et al., 2019) and the potential of *designing out* loneliness (Fried, 2020), there are very few interventions that address the structural neighbourhood or societal factors (e.g., Timmermans et al., 2020). Yet, there are some community-based interventions with the potential to support older adults' participation and social engagement, and to alleviate loneliness (e.g. Ristolainen et al., 2020, 2022; Fong et al., 2021).

In addition to community-level interventions, attention is needed at the policy-level shaping older adults' resources and opportunities for social and civic participation. In addition to deprivation and poverty, policies should aim to reduce ageism and discrimination at all levels of society. A key policy priority should be the prevention of old-age social exclusion, as it is known to have detrimental effects not only on individuals but also on communities and societies (Walsh et al., 2017). However, the lack of macro-level research on loneliness presents a significant gap in our understanding of its broader societal and structural determinants. Thus, we propose using the social exclusion perspective to capture multidimensional risk factors of loneliness and encourage researchers to consider factors and conditions at distinct levels to achieve a more comprehensive and integrated understanding of loneliness.

Acknowledgement Lena Dahlberg's research is funded by grants from the Swedish Research Council for Health, Working Life and Care (Forte; grant no. 2023-00164) and the Kamprad Family Foundation (grant no. 20210138). Research by Elisa Tiilikainen and Hanna Ristolainen has been funded by the Research Council of Finland (grant no. 342267).

Competing Interests The authors have no conflicts of interest to declare that are relevant to the content of this chapter.

References

Aartsen, M., Vasile, M., Tufa, L., Dumitrescu, D., Radogna, R., Wörn, J., & Precupetu, I. (2023). Patterns and correlates of old-age social exclusion in the Balkan states. *European Journal of Ageing, 20*(13). https://doi.org/10.1007/s10433-023-00762-1

Akhter-Khan, S. C., Hofmann, V., Warncke, M., Tamimi, N., Mayston, R., & Prina, M. A. (2023). Caregiving, volunteering, and loneliness in middle-aged and older adults: A systematic review. *Aging & Mental Health, 27*(7), 1233–1245. https://doi.org/10.1080/13607863.2022.2144130

Akhter-Khan, S. C., van Es, W., Prina, M., Lawrence, V., Piri, I., Rokach, A., Heu, L. C., & Mayston, R. (2024). Experiences of loneliness in lower- and middle-income countries: A systematic review of qualitative studies. *Social Science & Medicine, 340*, 116438. https://doi.org/10.1016/j.socscimed.2023.116438

Barbarella, F., Barlin, H., Barstad, J., Ferreira, C.C., Draulans, V., Hlebec, V., Lamura, G., Macleod, C., Maskeliunas, R., Siren, A. & ROSEnet Services Working Group (2020). Services exclusion in later life. In: K. Walsh and T. Scharf (series eds.), ROSEnet Briefing Paper Series: No. 4. CA 15122 Reducing Old-Age Exclusion: Collaborations in Research and Policy. ISBN: 978-1-908358-74-5.

Barnes, M., Blom, A., Cox, K., Lessof, C., & Walker, A. (2006). *The social exclusion of older people: Evidence from the first wave of the English Longitudinal Study of Ageing (ELSA): Final Report*. Retrieved February 23 2025, from https://ifs.org.uk/sites/default/files/output_url_files/odpm_social_exclusion.pdf

Barreto, M., van Breen, J., Victor, C., Hammond, C., Eccles, A., Richins, M. T., & Qualter, P. (2022). Exploring the nature and variation of the stigma associated with loneliness. *Journal of Social and Personal Relationships, 39*(9), 2658–2679. https://doi.org/10.1177/02654075221087

Barreto, M., Doyle, D. M., & Qualter, P. (2023). *Loneliness inequalities evidence review*. Wales Centre for Public Policy. Retrieved February 23, 2025, from https://wcpp.org.uk/publication/loneliness-inequalities-evidence-review/

Barreto, M., Doyle, D. M., & Qualter, P. (2024). Changing the narrative: Loneliness as a social justice issue. *Political Psychology, 45*(S1), 157–181. https://doi.org/10.1111/pops.12965

Barrett, P., Hale, B., & Gauld, R. (2012). Social inclusion through ageing-in-place with care? *Ageing & Society, 32*(3), 361–378. https://doi.org/10.1017/S0144686X11000341

Becker, E., Boreham, R., & National Centre for Social Research. (2009). *Understanding the risks of social exclusion across the life course: Older age*. Social Exclusion Task Force.

Beller, J. (2024). Social inequalities in loneliness: Disentangling the contributions of education, income, and occupation. *SAGE Open, 14*(3), 21582440241281408. https://doi.org/10.1177/2158244024128140

Burchardt, T., Le Grand, J., & Piachaud, D. (2009). Introduction. In J. Hills, J. Le Grand, & D. Piachaud (Eds.), *Understanding social exclusion* (pp. 1–12). Oxford University Press.

Burholt, V. (2023). Culture, social isolation and loneliness in later life. In A. Hajek, S. G. Riedel-Heller, & H. König (Eds.), *Loneliness and social isolation in old age* (pp. 50–60). Routledge.

Burholt, V. (2024a). Aging, place, and migration. In M. P. Cutchin & G. D. Rowles (Eds.), *Handbook on ageing and place* (pp. 405–424). Edward Elgar Publishing. https://doi.org/10.4337/9781802209983.00034

Burholt, V. (2024b). Contextualizing trends in the distribution of older people's rural support networks over two decades of social change. *The Journal of Aging and Social Change, 15*(1), 1–31. https://doi.org/10.18848/2576-5310/CGP/v15i01/1-31

Burholt, V. (2026). Non-evolutionary theories and models for explaining loneliness. In D. Perlman, C. Cutrona, & D. Russell (Eds.), *The Cambridge handbook of loneliness: Theory, research, and interventions*. Cambridge University Press.

Burholt, V., & Aartsen, M. (2021). Introduction: Framing exclusion from social relations. In K. Walsh, T. Scharf, S. Van Regenmortel, & A. Wanka (Eds.), *Social exclusion in later life. Interdisciplinary and policy perspectives* (pp. 77–82). Springer.

Burholt, V., Winter, B., Aartsen, M., Constantinou, C., Dahlberg, L., Feliciano, V., de Jong Gierveld, J., Van Regenmortel, S., Waldegrave, C., & The Working Group on Exclusion from Social Relations, part of the COST-finances Research Network (Reducing Old-Age Exclusion: Collaborations in Research and Policy' (ROSENet). (2020). A critical review and development of a conceptual model of exclusion from social relations for older people. *European Journal of Ageing, 17*(1), 3–19. https://doi.org/10.1007/s10433-019-00506-0

Chamberlain, S., Bronskill, S., Hsu, Z., Youngson, E., & Gruneir, A. (2022). Resident loneliness, social isolation and unplanned emergency department visits from supportive living facilities: A population-based study in Alberta, Canada. *BMC Geriatrics, 22*(21). https://doi.org/10.1186/s12877-021-02718-5

Chamberlain, S., Savage, R. D., Bronskill, S. E., Griffith, L. E., Rochon, P., Batara, J., & Gruneir, A. (2023). Retrospective cross-sectional study examining the association between loneliness and unmet healthcare needs among middle-aged and older adults using the Canadian Longitudinal Study of Aging (CLSA). *BMJ Open, 13*(3), e068769. https://doi.org/10.1136/bmjopen-2022-068769

Crystal, S., Shea, D. G., & Reyes, A. M. (2017). Cumulative advantage, cumulative disadvantage, and evolving patterns of late-life inequality. *The Gerontologist, 57*(5), 910–920. https://doi.org/10.1093/geront/gnw056

Dahl, H. M., Stoltz, P., & Willig, R. (2004). Recognition, redistribution and representation in capitalist global society: An interview with Nancy Fraser. *Acta Sociologica, 47*(4), 374–382. https://doi.org/10.1177/0001699304048

Dahlberg, L., & McKee, K. J. (2014). Correlates of social and emotional loneliness in older people: Evidence from an English community study. *Aging & Mental Health, 18*(4), 504–514. https://doi.org/10.1080/13607863.2013.856863

Dahlberg, L., & McKee, K. J. (2018). Social exclusion and well-being among older adults in rural and urban areas. *Archives of Gerontology and Geriatrics, 79*, 176–184. https://doi.org/10.1016/j.archger.2018.08.007

Dahlberg, L., McKee, K. J., Frank, A., & Naseer, M. (2022a). A systematic review of longitudinal risk factors for loneliness in older adults. *Aging & Mental Health, 26*(2), 225–249. https://doi.org/10.1080/13607863.2021.1876638

Dahlberg, L., McKee, K. J., Lennartsson, C., & Rehnberg, J. (2022b). A social exclusion perspective on loneliness in older adults in the Nordic countries. *European Journal of Ageing, 19*(2), 175–188. https://doi.org/10.1007/s10433-022-00692-4

Dannefer, D. (2003). Cumulative advantage/disadvantage and the life course: Cross-fertilizing age and social science theory. *The Journals of Gerontology Series B: Psychological Sciences and Social Sciences, 58*(6), S327–S337. https://doi.org/10.1093/geronb/58.6.S327

de Jong-Gierveld, J. (1998). A review of loneliness: Concepts and definitions, determinants and consequences. *Reviews in Clinical Gerontology, 8*(1), 73–80. https://doi.org/10.1017/S0959259898008090

de Jong-Gierveld, J., & Tesch-Römer, C. (2012). Loneliness in old age in Eastern and Western European societies: Theoretical perspectives. *European Journal of Ageing, 9*(4), 285–295. https://doi.org/10.1007/s10433-012-0248-2

Decker, P. D. (2023). Space as capital or why geography matters for ageing. *International Journal of Architecture and Planning, 3*(1), 61–71. https://doi.org/10.51483/IJARP.3.1.2023.61-71

Draulans, V., & Lamura, G. (2021). Introduction: Framing exclusion from services. In K. Walsh, T. Scharf, S. Van Regenmortel, & A. Wanka (Eds.), *Social exclusion in later life. Interdisciplinary and policy perspectives* (pp. 135–140). Springer.

Dykstra, P. A. (2009). Older adult loneliness: Myths and realities. *European Journal of Ageing, 6*(2), 91–100. https://doi.org/10.1007/s10433-009-0110-3

European Commission. (2014). *Tacking stock of the Europe 2020 strategy for smart, sustainable and inclusive growth.* European Commission. Retrieved September 20 2024, from https://commission.europa.eu/publications/taking-stock-europe-2020-strategy-smart-sustainable-and-inclusive-growth_en.

Fong, P., Cruwys, T., Robinson, S. L., Haslam, S. A., Haslam, C., Mance, P. L., & Fisher, C. L. (2021). Evidence that loneliness can be reduced by a whole-of-community intervention to increase neighbourhood identification. *Social Science & Medicine, 277*, 113909. https://doi.org/10.1016/j.socscimed.2021.113909

Fraser, N. (1998). *Social justice in the age of identity politics: redistribution, recognition, participation*. (Discussion Papers/Wissenschaftszentrum Berlin für Sozialforschung, Forschungsschwerpunkt Arbeitsmarkt und Beschäftigung, Abteilung Organisation und Beschäftigung, 98–108). Wissenschaftszentrum Berlin für Sozialforschung gGmbH. https://nbn-resolving.org/urn:nbn:de:0168-ssoar-126247

Fret, B., De Donder, L., Lambotte, D., Dury, S., Van Der Elst, M., De Witte, N., Switsers, L., Hoens, S., Van Regenmortel, S., & Verté, D. (2019). Access to care of frail community-dwelling older adults in Belgium: A qualitative study. *Primary Health Care Research & Development, 20*, e43. https://doi.org/10.1017/S1463423619000100

Fret, B., Mondelaers, B., De Donder, L., Switsers, L., Smetcoren, A.-S., Verté, D., & the D-SCOPE consortium. (2020). Exploring the cost of 'ageing in place': Expenditures of community-dwelling older adults in Belgium. *Ageing International, 45*(3), 209–229. https://doi.org/10.1007/s12126-018-9341-y

Frétigné, C. (1999). Sociologie de l'exclusion. *L'Harmattan*.

Fried, L. (2020). Designing a new social infrastructure to combat loneliness in aging adults. *Generations, 44*(3), 1–12.

Fusco, A., Guio, A.-C., & Marlier, E. (2010). *Income poverty and material deprivation in European countries (Theme: Population and social conditions, collection: Methodologies and Working Papers*, 2010, Cat. No. KS-RA-10-030-EN-N). Luxembourg: European Union.

Gibney, S., Moore, T., & Shannon, S. (2019). Loneliness in later life: A cross-sectional survey analysis of place-based factors in Ireland. *Quality in Ageing and Older Adults, 20*(2), 80–96. https://doi.org/10.1108/QAOA-04-2018-0015

Green, J., Jones, A., & Roberts, H. (2019). More than A to B: The role of free bus travel for the mobility and wellbeing of older citizens in London. *Ageing and Society, 34*(3), 472–494. https://doi.org/10.1108/QAOA-04-2018-0015

Guthmuller, S. (2022). Loneliness among older adults in Europe: The relative importance of early and later life conditions. *PLoS One, 17*(5), e0267562. https://doi.org/10.1371/journal.pone.0267562

Hagan, R., Manktelow, R., & Taylor, B. (2020). Loneliness, cumulative inequality and social capital in later life: Two stories. *Irish Journal of Sociology, 28*(2), 192–217. https://doi.org/10.1177/0791603520908764

Holt-Lunstad, J., Smith, T. B., Baker, M., Harris, T., & Stephenson, D. (2015). Loneliness and social isolation as risk factors for mortality: A meta-analytic review. *Perspectives on Psychological Science, 10*(2), 227–237. https://doi.org/10.1177/1745691614568

Hommerich, C. (2015). Feeling disconnected: exploring the relationship between different forms of social capital and civic engagement in Japan. *VOLUNTAS: International Journal of Voluntary and Nonprofit Organizations, 26*(1), 45–68. https://doi.org/10.1007/s11266-014-9525-3

Huxhold, O., Suanet, B., & Wetzel, M. (2022). Perceived social exclusion and loneliness: Two distinct but related phenomena. *Sociological Science, 9*, 430–453. https://doi.org/10.15195/v9.a17

Jentoft, E. E., Sandset, T., & Haldar, M. (2024). Problematizing loneliness as a public health issue: An analysis of policy in the United Kingdom. *Critical Policy Studies*, 1–18. https://doi.org/10.1080/19460171.2024.2306240

Jing, J., Dahlberg, L., Canter, D., & Plater-Zyberk, E. (2024). The role of third place concerning loneliness in the context of ageing in place: Three neighbourhoods in Stockholm. *Health & Social Care in the Community,* e4172682. https://doi.org/10.1155/2024/4172682

Kadowaki, L., Wister, A., & Chappel, N. (2015). Influence of home care on life satisfaction, loneliness, and perceived life stress. *Canadian Journal on Aging, 34*(1), 75–89. https://doi.org/10.1017/S0714980814000488

Kamiya, Y., Doyle, M., Henretta, J. C., & Timonen, V. (2014). Early-life circumstances and later-life loneliness in Ireland. *The Gerontologist, 54*(5), 773–783. https://doi.org/10.1093/geront/gnt097

Kemperman, A., van den Berg, P., Weijs-Perrée, M., & Uijtdewillegen, K. (2019). Loneliness of older adults: Social network and the living environment. *International Journal of Environmental Research and Public Health, 16*(3), 406. https://doi.org/10.3390/ijerph16030406

Kneale, D. (2012). *Is social exclusion still important for older people?* International Longevity Centre – UK.

Kröger, T (2022). *Care poverty. When older people's needs remain unmet*. Palgrave Macmillan.

Kröger, T., Puthenparambil, J., & Van Aerschot, L. (2019). Care poverty: Unmet care needs in a Nordic welfare state. *International Journal of Care and Caring, 3*(4), 485–500. https://doi.org/10.1332/239788219X15641291564296

Lam, J., & Wang, S. (2022). Built environment and loneliness among older adults in Southeast Queensland, Australia. *Journal of Applied Gerontology, 41*(11), 2382–2391. https://doi.org/10.1177/07334648221114345

Lam, J., Dickson, C., & Baxter, J. (2022). Ageing and loneliness: A life course and cumulative disadvantage approach. In J. Baxter, J. Lam, J. Povey, R. Lee, & S. R. Zubrick (Eds.), *Family dynamics over the life course. Life course research and social policies* (pp. 279–296). Springer. https://doi.org/10.1007/978-3-031-12224-8_13

Langenkamp, A. (2021). Lonely hearts, empty booths? The relationship between loneliness, reported voting behavior and voting as civic duty. *Social Science Quarterly, 102*(4), 1239–1254. https://doi.org/10.1111/ssqu.12946

Lee, S. (2022). Volunteering and loneliness in older adults: A parallel mediation model. *Aging & Mental Health, 26*(6), 1234–1241. https://doi.org/10.1080/13607863.2021.1913477

Lenoir, R. (1974). *Les Exclus: Un français sur dix*. Editions Du Seuil.

Levitas, R., Pantazis, C., Fahmy, E., Gordon, D., Lloyd, E., & Patsios, D. (2007). *The multi-dimensional analysis of social exclusion*. University of Bristol. https://dera.ioe.ac.uk/6853/1/multidimensional.pdf.

Lyu, Y., & Forsyth, A. (2022). Planning, aging, and loneliness: Reviewing evidence about built environment effects. *Journal of Planning Literature, 37*(1), 28–48. https://doi.org/10.1177/08854122211035131

MacLeavy, J. (2023). Austere futures: From hardship to hope? *The Geographical Journal*, geoj.12544. https://doi.org/10.1111/geoj.12544

Macleod, C. A., Ross, A., Sacker, A., Netuveli, G., & Windle, G. (2019). Re-thinking social exclusion in later life: A case for a new framework for measurement. *Ageing and Society, 39*(1), 74–111. https://doi.org/10.1017/S0144686X17000794

Martin, C., & Leaper, R. a. B. (1996). French review article: The debate in France over "Social Exclusion". *Social Policy & Administration, 30*(4), 382–392. https://doi.org/10.1111/j.1467-9515.1996.tb00567.x

Mcgrath, L., Griffin, V., Mundy, E., Curno, T., Weerasinghe, D., & Zlotowitz, S. (2016). The psychological impact of austerity: A briefing paper. *Educational Psychology Research and Practice, 2*(2), 46–57. https://doi.org/10.15123/uel.885xw

Meehan, D. E., Grunseit, A., Condie, J., HaGani, N., & Merom, D. (2023). Social-ecological factors influencing loneliness and social isolation in older people: A scoping review. *BMC Geriatrics, 23*(1), 726. https://doi.org/10.1186/s12877-023-04418-8

Miranti, R., & Yu, P. (2015). Why social exclusion persists among older people in Australia. *Social Inclusion, 3*(4), 112–126. https://doi.org/10.17645/si.v3i4.214

Moffatt, S., & Glasgow, N. (2009). How useful is the concept of social exclusion when applied to rural older people in the United Kingdom and the United States? *Regional Studies, 43*(10), 1291–1303. https://doi.org/10.1080/00343400903002697

Morgan, D., Dahlberg, L., Waldegrave, C., Mikulionienė, S., Rapolienė, G., Lamura, G., & Aartsen, M. (2021). Revisiting loneliness: Individual and country-level changes. In K. Walsh, T. Scharf,

S. Van Regenmortel, & A. Wanka (Eds.), *Social exclusion in ageing societies: Interdisciplinary and policy perspectives* (pp. 99–117). Springer.

Myck, M., Ogg, J., Aigner-Walder, B., Kareholt, I., Kostakis, I., Motel-Klingebiel, A., MarbanFlores, R., Murdock, E., Perek-Bialas, J., & Thelin, A. No 1 (2017). *Economic aspects of old age exclusion: A scoping report. Knowledge synthesis series.* Rosenet Cost Action (CA15122) Reducing Old-Age Social Exclusion: Collaborations in Research & Policy.

Myck, M., Waldegrave, C., & Dahlberg, L. (2021). Two dimensions of social exclusion: Economic deprivation and dynamics of loneliness in later life in Europe. In K. Walsh, T. Scharf, S. Van Regenmortel, & A. Wanka (Eds.), *Social exclusion in ageing societies: Interdisciplinary and policy perspectives* (pp. 311–326). Springer.

Niedzwiedz, C. L., Richardson, E. A., Tunstall, H., Shortt, N. K., Mitchell, R. J., & Pearce, J. R. (2016). The relationship between wealth and loneliness among older people across Europe: Is social participation protective? *Preventive Medicine, 91*, 24–31. https://doi.org/10.1016/j.ypmed.2016.07.016

Nissanholtz-Gannot, R., & Peretz-Dayan, H. (2023). Equal opportunities in aging: Income level moderates the relationship between infrequent participation in formal social activities and loneliness among older adults. *Journal of Applied Gerontology, 42*(9), 1982–1992. https://doi.org/10.1177/07334648231175429

Norlin, J., McKee, K. J., Lennartsson, C., & Dahlberg, L. (2025). Quantity and quality of social relationships and their associations with loneliness in older adults. *Aging & Mental Health*, 1–11. https://doi.org/10.1080/13607863.2025.2460068

Nyqvist, F., Nygård, M., & Scharf, T. (2019). Loneliness amongst older people in Europe: A comparative study of welfare regimes. *European Journal of Ageing, 16*(2), 133–143. https://doi.org/10.1007/s10433-018-0487-y

Nyqvist, F., McHugh Power, J., & Coll-Planas, L. (2025). Theorizing loneliness in later life: Micro, meso, and macro perspectives. In M. Aartsen, I. Precupetu, & B. Suanet (Eds.), *Macro social influences on loneliness in later life: Towards a better understanding of the loneliness paradox in later life*. Springer.

Ogg, J., & Myck, M. (2021). Introduction: Framing economic exclusion. In K. Walsh, T. Scharf, S. Van Regenmortel, & A. Wanka (Eds.), *Social exclusion in later life. Interdisciplinary and policy perspectives* (pp. 25–30). Springer.

Pan, H., Qualter, P., Barreto, M., Stegen, H., & Dury, S. (2023). Loneliness in older migrants: Exploring the role of cultural differences in their loneliness experience. *International Journal of Environmental Research and Public Health, 20*(4), 2785. https://doi.org/10.3390/ijerph20042785

Peiponen, J., Tiilikainen, E., Kinni, R. L., & Rissanen, S. (2024). Navigating social services from the perspective of Finnish older adults with complex needs: An examination of different dimensions of access. *Journal of Social Service Research, 51*(1), 144–161. https://doi.org/10.1080/01488376.2024.2388627

Perlman, D., & Peplau, L. A. (1981). Toward a social psychology of loneliness. *Personal Relationships, 3*, 31–56.

Pikhartova, J., Bowling, A., & Victor, C. (2016). Is loneliness in later life a self-fulfilling prophecy? *Aging & Mental Health, 20*(5), 543–549. https://doi.org/10.1080/13607863.2015.1023767

Rhubart, D., Sun, Y., Pendergrast, C., & Monnat, S. (2022). Sociospatial disparities in "third place" availability in the United States. *Socius, 8*, 23780231221090301. https://doi.org/10.1177/23780231221090

Ristolainen, H., Kannasoja, S., Tiilikainen, E., Hakala, M., Närhi, K., & Rissanen, S. (2020). Effects of 'participatory group-based care management' on wellbeing of older people living alone: A randomized controlled trial. *Archives of Gerontology and Geriatrics, 89*, 104095. https://doi.org/10.1016/j.archger.2020.104095

Ristolainen, H., Tiilikainen, E., & Rissanen, S. (2022). Pragmatic randomized controlled study of the effectiveness of participatory group-based care management. *Journal of Social Medicine, 59*(4), 429–446. https://doi.org/10.23990/sa.102338

Ristolainen, H., Tiilikainen, E., & Forma, L. (2024a). Social exclusion among older people receiving formal home care services in Finland: Prevalence and associated factors. *International Journal of Care and Caring*, 1–26. https://doi.org/10.1332/23978821Y2024D000000075

Ristolainen, H., Van Regenmortel, S., De Donder, L., Vercauteren, T., Lehtiö, J., & Tiilikainen, E. (2024b). Patterns of multidimensional social exclusion among older home care services recipients. *The Journals of Gerontology, Series B: Psychological Sciences and Social Sciences, 79*(9), gbae118. https://doi.org/10.1093/geronb/gbae118

Ruan, Y., & Cheung, M. (2024). Systematic review of factors influencing loneliness in older-adult migrants. *Aging & Mental Health, 28*(8), 1129–1141. https://doi.org/10.1080/13607863.2024.2340736

Scharf, T., Phillipson, C., & Smith, A. E. (2005). Social exclusion of older people in deprived urban communities of England. *European Journal of Ageing, 2*(2), 76–87. https://doi.org/10.1007/s10433-005-0025-6

Serrat, R., Scharf, T., & Villar, F. (2021). Reconceptualising exclusion from civic engagement in later life: Towards a new research agenda. In K. Walsh, T. Scharf, S. Van Regenmortel, & A. Wanka (Eds.), *Social exclusion in later life. Interdisciplinary and policy perspectives* (pp. 245–257). Springer.

Shiovitz-Ezra, S., Shemesh, J., & McDonnell/Naughton, M. (2018). Pathways from ageism to loneliness. In L. Ayalon & C. Tesch-Römer (Eds.), *Contemporary perspectives on ageism. International perspectives on aging* (pp. 131–147). Springer. https://doi.org/10.1007/978-3-319-73820-8_9

Shiovitz-Ezra, S., Erlich, B., & Ayalon, L. (2023). Short- and medium-term effects of ageism on loneliness experienced during the COVID-19 pandemic. *Journal of Applied Gerontology, 42*(6), 1255–1266. https://doi.org/10.1177/07334648231159372

Silver, H. (1994). Social exclusion and social solidarity: Three paradigms. *International Labour Review, 133*(5–6), 531–578.

Smith, K., & Victor, C. (2022). The association of loneliness with health and social care utilization in older adults in the general population: A systematic review. *The Gerontologist, 62*(10), e578–e596. https://doi.org/10.1093/geront/gnab177

Smith, M. L., Racoosin, J., Wilkerson, R., Ivey, R. M., Hawkley, L., Holt-Lunstad, J., & Cudjoe, T. K. M. (2023). Societal- and community-level strategies to improve social connectedness among older adults. *Frontiers in Public Health,* 11. https://doi.org/10.3389/fpubh.2023.1176895

Social Exclusion Unit. (2006). *A sure start to later life: Ending inequalities for older people*. Social Exclusion Unit.

Suanet, B., & Pavlidis, G. (2025). *And, you know: There's such a thing as society*: Towards a clarification of the 'loneliness paradox' by a macrofication of loneliness studies. In M. Aartsen, I. Precupetu, & B. Suanet (Eds.), *Macro social influences on loneliness in later life: Towards a better understanding of the loneliness paradox in later life*. Springer.

Sutin, A. R., Stephan, Y., Carretta, H., & Terracciano, A. (2015). Perceived discrimination and physical, cognitive, and emotional health in older adulthood. *The American Journal of Geriatric Psychiatry, 23*(2), 171–179. https://doi.org/10.1016/j.jagp.2014.03.007

Tang, V. F. Y., & Chou, K. L. (2024). An exploratory study on material deprivation and loneliness among older adults in Hong Kong. *BMC Geriatrics, 24*(1), 400. https://doi.org/10.1186/s12877-024-05013-1

Tesch-Roemer, C., & Huxhold, O. (2019). Social isolation and loneliness in old age. *Oxford Research Encyclopedia of Psychology*.

Tiilikainen, E., Aartsen, M., & Kraav, S. L. (2024). Early-life circumstances and late life loneliness trajectories among Finnish older adults. *BMC Geriatrics, 24*, 459. https://doi.org/10.1186/s12877-024-04967-6

Timmermans, E. J., Reinhard, E., Ruijsbroek, A., Huisman, M., & Avendano, M. (2020). Regeneration of deprived neighbourhoods and indicators of functioning in older adults: A quasi-experimental evaluation of the Dutch District Approach. *Health & Place, 64*, 102359. https://doi.org/10.1016/j.healthplace.2020.102359

Torres, S. (2021). Introduction: Framing civic exclusion. In K. Walsh, T. Scharf, S. Van Regenmortel, & A. Wanka (Eds.), *Social exclusion in later life. Interdisciplinary and policy perspectives* (pp. 239–243). Springer.

Torres, S., Bilfeldt, A., Conroy, P., Gallist, V., Gerdina, O., Larragy, J., et al. (2020) *Civic exclusion in later life: Ageism excludes everyone and harms our societies! COST, ROSEnet Briefing Paper Series No. 3*. Retrieved 6th of September 2024 from https://rosenetcost.com/wp-content/uploads/2017/01/cost_rosenet_actionpolicy3_web.pdf

Tournier, I., & Vidovićová, L. (2021). Introduction: Framing community and spatial exclusion. In K. Walsh, T. Scharf, S. Van Regenmortel, & A. Wanka (Eds.), *Social exclusion in later life. Interdisciplinary and policy perspectives* (pp. 185–192). Springer.

van den Berg, P., Kemperman, A., de Kleijn, B., & Borgers, A. (2016). Ageing and loneliness: The role of mobility and the built environment. *Travel Behaviour and Society, 5*, 48–55. https://doi.org/10.1016/j.tbs.2015.03.001

Van Regenmortel, S., De Donder, L., Dury, S., Smetcoren, A.-S., De Witte, N., & Verté, D. (2016). Social exclusion in later life: A systematic review of the literature. *Journal of Population Ageing, 9*(4), 315–344. https://doi.org/10.1007/s12062-016-9145-3

Van Regenmortel, S., De Donder, L., Smetcoren, A.-S., Lambotte, D., De Witte, N., & Verté, D. (2018). Accumulation of disadvantages: Prevalence and categories of old-age social exclusion in Belgium. *Social Indicators Research, 140*(3), 1173–1194. https://doi.org/10.1007/s11205-017-1817-8

Van Regenmortel, S., Smetcoren, A.-S., Marsillas, S., Lambotte, D., Fret, B., & De Donder, L. (2021). Exploring underexposed stories: The experienced lifecourse of financially excluded older adults. *Ageing and Society, 41*(4), 724–745. https://doi.org/10.1017/S0144686X19001235

van Tilburg, T. G., & de Jong Gierveld, J. (2024). The concepts and measurements of social isolation and loneliness. In A. Hajek, S. G. Riedel-Heller, & H.-H. König (Eds.), *Loneliness and social isolation in old age: Correlates and implications* (pp. 3–12). Routledge.

Vercauteren, T., Regenmortel, S. V., Näsman, M., Nyqvist, F., Brosens, D., Serrat, R., & Dury, S. (2024). Multi-dimensional civic engagement of older Europeans: A latent class analysis. *Ageing & Society*, 1–26. https://doi.org/10.1017/S0144686X2400062X

Victor, C. R., Rippon, I., Barreto, M., Hammond, C., & Qualter, P. (2022). Older adults' experiences of loneliness over the lifecourse: An exploratory study using the BBC loneliness experiment. *Archives of Gerontology and Geriatrics, 102*, 104740. https://doi.org/10.1016/j.archger.2022.104740

von Humboldt, S., Costa, A., Ilyas, N., & Leal, I. (2024). Older adults, perceived ageism, civic participation and mental health: A qualitative study. *Aging & Mental Health, 28*(11), 1489–1501. https://doi.org/10.1080/13607863.2024.2348611

Wagner, M., & Brandt, M. (2018). Long-term care provision and the well-being of spousal caregivers: An analysis of 138 European regions. *The Journals of Gerontology: Series B, 73*(4), e24–e34. https://doi.org/10.1093/geronb/gbx133

Waldegrave, C., Aartsen, M., Lowenstein, A., Seppänen, M., Niemi, M., Melchiorre, M. G., & Lamura, G. (2021). Conflicting relations, abuse and discrimination experienced by older adults. In K. Walsh, T. Scharf, A. Wanka, & S. Van Regenmortel (Eds.), *Social exclusion in ageing societies: Interdisciplinary and policy perspectives* (pp. 119–132). Springer.

Walsh, K., Scharf, T., & Keating, N. (2017). Social exclusion of older persons: A scoping review and conceptual framework. *European Journal of Ageing, 14*(1), 81–98. https://doi.org/10.1007/s10433-016-0398-8

Walsh, K., Scharf, T., Van Regenmortel, S., & Wanka, A. (2021). The intersection of ageing and social exclusion. In K. Walsh, T. Scharf, S. Van Regenmortel, & A. Wanka (Eds.), *Social exclusion in later life. Interdisciplinary and policy perspectives* (pp. 3–21). Springer.

Weiss, R. S. (1973). *Loneliness: The experience of emotional and social isolation*. MIT Press.

Wilkinson, E. (2022). Loneliness is a feminist issue. *Feminist Theory, 23*(1), 23–38. https://doi.org/10.1177/14647001211062739

Williams, A. J., McHale, C., Chow, C., Van Ry, R., & Cope, A. (2024). Systematic review of the associations between transport and loneliness. *Health on the Move 3: The Reviews*, 283–342. https://doi.org/10.1016/bs.atpp.2023.11.005

Wu, J., Zhang, J., & Fokkema, T. (2022). The micro-macro interplay of economic factors in late-life loneliness: Evidence from Europe and China. *Frontiers in Public Health, 10*. https://doi.org/10.3389/fpubh.2022.968411

Yarker, S., Doran, P., & Buffel, T. (2023). Theorizing "place" in aging in place: The need for territorial and relational perspectives. *The Gerontologist*, gnad002. https://doi.org/10.1093/geront/gnad002

Zeng, Y., Mao, S., Lu, N., & Chen, M. (2023). Activity patterns and loneliness in later life: The Mediating effects of social support and attitudes toward aging. *Journal of Gerontological Social Work, 66*(2), 303–318. https://doi.org/10.1080/01634372.2022.2103761

Sofie Van Regenmortel works as a postdoctoral researcher within the Society and Ageing Research Lab since 2022. Sofie provides methodological support to various research projects (e.g. CIVEX, HOUSE), conducts research on social exclusion in later life and was postdoctoral researcher on the FWO-SBO project 'A Lonely Planet? addressing loneliness from a neighbourhood perspective'. In 2017 she obtained her PhD, titled 'Research on Social Exclusion in Later Life (SELL). Measurement and drivers of social exclusion among older adults'.

Elisa Tiilikainen works as an Associate Professor of Social Work at University of Eastern Finland (UEF). Her research has focused on loneliness and social exclusion in later life and how they are acknowledged and addressed in social and healthcare services. Currently Tiilikainen leads research projects on social exclusion among older adults receiving home care (SOLDEX) and older men's driving cessation (DRIVEX).

Hanna Ristolainen obtained a PhD in social work and is a University Lecturer in the Department of Social Sciences at University of Eastern Finland (UEF). Her background is in gerontological social work and nursing, and she has expertise in effectiveness research of social care services. Her research has focused on eldercare services, such as community case management and home care, and issues related to older adults' wellbeing.

Vanessa Burholt is Emeritus Professor at Swansea University, Wales, UK and holds an honorary position as Professor of Gerontology in the School of Nursing/School of Population Health, Faculty of Health and Medicine at the University of Auckland. She has overseen the integration of transdisciplinary research in ageing and dementia, and is committed to co-production of research on ageing. She has published on dementia, rurality, social exclusion, loneliness, support networks, intergenerational relationships, ethnicity and migration.

Lena Dahlberg is professor in social work at Dalarna University, Sweden, and affiliated to Karolinska Institutet. She has previously worked at research and development units in Sweden and at Sheffield Hallam University in the United Kingdom. Her primary research interests are loneliness, social exclusion and informal care in later life.

Open Access This chapter is licensed under the terms of the Creative Commons Attribution 4.0 International License (http://creativecommons.org/licenses/by/4.0/), which permits use, sharing, adaptation, distribution and reproduction in any medium or format, as long as you give appropriate credit to the original author(s) and the source, provide a link to the Creative Commons license and indicate if changes were made.

The images or other third party material in this chapter are included in the chapter's Creative Commons license, unless indicated otherwise in a credit line to the material. If material is not included in the chapter's Creative Commons license and your intended use is not permitted by statutory regulation or exceeds the permitted use, you will need to obtain permission directly from the copyright holder.

Part III
Empirical Dimensions

Chapter 5
Loneliness Prevalence in Different Age Groups in Europe

Marian Vasile and Marja Aartsen

5.1 Introduction

In this chapter, we understand loneliness in line with the cognitive approach to loneliness as the subjectively experienced discrepancy between the desired and actual quantity and quality of social relationships (Peplau & Perlman, 1982). Loneliness embodies societal changes that disconnect individuals both from each other and from institutions and society (Alberti, 2019). Loneliness is frequently discussed in conjunction with social isolation (Walsh et al., 2017), and while they are highly correlated, they are not the same. In contrast to loneliness, social isolation refers to an objective lack of interactions with other people. People can feel lonely in the middle of the crowd, and not all people that are socially isolated also feel lonely. Loneliness and social isolation are different from solitude, which is experienced when people purposefully withdraw from the social world to be creative, recharge their batteries or, simply, be with oneself (Buetow, 2023; Deresiewicz, 2022).

In recent times, attention to loneliness has been booming, not only in the press but also among academics and policy makers. The World Health Organization acknowledges loneliness and social isolation as public health priorities and launched the "Commission on Social Connection" to identify solutions. Some authors use a dark tone, announcing the doom days of a "loneliness century" (Hertz, 2020) or "anti-social century" (Thompson, 2025). This perspective is mostly about United States of America, but there are European voices echoing the same labeling (Spitzer, 2019). Nevertheless, loneliness is on the public agenda and has become a major

M. Vasile (✉)
Department of Sociology, Faculty of Sociology and Social Work, University of Bucharest, Bucharest, Romania
e-mail: marian.vasile@unibuc.ro

M. Aartsen
Norwegian Social Research (NOVA), Oslo Metropolitan University, Oslo, Norway

© The Author(s) 2025

M. Aartsen et al. (eds.), *Macro Social Influences on Loneliness in Later Life*, International Perspectives on Aging 47,
https://doi.org/10.1007/978-3-031-94565-6_5

public health issue (Meisters et al., 2021; Mihalopoulos et al., 2020) because of its associations with a range of negative health outcomes such as depression, anxiety, cognitive decline (Park et al., 2020), cardiovascular diseases (Valtorta et al., 2018), and increased mortality (Holt-Lunstad et al., 2015). Loneliness can even be a source of political radicalization (Peterson et al., 2025). At the same time, interventions to reduce loneliness have been little effective so far (Hickin et al., 2021).

"Loneliness epidemic" is a popular term generating hundreds of thousands of results when searched on Google, but what is the loneliness epidemic? An epidemic refers to spread, rapid increase, and contagion but not necessarily in the same definition or explicitly stated. Its users discuss the ubiquity of loneliness, adding a sense of unease due to its 'alarming' prevalence. In terms of data, this should be reflected in high percentages of people reporting feelings of loneliness or exhibiting symptoms of loneliness across age groups and different social categories. Another aspect is the surge or rapid increase of loneliness compared to the recent past. Data should reflect this through higher percentages of lonely individuals across different generations. Finally, an epidemic of loneliness suggests the possibility of contagion, not in a biological sense but in a psychosocial sense, through social influence. An interesting study by Cacioppo and others indeed suggest that loneliness spreads through a contagious process (Cacioppo et al., 2009). Advocates of the loneliness epidemic attribute its developments to global processes such as the increasing popularity of neoliberal policies assuming people are solely responsible for their well-being while the welfare state and social protection is less and less prominent, therefore favoring or complementing individualization (Beck & Beck-Gernsheim, 2002), the use of social media and large-scale migration. Between 2014 and 2023 Europe went through at least two major events, which are the COVID-19 pandemic and the Russia-Ukraine conflict, followed by important political and economic developments. The COVID-19 pandemic can be viewed as a natural experiment (Leatherdale, 2019) to examine whether mobility restrictions and appeals to solidarity with vulnerable groups, particularly older people affect levels of loneliness. There are studies showing that at least young adults felt lonely more often during the pandemic (Baarck et al., 2021; European Foundation for the Improvement of Living and Working Conditions, 2021). If there is indeed a surge of loneliness, we should find empirical support in the form of higher percentages in 2023 as compared to the data from 2014, at least for the younger age groups.

However, the popular view of high and increasing levels of loneliness in older adults is challenged by various recent studies in Europe, such as in Norway (Aunsmo et al., 2023), Sweden (Dahlberg et al., 2024), and Germany (Suanet et al., 2024), suggesting that although the absolute number of lonely older people may rise in the years to come, the prevalence in subsequent birth cohorts is rather stable or even declining. One explanation for lower levels of loneliness in today's older people is the improved access to resources and social values that enhance control and choice in social relationships (Suanet et al., 2024), as well as improved psychological resources such as mastery and self-efficacy (Suanet & van Tilburg, 2019). However, life changes over the individual's life course suggest that, regardless of cohort, loneliness does increase with a person's age (de Jong Gierveld et al., 2006; Pagan &

Malo, 2024; Suanet et al., 2024), most likely due to the increasing number of social losses and health issues with ageing.

5.2 The Measurement of Loneliness

Loneliness is a subjective experience, typically measured through self-reports, where people describe their situation using at least one item in a questionnaire. Most single-item measures are direct measures because they use words such as "lonely" or "loneliness." Single-item measures are frequently used in loneliness research, but they are also criticized for being prone to response bias, as people must admit that they are lonely, which is taboo in many countries (Barreto et al., 2022; Lau & Gruen, 1992; Schoenmakers, 2020). However, empirical data also indicate that classifying respondents as lonely based on their frequent or constant feelings of loneliness yields remarkably similar results for both single-item questions and aggregated scales (Victor et al., 2005), which mitigates the potential underestimation of loneliness when loneliness is more severe. Multi-item measures often use indirect questions avoiding the word lonely but infer loneliness from self-perceived manifestations of different feelings. Multi-item measures can be unidimensional such as the UCLA scale (Russell et al., 1980) tackling overall or global loneliness, or multidimensional, such as the de Jong Gierveld loneliness scale (de Jong Gierveld et al., 2006) and the Social and Emotional Loneliness scale (DiTommaso & Spinner, 1993), measuring emotional and social loneliness.

Both direct and indirect measures of loneliness provide valid estimations of loneliness and can be used with general populations to assess loneliness (Mund et al., 2023). However, there are some precautions. Multi-item measures can include items that measure other constructs related to loneliness, and there are indications that loneliness scales are not invariant across populations (Maes et al., 2022; van Tilburg & Fokkema, 2021). Single item questions are criticized for being inappropriate for screening in clinical populations due to their inability to capture the complexity of loneliness (Mund et al., 2023). Hence, conclusions on loneliness prevalence and comparison of loneliness between groups or countries and over time are compromised due to the limited use of the same loneliness measures (Surkalim et al., 2022).

There are different methods to evaluate measurement invariance. Putnick and Bornstein (2016) describe four steps, including the testing of configural invariance (whether the number of factors and factor loadings are similar across the groups), metric invariance (whether each item of the scale contributes equally to loneliness across groups), scalar invariance (whether the starting points of the items are the same across groups), and checking the residual invariance (whether the unaccounted-for variance (error) in items is the same across culture, gender, education, socio-economic groups. All these steps can be evaluated with multi-group confirmatory factor analyses or similar techniques. Hawkley et al. (2016) published a working paper to assist other researchers with research on measurement invariance. In this paper, they evaluate the measurement invariance and validity of the 3-item UCLA scale as used in two American surveys (the Health and Retirement Study and the National Social Life, Health and Ageing Project) and one German survey (German Socio-Economic Panel). They conclude that the three items of the UCLA scale are good indicators of the latent loneliness factor and that there is strong invariance of the three items across the three populations, allowing for valid and meaningful comparisons of mean loneliness levels across the three surveys. Given that the issue of measurement invariance has only recently garnered the attention of researchers, further investigation is required to extend the evaluation of invariance across various social groups, including gender (men and women), educational attainment (high and low education), and marital status.

In this chapter we will evaluate whether the "loneliness epidemic" hypothesis has empirical support. We build on the assumption of the ubiquity of loneliness on the one hand, and sharp increase of loneliness on the other hand, in a significant social space. Therefore, we compare percentages of people reporting feeling lonely at two time points, 2014 and 2023, in several European countries for overall populations and for age groups. Studies show age differences in loneliness patterns, usually as a U-shaped relationship, with higher levels among youngest and oldest age groups, due to life-stage specific social needs and social experiences such as peer pressure, career stage, family roles, retirement, declining health and mobility, and the formation or shrinking of social networks (Luhmann & Hawkley, 2016; Pinquart & Sorensen, 2001; Qualter et al., 2015; Victor & Yang, 2015). In short, there are good reasons to identify prevalences of loneliness in different age groups and countries so that policies can be tailored accordingly. If there is indeed a loneliness epidemic, we should see large prevalences of loneliness in 2023, at least for some of these countries and age groups and a sharp increase since 2014. If not, then loneliness might be more a "trait-like feature" influenced by developmental and idiosyncratic experiences (Mund et al., 2020) than by global societal changes, as advocates of the loneliness epidemic argue.

Before presenting the numbers, we first provide an overview of several social surveys popular in Europe that include questions on loneliness and describe how loneliness is measured. We will describe the strengths and limitations of each survey with respect to the loneliness measures and this chapter's objectives.

5.3 European Surveys Including Measures of Loneliness

Evaluating if there is indeed a loneliness epidemic in Europe requires assessments of loneliness that are invariant across groups, and data that come from different countries, reflecting different economic realities, different social protection systems, different cultures and social values. Therefore, we need representative data from a large cross-national survey that includes measures of loneliness. Below, we describe such projects, emphasize their strengths and weaknesses relative to our intentions, and conclude which of the surveys can be best used for our purpose.

5.3.1 European Union Loneliness Survey

The European Union Loneliness Survey (EULS) is specifically developed to provide data on the prevalence, risk factors, and outcomes of loneliness across European Union (EU) Member States (European Commission, Joint Research Centre, 2024; Mauri et al., 2024). The EULS is a project of the Joint Research Centre (JRC) of the European Commission. Data were collected only once so far, in November and December 2022, in each of the European Union's 27 (EU27) countries (European Commission, Joint Research Centre, 2024). There are two samples: one non-probabilistic online survey targeting the general population aged 16 and above in all 27 EU Member States and one random probability-based sample drawn in four countries (EU4), including France, Italy, Poland, and Sweden, targeting the same population. The country samples included approximately 1000 cases for most countries. Using quotas for age, gender, education, geographical distribution and economic characteristics, researchers selected respondents from consumer panels who were not involved in other surveys during the last two weeks. Survey weights are provided with the dataset.

The EULS questionnaire includes several measures of loneliness (Mauri et al., 2024). Two are direct measures, that is, use the words "loneliness" or "lonely". One direct measure asks about the frequency of loneliness: "How much of the time, during the past four weeks, have you been feeling lonely?". The other asks about the intensity of loneliness: "How intense was this feeling of loneliness?". Two are indirect measures. Indirect measures usually are multi-item scales, asking about different facets of being lonely but without using the words "loneliness" or "lonely". One indirect measure is the De Jong Gierveld (DJG) 6-item scale (de Jong Gierveld & van Tilburg, 2006). Examples of items are "I miss having people around", "I often feel rejected" and "There are many people I can trust completely". The other indirect measure is the 3-item UCLA loneliness scale, with the following items: "Feel that you lack companionship", "Feel left out", and "Feel isolated from others" (Russell, 1982). The DJG scale allows for differentiation between social and emotional loneliness. Emotional loneliness is the result of the absence of a close, intimate relationship, while social loneliness is the result of not being part of a community (Weiss, 1973).

The strength of the EULS is the large sample size, the wide variety of loneliness measures, the inclusion of all EU countries, and the possibility for evaluating the quality of existing loneliness measures. However, while the EU4 is a probabilistic sample, the EU27 is not, making it more complicated to estimate loneliness prevalence. For example, for the Romanian sample, there is a major difference between the sampling framework and population regarding the percentage of people aged between 56 and 80 years, which is around 4% in the source consumer panel, whereas this percentage is approximately 32% in the Romanian population. The survey weights that are provided cannot fully correct for the underrepresentation of people aged 65+ and people with lower education. This compromises the comparability of loneliness prevalence between all EU countries and reduces the generalizability of the findings.

5.3.2 European Social Survey

The European Social Survey (ESS) is an academically driven, repeated cross-sectional survey, measuring attitudes, beliefs, and behaviors on different topics. The ESS target population is persons aged 15 and over, residents in private households in participating countries. ESS is not focused only on European Union countries, including countries like Norway, Serbia, or United Kingdom. The list of participating countries, unfortunately, is not the same for each wave. ESS uses random probability sampling. ESS aims for minimum effective sample sizes of 1500 respondents per country for most participating nations. For countries with populations smaller than two million, the target is reduced to 800 respondents (European Social Survey website). In this chapter, we will use data from ESS7 and ESS11, waves from 2014/2015 and 2023/2024 (hereafter referred to as 2014 and 2023).

Loneliness is not a standard item in the core questionnaires, but it is included in the questionnaires from years 2006, 2010, 2012, 2014, and 2023. In 2023 the question about loneliness is a direct measure of loneliness that is part of the 8-item version of the Centre of Epidemiological Studies Depression Scale (CES-D) (Balaj et al., n.d.): "Please tell me how much of the time during the past week you felt lonely? None or almost none of the time; Some of the time; Most of the time; All or almost all of the time."

The strength of the ESS is its sound methodological design, use of probabilistic samples, and availability of several waves. Since the ESS is not a panel study, it cannot be used to study within-person changes in loneliness but can be used to trace overall changes at the country level and for different social groups. A limitation of the ESS is that it is not developed as a loneliness survey, which means that it includes only one measure of loneliness, which is a direct question of which studies have indicated that it might lead to an underestimation of the loneliness prevalence (Stegen et al., 2024; Victor et al., 2005). Also, not all predictors and outcomes in which the researcher is interested will be available. However, as we will see from the rest of this section, the ESS is the best option available to meet this chapter's purpose.

5.3.3 European Quality of Life Survey

The European Quality of Life Survey (EQLS) is a repeated cross-sectional survey with waves in the years 2003, 2007, 2011, and 2016 (Leoncikas, 2018). It examines the objective and subjective quality of life of European Union citizens. For each wave, a multi-stage random probability sample between 1000 and 2000 respondents was extracted from the population of persons aged at least 18 years who reside in private households in European Union member countries and also candidate countries at that time, such as Albania, the former Yugoslav Republic of Macedonia, Montenegro, Serbia, and Turkey.

The EQLS questionnaire contains one direct indicator of loneliness: "Please indicate which is the closest to how you have been feeling over the last two weeks: I have felt lonely," and several possible indirect indicators.

The strength of EQLS is its sound methodological design, use of probabilistic samples, and availability of several waves allowing for analyzing change over time for countries and specific social groups. The weaknesses of the EQLS are the same as for ESS, most importantly that the last wave available is from 2016 and there has not been a registration after the COVID-19 pandemic to see a change in loneliness prevalences.

5.3.4 Living and Working in the EU e-Survey (LWEU)

The Living and Working in the EU e-survey (LWEU) is an on-line survey done by the European Foundation for the Improvement of Living and Working Conditions (Eurofound), the same organization responsible for EQLS. This project was launched at the beginning of COVID-19 pandemic, in spring 2020, to measure its impact on people's life and work. Towards the end of the COVID-19 pandemic, in spring 2022, the questionnaire was adapted to reflect new challenges EU countries face, such as the situation in Ukraine and its aftermaths. In total, there are seven rounds, the latest being conducted in spring 2024. In later rounds, the e-survey was extended to non-EU countries such as Albania or Armenia, and non-European countries such as Egypt and Lebanon.

The LWEU questionnaire contains the same direct indicator of loneliness as in the EQLS. LWEU uses a non-probability sampling method, respondents being recruited by availability through social media and snowball sampling. However, weighting variables are available to adjust for gender, age, education, self-defined urbanization level, and, in the last rounds, for employment status.

Nevertheless, as in the case of the EULS, the weighting system cannot resolve the fact that specific categories of the target population are excluded, such as people with no internet access, people not using social media, and people with low digital literacy. These factors affect the representativity of the survey for social categories such as older people, who are known to have lower usage of internet or lower digital literacy, and people with low education.

5.3.5 Survey of Health, Ageing and Retirement in Europe (SHARE)

The Survey of Health, Ageing and Retirement in Europe (SHARE) is another European-wide survey that includes information on loneliness. SHARE is devoted to understanding the effects of diverse factors over the life course of European citizens aged 50 years and over (Börsch-Supan et al., 2013). Data have been collected from 27 European countries and Israel, although not all countries are included in every round. The first wave was held in 2004, and a follow-up was held every second year, bringing the total to nine regular waves. Partners are also included in the target population, even if they are younger than 50 years, making it possible to define the target population in terms of households with at least one member. Two additional waves were conducted during the COVID-19 pandemic. The first SHARE Corona Survey (SCS) was held between June and August in 2020, and the second in June and August 2021. SHARE includes people living in nursing homes and residential care. In contrast with the ESS and the EQLS, SHARE is designed as a panel survey.

SHARE uses probability-based sampling procedures and includes in waves 5, 6, 8, and 9, the three-item UCLA loneliness scale, with the items "How often do you feel that you lack companionship?", "How often do you feel left out?", and "How often do you feel isolated from others?". In some waves a direct measure of loneliness was used: "How much of the time do you feel lonely?" (Gruber et al., 2024; Hughes et al., 2004).

A major strength of the SHARE study is its panel design, long follow-up, and large sample size, allowing for studies on causality. A weakness of SHARE, from the perspective of this chapter, is its target population, people with a minimum age of 50 years, which does not allow for comparison of loneliness prevalences among different age groups such as young adults, and middle-aged adults.

5.3.6 Comparing the Strengths and Weaknesses of the European Surveys

Both the EU27 sample of the EULS and LWEU data use non-probabilistic samples that deviate from population distribution for important socio-demographic characteristics. The weighting systems are not able to fully balance these samples. However, the EU4 sample of the EULS contains probabilistic samples, albeit with only four European countries, which is a weakness relative to our intentions. EQLS, ESS, and SHARE have sound sampling designs, using probabilistic samples, which is important for the estimation of loneliness prevalence. The slight deviation from population distribution for important socio-demographic characteristics can be balanced by the weighting system. SHARE is so far the only study with a panel design covering several European countries, which can be used to study trajectories of loneliness for older people. However, SHARE's target population includes people from 50 years of age, not allowing comparisons between older and younger age groups.

EULS provides the most diverse range of loneliness measures among large-scale European surveys. All studies discussed in this chapter include a direct measure of loneliness, versions that are similar. These questions ask about occurrences of feeling lonely in the last week (ESS), the last two (EQLS, LWEU), or four weeks (EULS), or do not frame the period (SHARE). The response scale is common for some surveys (EQLS, LWEU) or overlaps for certain categories (EULS, EQLS, ESS, LWEU) allowing at least for identifying very lonely people (i.e. feeling lonely all the time or most of the time). Direct, single-item questions about loneliness have the benefit that they do not take much time in the interview and, therefore, are often used in surveys where interview time is scarce. Single-item direct measures are considered adequate as "benchmarks" for "real" loneliness even by scholars who advocate for the demise of the current system of researching loneliness (Mund et al., 2024) because they are easy to include in every study and economical, letting people appreciate what lonely or loneliness is more in tune with the idiographic recommended perspective, their better discriminant validity and, in fact, their better overall validity and reliability than multi-item indirect measures.

There are, however, clear caveats with direct questions. Firstly, the periods in the direct questions vary from one to four weeks, and sometimes no time limit is mentioned. Second, people may not have a unified understanding of loneliness (Stein & Tuval-Mashiach, 2015). Some may think of loneliness as the "disintegrative" feeling leading to "psychotic states," letting people feel "helpless," an undesirable stigmatizing state (Mauri et al., 2024; Fromm-Reichmann, 1959). Others may think of loneliness as a situation of being alone, or even as solitude, which is a positive period of aloneness, when people redraw from the fast life to recharge their batteries or explore inner self, being creative or contemplating (Buetow, 2023). Third, a single question cannot differentiate between types of loneliness, such as social and emotional loneliness (Weiss, 1973). Fourth, since there is often a brief period in the question, for example "I felt lonely during the last week," we do not know whether the loneliness measured is transient, situational, or chronic (Mauri et al., 2024). Direct questions may reflect mainly the effect of temporarily negative events, such as a good friend or spouse may have died, children leaving the house, or other similar events. Feelings produced by negative events will take a longer time to heal; however, healing is expected due to a protective homeostatic process that reverts the state of mind towards its set point (Cummins et al., 2012).

Researchers interested in differentiating between loneliness types should use the EULS, as it is the only European wide survey that also includes the 11-item, or the shorter 6-item De Jong Gierveld loneliness scale (de Jong-Gierveld & Kamphuis, 1985; de Jong Gierveld & van Tilburg, 2006) that can differentiate between social and emotional loneliness. Also, for evaluating the validity and reliability of assessments of loneliness, the EULS is the only alternative because of its wide selection of measurement scales. Researchers interested in the dynamic nature of loneliness among older people can only use the SHARE dataset, as it is the only large-scale

European survey including panel data on loneliness in older adults. Moreover, panel data are indispensable for causal research because they allow researchers to control unobserved and time-varying confounders and can address issues of reverse causality.

In conclusion, none of these surveys are perfect for this chapter's purpose. For a valid estimation of loneliness prevalence among older adults in the general population, study designs must adhere to specific prerequisites that ensure representativeness, reliability, and validity of the findings. This means that all people representative of the population under study need a chance different from zero to be included, which is achieved with a probability sampling method. This is possible with ESS, EQLS, and SHARE. The sample size needs to be sufficiently large to account for the population diversity (e.g., minorities, people with functional limitations) and to assure sufficient precision in the prevalence estimate. This is possible for older people only with SHARE. Questionnaires should include different measures for overall loneliness and its types, like emotional and social loneliness. This is the case with EULS. The ESS serves our purposes the best because it has a probabilistic sampling design, and an overall sound methodological approach, covering a large range of ages, starting from 15 years, allowing comparisons between age groups. Table 5.1 summarizes the measurement of loneliness in these surveys.

Table 5.1 Overview of loneliness measurements in EULS, EQLS, ESS, SHARE, and LWEU

Survey	Direct questions (answering categories)	Indirect questions (answering categories)
EULS	How much of the time, during the past 4 weeks, have you been feeling lonely? (All of the time; Most of the time; Some of the time; A little bit of the time; None of the time). How intense was this feeling of loneliness? (Not very intense (1) … Very intense (10)).	3 item UCLA scale: Please indicate how often you feel each of the following. _a. Feel that you lack companionship; _b. Feel left out; _c. Feel isolated from others. (Hardly ever or never; Some of the time; Often) 6-item DJG scale: Please indicate for each of the statements, the extent to which they apply to your situation and the way you feel now. _a. I experience a general sense of emptiness; _b. I miss having people around; _c. I often feel rejected; _d. There are plenty of people I can rely on when I have problems; _e. There are many people I can trust completely; _f. There are enough people that I feel close to. (Yes; More or less; No).

(continued)

Table 5.1 (continued)

Survey	Direct questions (answering categories)	Indirect questions (answering categories)
EQLS	Please indicate which is the closest to how you have been feeling over the last two weeks: I have felt lonely. (All of the time; Most of the time; More than half of the time; Less than half of the time; Some of the time; At no time).	To what extent do you agree or disagree with: I feel left out of society. Strongly agree; Agree; Neither agree nor disagree; Disagree; Strongly disagree. To what extent do you agree or disagree with: I feel close to people in the area where I live. Strongly agree; Agree; Neither agree nor disagree; Disagree; Strongly disagree. Note: these are items similar with some of those available in different multi-item scales measuring loneliness. They are not specifically attributed as measures of loneliness in this survey.
ESS	Please tell me how much of the time during the past week you felt lonely? (None or almost none of the time; Some of the time; Most of the time; All or almost all of the time).	Not available
SHARE	How much of the time do you feel lonely? (Often; Some of the time; Hardly ever or never).	I will now read some statements and would like to ask you to answer how much of the time you feel certain ways: (i) Lack companionship; (ii) Left out; (iii) Isolated from others. (Often; Some of the time; Hardly ever or never)
LWEU	Please indicate which is the closest to how you have been feeling over the last two weeks: I have felt lonely. (All of the time; Most of the time; More than half of the time; Less than half of the time; Some of the time; At no time).	To what extent do you agree or disagree with: I feel left out of society. (Strongly agree; Agree; Neither agree nor disagree; Disagree; Strongly disagree). To what extent do you agree or disagree with: I feel close to people in the area where I live. (Strongly agree; Agree; Neither agree nor disagree; Disagree; Strongly disagree). Note: these are items similar to some of those available in different multi-item scales measuring loneliness. They are not specifically attributed as measures of loneliness in this survey.

Notes: EULS = EU-Loneliness Survey; EQLS = European Quality of Life Survey, ESS = European Social Survey; SHARE = Survey of Health and Retirement Europe; LWEU = Living and working in the EU e-survey

5.4 Loneliness Prevalences in European Countries Before and After COVID-19 Pandemic

5.4.1 Loneliness Prevalence in 2014 and 2023: An Overall Picture

We use European Social Survey waves 7 and 11 from 2014 and 2023. Samples are probabilistic representative for the resident population aged at least 15 years. Sample sizes allow for analyzing different age groups (Table 5.2). In both waves, respondents were asked "Please tell me how much of the time during the past week you felt lonely?" and the following answering categories were provided: none or almost none of the time (1), some of the time (2), most of the time (3), all or almost all of the time (4). Since we are interested in country-level changes, we focus on countries participating in both ESS7 and ESS11, which are Austria, Belgium, Finland, France, Germany, Hungary, Ireland, Lithuania, Netherlands, Norway, Poland, Portugal, Slovenia, Spain, Sweden, Switzerland, and the United Kingdom (Table 5.2).

In our first step, we merge all countries per measurement round (ESS7 and ESS11) and examine the loneliness prevalences for each pooled sample, stratified by 10-year age groups. Very severe loneliness, that is feeling lonely "all or almost all of the time" is rare, only 3% felt like this in 2023, while severe loneliness, that is feeling lonely "most of the time," occurs in 4% of the cases (Table 5.3). Two out of ten people (21%) report moderate loneliness, that is feeling lonely "some of the time." The oldest old people (age 80+) have the highest prevalence in 2023 of

Table 5.2 Unweighted sample size for each country participating in European Social Survey round 7 (2014) and/or European Social Survey round 11 (2023)

Country	ESS7, 2014/2015	ESS11, 2023/2024
Austria	1795	2354
Belgium	1769	1594
Finland	2087	1563
France	1917	1771
Germany	3045	2420
Hungary	1698	2118
Ireland	2390	2017
Lithuania	2250	1365
Netherlands	1919	1695
Norway	1436	1337
Poland	1615	1442
Portugal	1265	1373
Slovenia	1224	1248
Spain	1925	1844
Sweden	1791	1230
Switzerland	1532	1384
United Kingdom	2264	1684
Total	31,922	28,439

Table 5.3 Age and loneliness in European countries 2023, pooled sample with countries participating in ESS7 and ESS11

Age group	None or almost none of the time	Some of the time	Most of the time	All or almost all of the time	Total
15–19	66%	27%	4%	2%	100%
20–29	64%	28%	5%	2%	100%
30–39	72%	22%	4%	2%	100%
40–49	75%	19%	4%	2%	100%
50–59	75%	19%	3%	2%	100%
60–69	77%	17%	4%	3%	100%
70–79	74%	18%	5%	3%	100%
80 +	65%	21%	8%	5%	100%
Total	72%	21%	4%	3%	100%

Note: Percentages may not add up to 100% due to rounding errors

Table 5.4 Age and loneliness in European countries 2014, pooled sample with countries participating in ESS7 and ESS11

Age group	None or almost none of the time	Some of the time	Most of the time	All or almost all of the time	Total
15–19	77%	20%	3%	1%	100%
20–29	70%	23%	5%	2%	100%
30–39	73%	22%	4%	2%	100%
40–49	76%	19%	3%	2%	100%
50–59	73%	19%	5%	3%	100%
60–69	74%	19%	4%	3%	100%
70–79	73%	18%	5%	3%	100%
80 +	58%	26%	9%	6%	100%
Total	73%	20%	4%	2%	100%

Note: Percentages may not add up to 100% due to rounding errors

feeling severely or very severely lonely (13% in total), whereas the youngest age groups (15–19 and 20–29 years) have the highest prevalence of moderate loneliness. Interestingly, the proportion of young people (aged 15–19) feeling lonely "some of the time" or more often increased from 2014 to 2023 by 9%, whereas for the oldest old the percentage of lonely people declined by 7% in the same period (Tables 5.3 and 5.4). The loneliness prevalence remained rather stable for the other age groups during the last decade.

Figure 5.1 depicts the absolute change in loneliness prevalence for the age groups. Each bar represents the % change per age group between 2014 and 2023 in such a way that a negative value indicates a decrease, and a positive value an increase of the prevalence in the relevant category. For example, in 2023, the prevalence of not feeling lonely among 15–19 years old was 11% lower than in 2014, indicating

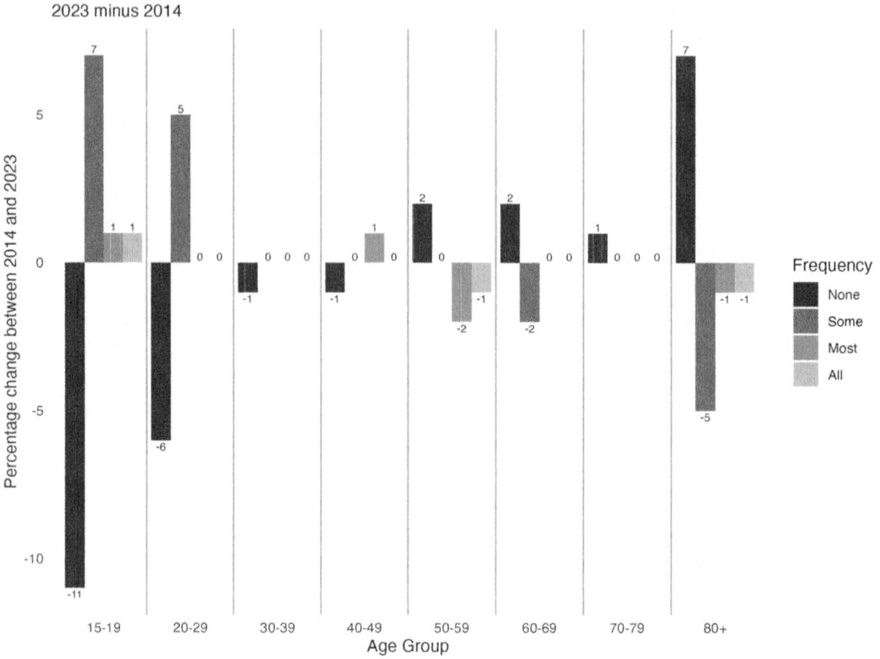

Fig. 5.1 Difference between loneliness levels within age groups 2023 versus 2014 in European countries participating in ESS7 and ESS11

an increase in loneliness prevalence. For 80+ people the prevalence of people feeling lonely none or almost none of the time was 7% higher in 2023 than in 2014. Changes in loneliness prevalence between 2014 and 2023 are negligible in the age groups between 30 and 70 years.

5.4.2 *Loneliness Prevalence in 2014 and 2023: A Country Perspective*

We will now examine whether the same patterns are present within countries. Due to the small number of cases in the categories "all or almost all of the time" and "most of the time" of a direct loneliness measure, we have combined them into a single category, "severe lonely", while keeping categories "some of the time" and "none or almost none of the time" as they are.

The first two groups of columns in Table 5.5 provide the prevalences for the three categories of loneliness for 2014 and 2023 for the countries participating in both ESS-rounds. In 2014, 27% of all people in these European countries felt lonely

Table 5.5 Loneliness prevalence for each European country participating in ESS7 and ESS11

Survey, year	ESS7, 2014			ESS11, 2023			Change from 2014 to 2023		
Indicator	Feeling lonely in the past week			Feeling lonely in the past week			Feeling lonely in the past week		
Country	(Almost) none of the time	Some of the time	Most or all of the time	(Almost) none of the time	Some of the time	Most or all of the time	(Almost) none of the time	Some of the time	Most or all of the time
Austria	73%	21%	6%	80%	16%	4%	7%	−5%	−2%
Belgium	74%	20%	7%	70%	22%	8%	−4%	2%	1%
Switzerland	79%	17%	4%	75%	21%	5%	−4%	4%	1%
Germany	78%	18%	4%	78%	17%	5%	0%	−1%	1%
Spain	69%	22%	8%	70%	22%	7%	1%	0%	−1%
Finland	81%	16%	3%	77%	18%	4%	−4%	2%	1%
France	66%	24%	10%	66%	26%	9%	0%	2%	−1%
United Kingdom	75%	20%	5%	70%	23%	7%	−5%	3%	2%
Hungary	62%	27%	11%	64%	25%	11%	2%	−2%	0%
Ireland	72%	24%	5%	72%	23%	4%	0%	−1%	−1%
Lithuania	55%	37%	8%	57%	34%	8%	2%	−3%	0%
Netherlands	82%	16%	3%	78%	19%	3%	−4%	3%	0%
Norway	78%	18%	4%	74%	22%	4%	−4%	4%	0%
Poland	74%	15%	12%	76%	15%	9%	2%	0%	−3%
Portugal	65%	25%	10%	63%	26%	11%	−2%	1%	1%
Sweden	72%	23%	5%	72%	23%	5%	0%	0%	0%
Slovenia	75%	19%	6%	77%	19%	5%	2%	0%	−1%
Total	73%	20%	7%	72%	21%	7%	−1%	1%	0%

some or most of the time, but variations between countries are substantial. The highest prevalence of severe loneliness is in the East and South-East of Europe (Hungary, Poland, Portugal) and France. The lowest loneliness prevalence is in Finland and the Netherlands. In 2023, 28% of all people in the analyzed European countries felt lonely some or most of the time. Hungary, Portugal, and France still have the highest proportions of severely lonely people, while the prevalence of severe lonely people in Poland declined slightly. In 2024, the lowest loneliness prevalence is in Austria, followed closely by Finland, Germany, and the Netherlands. Lithuania is with 45% (2014) and 42% (2023) of the people some or most of the time lonely an exceptional case.

The last three columns of Table 5.5 indicate the stability and change in loneliness prevalence for each country from 2014 to 2023. While most of the change is negligible, there were some larger changes in Austria, where loneliness became less prevalent over the years, and Switzerland, United Kingdom, Norway and the Netherlands, where loneliness became more prevalent.

We now look at the prevalence of loneliness for different age groups in each country. Although ESS samples are quite large, we considered it necessary to recategorize age into six categories (15–29 years, 30–39, 40–49, 50–59, 60–69, 70+). Due to the shortage of space, we focus on countries for which the association between age and loneliness is statistically significant at the 95% confidence level in both ESS waves which are Germany, Spain, France, United Kingdom, Hungary, Poland, and Portugal. In 2023, in general, the oldest old, people from 70 years of age, have a higher probability to experience severe or extremely severe loneliness except for United Kingdom, where this is the case for the youngest people, aged between 15–29 years. In Germany, those aged between 15–29 years and 70+ are similar in this aspect. The youngest group, 15–29 years, and sometimes people between 30–39, have a higher probability of experiencing moderate loneliness in almost all these countries, except for Hungary and Portugal.

Figure 5.2 shows the difference between percentages in 2023 and 2014 for people experiencing severe loneliness (i.e., most of the time) combined with people experiencing very severe loneliness (i.e., almost all or all of the time). Fig. 5.3 shows the same but for people experiencing moderate loneliness (i.e., some of the time). If there is a change for (very) severe loneliness we see a mix of situations; for some age groups there is an increase, the most obvious one being in United Kingdom, +6%, for those aged 15–29 years, while for some age groups there is a decrease, the most obvious one being in Poland, −13%, for those aged 70+. The same happens for moderate loneliness, although the change seems to be more pronounced for this level of loneliness. A point to note is that patterns of change for (very) severe loneliness and moderate loneliness are not similar; in general, it is a small change, and if it is a larger change, it is a decrease in the (very) severe loneliness population, while for (moderate) loneliness we see a larger decrease or increase for different age groups.

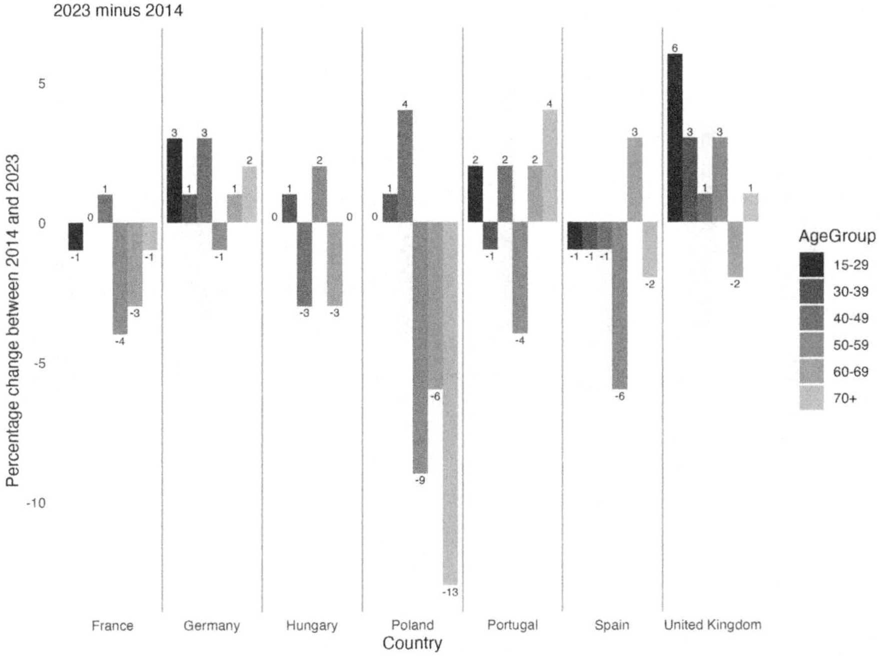

Fig. 5.2 Difference between percentages of severe and very severe loneliness in 2023 and 2014 in European countries for which the relationship between age and loneliness is statistically significant in ESS11 and ESS7

5.4.3 Loneliness Prevalence in 2014 and 2023 for the Older Population

So far, we have provided information about loneliness prevalence and changes in the prevalence over the last decade for the entire 15+ population. Since the book has a particular focus on the older population, we present additional tables for people aged 60 years and over, also participating in ESS round 7 and 11. Substantial variation in loneliness prevalence across countries is also visible in the 60+ subgroup (Table 5.6).

Finally, we represent the loneliness prevalences for people aged 60+ for all countries participating in ESS7 or ESS11. For these maps, we combine the initial categories of "some of the time," "most of the time," and "all or almost all of the time" into a single category of loneliness. According to ESS data from both 2014 and 2023, there is a divide between Southern and Northern Europe, as well as between East and West, in line with the literature (Fig. 5.4).

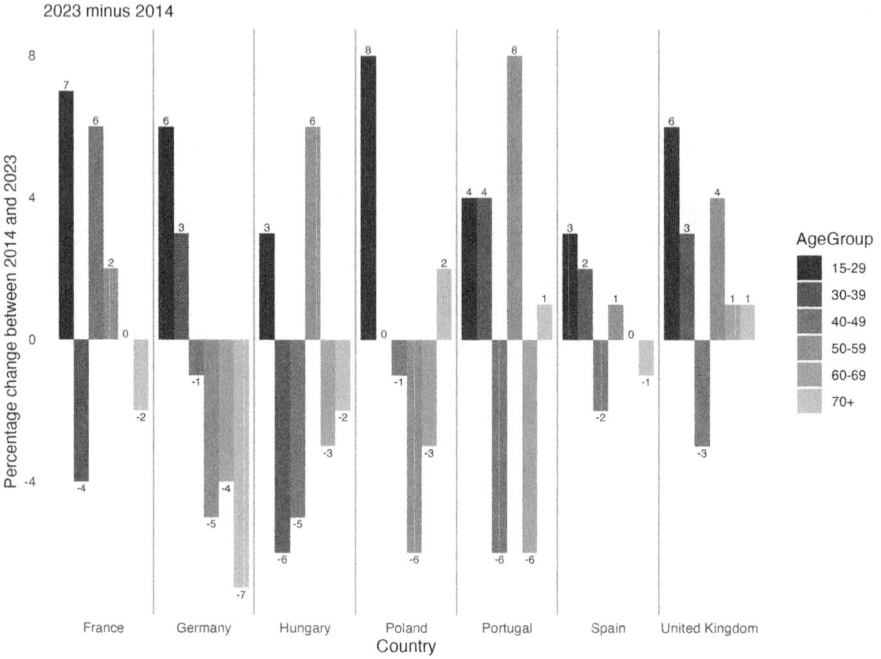

Fig. 5.3 Difference between percentages of moderate loneliness in 2023 and 2014 in European countries for which the relationship between age and loneliness is statistically significant in ESS11 and ESS7

5.5 Discussion

In this chapter, we presented updated information on loneliness prevalence to determine if the "loneliness epidemic" has empirical support in the European Social Survey data. Our findings indicate that, overall, the percentage of lonely people was around 25% in people aged 15 years and over in 2014 and 2023, providing no support for an increase in loneliness prevalence over the last 10 years in Europe. However, when examining different age groups, we observed some differences. When examining both the pooled sample of countries in 2014 and 2023 and each country sample, loneliness increased among the youngest age groups, those below 30 years of age, and less among the older groups and especially the oldest old, aged 70 years and above.

Why the prevalence of loneliness increased in the youngest age groups is not clear. Between ESS7, 2014/2015, and ESS11, 2023/2024, the COVID-19 pandemic happened with significant mobility restrictions that probably affected mostly younger age groups. At the same time, older people, identified as the main vulnerable group in front of the virus, received increased attention through political and media channels, which likely enhanced the support they received within families as well as in the neighborhood. Some studies indeed support the claim that the

Table 5.6 Loneliness among 60 years and older people in European countries

Survey, Year	ESS7, 2014			ESS11, 2023			Change from 2014 to 2023		
Indicator	Felt lonely last week			Felt lonely last week			Felt lonely last week		
Country	(Almost) none of the time	Some of the time	Most or all of the time	(Almost) none of the time	Some of the time	Most or all of the time	(Almost) none of the time	Some of the time	Most or all of the time
Austria	69%	23%	8%	75%	20%	4%	6%	−3%	−4%
Belgium	72%	20%	9%	74%	18%	8%	2%	−2%	−1%
Switzerland	82%	15%	3%	79%	17%	3%	−3%	2%	0%
Germany	79%	17%	5%	83%	11%	6%	4%	−6%	1%
Spain	71%	18%	11%	71%	18%	11%	0%	0%	0%
Finland	82%	14%	4%	79%	16%	6%	−3%	2%	2%
France	64%	24%	12%	67%	22%	11%	3%	−2%	−1%
United Kingdom	74%	19%	6%	73%	21%	6%	−1%	2%	0%
Hungary	50%	30%	20%	56%	27%	18%	6%	−3%	−2%
Ireland	67%	26%	7%	71%	24%	4%	4%	−2%	−3%
Lithuania	37%	48%	15%	55%	32%	12%	18%	−16%	−3%
Netherlands	82%	14%	4%	80%	15%	5%	−2%	1%	1%
Norway	81%	15%	4%	80%	16%	3%	−1%	1%	−1%
Poland	62%	18%	20%	72%	17%	11%	10%	−1%	−9%
Portugal	57%	28%	14%	56%	26%	18%	−1%	−2%	4%
Sweden	75%	19%	6%	77%	17%	6%	2%	−2%	0%
Slovenia	70%	18%	12%	77%	18%	5%	7%	0%	−7%

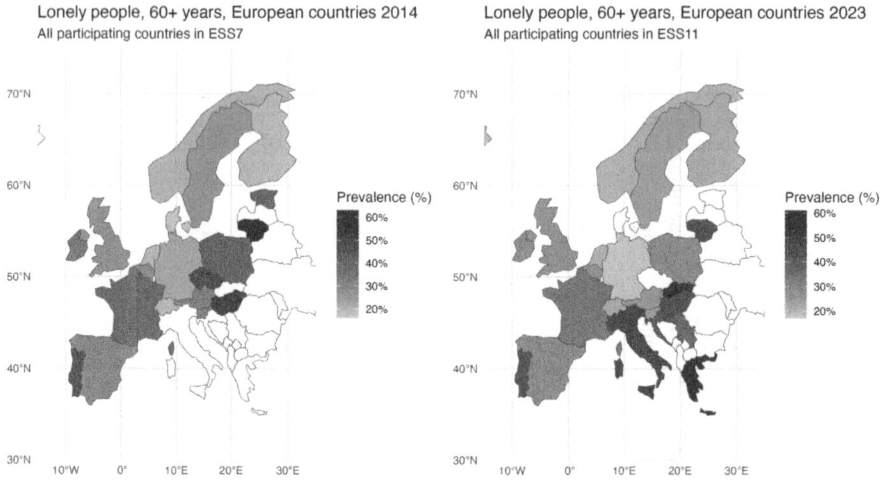

Fig. 5.4 Lonely people aged 60+, in European countries, 2014 and 2023

youngest people were hit hardest by the COVID pandemic (Herpertz-Dahlmann et al., 2022), which may explain the still increased loneliness prevalence in 2023. However, other predictors of (change in) loneliness among adolescents may have shifted as well, such as leaving the parental home before the age of 18, not having at least one close friend, and not having siblings (Von Soest et al., 2020). It is difficult to retrospectively assess these assumptions, especially when using survey data not designed for this purpose. The COVID-19 pandemic and the Russia-Ukraine conflict generated political change due to economic instability, with more people – previously a silent population– finding their voice in a different type of leadership than the one popular before these events. On the other hand, if the act of reporting loneliness is country-dependent, then future studies should investigate cultural norms about reporting feelings, and especially negative feelings.

Data further offer support for the hypothesis of a Northwestern—Southeastern loneliness divide among population aged 60 years and above (Hansen & Slagsvold, 2016; Yang & Victor, 2011). There are more lonely older people in Southern and Eastern European countries. The countries with the highest prevalence of older (60+) people in Europe are Lithuania, Hungary, France, and Portugal. For some of these countries, an explanation for the high loneliness prevalence may lie in their history of being ruled by dictatorial regimes during a substantial part of the older people's life, which may have eroded trust leading to higher prevalence of loneliness (Rapolienė & Aartsen, 2022). These countries were also among those with the highest loneliness prevalence in 2023, albeit with somewhat lower prevalences. Differences between countries do not validate the replacement of the standard nomothetic perspective with the idiographic perspective of loneliness suggested by Mund et al. (2024). Our analysis suggests the importance of contextual covariates for loneliness, and we advocate, instead of completely switching to the idiographic perspective, for exploring this pathway while also putting more effort into a multilevel perspective of loneliness, assessing covariation between loneliness and personal, neighborhood, locality, country, and other social unit characteristics, as well cross-level interactions (for an analysis using a combination of country indicators, see Chap. 11 of this book; Precupetu et al., 2025).

In conclusion, we did not find support for a "loneliness epidemic" in the European Social Survey data. There are around 7% of very lonely people in European countries, and around 20% of moderately lonely people, but these percentages are rather similar 10 years later so the idea of an epidemic which should manifest in important percentage increase across time could not be observed. We should be reluctant with using the term "loneliness epidemic" because, as with every exaggeration, at some point it can make the real problem of loneliness questionable. Frank Furedi, for example, when talking about "therapy culture" (Furedi, 2004), argues that when a (psychological) medical act goes beyond its purpose and starts to shape public perceptions it becomes a social problem. In other words, chronic loneliness is a medical act indeed, but it does not affect large portions of the population to consider it a general problem, an epidemic. It is an exaggeration which, in time, if we see loneliness everywhere and in every temporary discomfort we have with our relationships then we devoid loneliness from its content. We should not create a "culture of fear" (Furedi, 2006) around loneliness and other mental well-being issues.

Our analyses are based on repeated cross-sectional analyses, which supports valid conclusions about changing prevalences on loneliness. However, this type of analyses does not allow conclusions on within-person changes as that would require panel data. Hence, we cannot draw conclusions about age-related changes. Moreover, we used a single-item direct measure of loneliness which can underestimate moderate levels of loneliness. Future research should take these limitations into account and compare results obtained with the approach from this chapter and more complex statistical techniques such as multilevel modeling possible into a structural equation framework if multi-item indirect measures and panel data of loneliness are available.

Competing Interests The authors have no conflicts of interest to declare that are relevant to the content of this chapter.

References

Alberti, F. B. (2019). *A biography of loneliness: The history of an emotion* (First edition). Oxford University Press.

Aunsmo, R. H., Langballe, E. M., Hansen, T., Selbæk, G., & Strand, B. H. (2023). Time trends in loneliness from 1984 to 2019 among 27,032 older adults in Norway: A HUNT study. *Preventive Medicine, 175*, 107659. https://doi.org/10.1016/j.ypmed.2023.107659

Baarck, J., Balahur, A., Cassio, L., d'Hombres, B., Pásztor, Z., & Tintori, G. (2021). *Loneliness in the EU: Insights from surveys and online media data*. Publications Office of the European Union.

Balaj, M., Eikemo, T., Huijts, T., Haggebø, K., & Bambra, C. (n.d.). ESS Round 11 question module design template. *Module Title: Social inequalities in health and their determinants*. https://www.europeansocialsurvey.org/methodology/ess-methodology/source-questionnaire

Barreto, M., Van Breen, J., Victor, C., Hammond, C., Eccles, A., Richins, M. T., & Qualter, P. (2022). Exploring the nature and variation of the stigma associated with loneliness. *Journal of Social and Personal Relationships, 39*(9), 2658–2679. https://doi.org/10.1177/02654075221087190

Beck, U., & Beck-Gernsheim, E. (2002). *Individualization: Institutionalized individualism and its social and political consequences*. SAGE.

Börsch-Supan, A., Brandt, M., Hunkler, C., Kneip, T., Korbmacher, J., Malter, F., Schaan, B., Stuck, S., & Zuber, S. (2013). Data resource profile: The Survey of Health, Ageing and Retirement in Europe (SHARE). *International Journal of Epidemiology, 42*(4), 992–1001. https://doi.org/10.1093/ije/dyt088

Buetow, S. (2023). *From loneliness to solitude in person-centred health care*. Routledge, Taylor & Francis Group.

Cacioppo, J. T., Fowler, J. H., & Christakis, N. A. (2009). Alone in the crowd: The structure and spread of loneliness in a large social network. *Journal of Personality and Social Psychology, 97*(6), 977–991. https://doi.org/10.1037/a0016076

Cummins, R. A., Lau, A. L. D., & Davern, M. T. (2012). Subjective wellbeing homeostasis. In K. C. Land, M. J. Sirgy, & A. C. Michalos (Eds.), *Handbook of social indicators and quality-of-life research* (pp. 79–98). Springer.

Dahlberg, L., Von Saenger, I., Naseer, M., Lennartsson, C., & Agahi, N. (2024). National trends in loneliness and social isolation in older adults: An examination of subgroup trends over three decades in Sweden. *Frontiers in Public Health, 12*, 1444990. https://doi.org/10.3389/fpubh.2024.1444990

Deresiewicz, W. (2022). *The end of solitude: Selected essays on culture and society* (1st ed.). Henry Holt and Company.

DiTommaso, E., & Spinner, B. (1993). The development and initial validation of the Social and Emotional Loneliness Scale for Adults (SELSA). *Personality and Individual Differences, 14*(1), 127–134. https://doi.org/10.1016/0191-8869(93)90182-3

European Commission. Joint Research Centre. (2024). EU loneliness survey*: Methodological report*. Publications Office. https://data.europa.eu/doi/10.2760/2083329.

European Foundation for the Improvement of Living and Working Conditions. (2021). *Living, working and COVID-19 (Update April 2021): Mental health and trust decline across EU as pandemic enters another year*. Publications Office. https://data.europa.eu/doi/10.2806/76802

Fromm-Reichmann, F. (1959). Loneliness. *Psychiatry, 22*(1), 1–15. https://doi.org/10.1080/00332747.1959.11023153

Furedi, F. (2004). *Therapy culture: Cultivating vulnerability in an uncertain age*. Routledge.

Furedi, F. (2006). *Culture of fear revisited: Risk-taking and the morality of low expectation* (4th ed). Continuum.

Gruber, S., Wagner, M., & Batta, F. (2024). *Scales and multi-item indicators in the Survey of Health, Ageing and Retirement in Europe*. SHARE Berlin Institute.

Hansen, T., & Slagsvold, B. (2016). Late-life loneliness in 11 European countries: Results from the generations and gender survey. *Social Indicators Research, 129*(1), 445–464. https://doi.org/10.1007/s11205-015-1111-6

Hawkley, L. C., Duvoisin, R., Ackva, J., Murdoch, J. C., & Luhmann, M. (2016). *Loneliness in older adults in the USA and Germany: Measurement invariance and validation*. NORC at the University of Chicago.

Herpertz-Dahlmann, B., Dempfle, A., & Eckardt, S. (2022). The youngest are hit hardest: The influence of the COVID-19 pandemic on the hospitalization rate for children, adolescents, and young adults with anorexia nervosa in a large German representative sample. *European Psychiatry, 65*(1), e84. https://doi.org/10.1192/j.eurpsy.2022.2345

Hertz, N. (2020). *The lonely century: Coming together in a world that's pulling apart*. Sceptre.

Hickin, N., Käll, A., Shafran, R., Sutcliffe, S., Manzotti, G., & Langan, D. (2021). The effectiveness of psychological interventions for loneliness: A systematic review and meta-analysis. *Clinical Psychology Review, 88*, 102066. https://doi.org/10.1016/j.cpr.2021.102066

Holt-Lunstad, J., Smith, T. B., Baker, M., Harris, T., & Stephenson, D. (2015). Loneliness and social isolation as risk factors for mortality: A meta-analytic review. *Perspectives on Psychological Science, 10*(2), 227–237. https://doi.org/10.1177/1745691614568352

Hughes, M. E., Waite, L. J., Hawkley, L. C., & Cacioppo, J. T. (2004). A short scale for measuring loneliness in large surveys: Results from two population-based studies. *Research on Aging, 26*(6), 655–672. https://doi.org/10.1177/0164027504268574

de Jong Gierveld, J., & van Tilburg, T. (2006). A 6-item scale for overall, emotional, and social loneliness: Confirmatory tests on survey data. *Research on Aging, 28*(5), 582–598. https://doi.org/10.1177/0164027506289723

de Jong Gierveld, J., van Tilburg, T., & Dykstra, P. A. (2006). Loneliness and social isolation. In A. L. Vangelisti & D. Perlman (Eds.), *The Cambridge handbook of personal relationships* (1st ed., pp. 485–500). Cambridge University Press. https://doi.org/10.1017/9781316417867

de Jong-Gierveld, J., & Kamphuis, F. (1985). The development of a Rasch-type loneliness scale. *Applied Psychological Measurement, 9*(3), 289–299. https://doi.org/10.1177/014662168500900307

Lau, S., & Gruen, G. E. (1992). The social stigma of loneliness: Effect of target Person's and Perceiver's Sex. *Personality and Social Psychology Bulletin, 18*(2), 182–189. https://doi.org/10.1177/0146167292182009

Leatherdale, S. T. (2019). Natural experiment methodology for research: A review of how different methods can support real-world research. *International Journal of Social Research Methodology, 22*(1), 19–35. https://doi.org/10.1080/13645579.2018.1488449

Leoncikas, T. (2018). *European Quality of Life Survey 2016: Technical and fieldwork report. On-line working paper*. European Foundation for the Improvement of Living and Working Conditions (Eurofound). Eurofound reference number: WPEF18016. https://www.eurofound.europa.eu/sites/default/files/wpef18016.pdf

Luhmann, M., & Hawkley, L. C. (2016). Age differences in loneliness from late adolescence to oldest old age. *Developmental Psychology, 52*(6), 943–959. https://doi.org/10.1037/dev0000117

Maes, M., Qualter, P., Lodder, G. M. A., & Mund, M. (2022). How (not) to measure loneliness: A review of the eight most commonly used scales. *International Journal of Environmental Research and Public Health, 19*(17), 10816. https://doi.org/10.3390/ijerph191710816

Mauri, C., Barjakovà, M., & Berlingieri, F. (2024). Measuring loneliness: The European union loneliness survey covering 27 European Countries. In S. V. Schnepf, B. d'Hombres, & C. Mauri (Eds.), *Loneliness in Europe: Determinants, risks and interventions*. Springer Nature Switzerland. https://doi.org/10.1007/978-3-031-66582-0

Meisters, R., Westra, D., Putrik, P., Bosma, H., Ruwaard, D., & Jansen, M. (2021). Does loneliness have a cost? A population-wide study of the association between loneliness and healthcare expenditure. *International Journal of Public Health, 66*, 581286. https://doi.org/10.3389/ijph.2021.581286

Mihalopoulos, C., Le, L. K.-D., Chatterton, M. L., Bucholc, J., Holt-Lunstad, J., Lim, M. H., & Engel, L. (2020). The economic costs of loneliness: A review of cost-of-illness and economic evaluation studies. *Social Psychiatry and Psychiatric Epidemiology, 55*(7), 823–836. https://doi.org/10.1007/s00127-019-01733-7

Mund, M., Freuding, M. M., Möbius, K., Horn, N., & Neyer, F. J. (2020). The stability and change of loneliness across the life span: A meta-analysis of longitudinal studies. *Personality and Social Psychology Review, 24*(1), 24–52. https://doi.org/10.1177/1088868319850738

Mund, M., Maes, M., Drewke, P. M., Gutzeit, A., Jaki, I., & Qualter, P. (2023). Would the real loneliness please stand up? The validity of loneliness scores and the reliability of single-item scores. *Assessment, 30*(4), 1226–1248. https://doi.org/10.1177/10731911221077227

Mund, M., Maurer, L., Schultz, A., & Maes, M. (2024). The measurement of loneliness: An obituary (and how to move on). *Open Science Framework*. https://doi.org/10.31219/osf.io/wa8n6

Pagan, R., & Malo, M. A. (2024). Dynamic analysis of loneliness at older ages in Europe by gender. *Applied Research in Quality of Life, 19*(4), 1601–1630. https://doi.org/10.1007/s11482-024-10300-5

Park, C., Majeed, A., Gill, H., Tamura, J., Ho, R. C., Mansur, R. B., Nasri, F., Lee, Y., Rosenblat, J. D., Wong, E., & McIntyre, R. S. (2020). The effect of loneliness on distinct health outcomes: A comprehensive review and meta-analysis. *Psychiatry Research, 294*, 113514. https://doi.org/10.1016/j.psychres.2020.113514

Peplau, L. A., & Perlman, D. (Eds.). (1982). *Loneliness: A sourcebook of current theory, research, and therapy*. Wiley.

Peterson, D., Rooduijn, M., Hopp, F. R., Schumacher, G., & Bakker, B. N. (2025). Loneliness is positively associated with populist radical right support. *Social Science & Medicine, 117676*. https://doi.org/10.1016/j.socscimed.2025.117676

Pinquart, M., & Sorensen, S. (2001). Influences on loneliness in older adults: A meta-analysis. *Basic and Applied Social Psychology, 23*(4), 245–266. https://doi.org/10.1207/S15324834BASP2304_2

Precupetu, I., Pop, C., & Aartsen, M. (2025). Macro-level influences on loneliness in later life: An fsQCA analysis. In M. Aartsen, I. Precupetu, & B. Suanet (Eds.), *Macro social influences on loneliness in later life: Towards a better understanding of the loneliness paradox in later life*. Springer.

Putnick, D. L., & Bornstein, M. H. (2016). Measurement invariance conventions and reporting: The state of the art and future directions for psychological research. *Developmental Review, 41*, 71–90. https://doi.org/10.1016/j.dr.2016.06.004

Qualter, P., Vanhalst, J., Harris, R., Van Roekel, E., Lodder, G., Bangee, M., Maes, M., & Verhagen, M. (2015). Loneliness across the life span. *Perspectives on Psychological Science, 10*(2), 250–264. https://doi.org/10.1177/1745691615568999

Rapolienė, G., & Aartsen, M. (2022). Lonely societies: Low trust societies? Further explanations for national variations in loneliness among older Europeans. *European Journal of Ageing, 19*(3), 485–494. https://doi.org/10.1007/s10433-021-00649-z

Russell, D. (1982). The measurement of loneliness. In L. A. Peplau & D. Perlman (Eds.), *Loneliness: A sourcebook of current theory, research, and therapy* (p. 71). Wiley.

Russell, D., Peplau, L. A., & Cutrona, C. E. (1980). The revised UCLA Loneliness Scale: Concurrent and discriminant validity evidence. *Journal of Personality and Social Psychology, 39*(3), 472–480. https://doi.org/10.1037/0022-3514.39.3.472

Schoenmakers, E. (2020). Why and how to talk about loneliness. *Journal of Social Intervention: Theory and Practice, 29*(4), 4. https://doi.org/10.18352/jsi.646

Spitzer, M. (2019). *Einsamkeit: Die unerkannte Krankheit* (Vollständige Taschenbuchausgabe). Droemer Taschenbuch.

Stegen, H., Duppen, D., Savieri, P., Stas, L., Pan, H., Aartsen, M., Callewaert, H., Dierckx, E., & De Donder, L. (2024). Loneliness prevalence of community-dwelling older adults and the impact of the mode of measurement, data collection, and country: A systematic review and meta-analysis. *International Psychogeriatrics, 36*(9), 747–761. https://doi.org/10.1017/S1041610224000425

Stein, J. Y., & Tuval-Mashiach, R. (2015). The social construction of loneliness: An integrative conceptualization. *Journal of Constructivist Psychology, 28*(3), 210–227. https://doi.org/10.1080/10720537.2014.911129

Suanet, B., & van Tilburg, T. G. (2019). Loneliness declines across birth cohorts: The impact of mastery and self-efficacy. *Psychology and Aging, 34*(8), 1134–1143. https://doi.org/10.1037/pag0000357

Suanet, B., Drewelies, J., Duezel, S., Eibich, P., Demuth, I., Steinhagen-Thiessen, E., Wagner, G. G., Lindenberger, U., Ram, N., Ghisletta, P., & Gerstorf, D. (2024). Historical change in trajectories of loneliness in old age: Older adults today are less lonely, but do not differ in their age trajectories. *Psychology and Aging, 39*(4), 350–363. https://doi.org/10.1037/pag0000803

Surkalim, D. L., Luo, M., Eres, R., Gebel, K., Van Buskirk, J., Bauman, A., & Ding, D. (2022). The prevalence of loneliness across 113 countries: Systematic review and meta-analysis. *BMJ*, e067068. https://doi.org/10.1136/bmj-2021-067068

Thompson, D. (2025, January 8). The anti-social century. Americans are now spending more time alone than ever. It's changing our personalities, our politics, and even our relationship to reality. *The Atlantic*. https://www.theatlantic.com/magazine/archive/2025/02/

american-loneliness-personality-politics/681091/?gift=4Uv8fRpVF1qRXq8TaWY_R9O2tP_ogf3c0kE3H4-TMuM&utm_source=copy-link&utm_medium=social&utm_campaign=share

Valtorta, N. K., Kanaan, M., Gilbody, S., & Hanratty, B. (2018). Loneliness, social isolation and risk of cardiovascular disease in the English Longitudinal Study of Ageing. *European Journal of Preventive Cardiology, 25*(13), 1387–1396. https://doi.org/10.1177/2047487318792696

van Tilburg, T. G., & Fokkema, T. (2021). Stronger feelings of loneliness among Moroccan and Turkish older adults in the Netherlands: In search for an explanation. *European Journal of Ageing, 18*(3), 311–322. https://doi.org/10.1007/s10433-020-00562-x

Victor, C. R., & Yang, K. (2015). The prevalence of loneliness among adults: A case study of the United Kingdom. In A. Rokach (Ed.), *Loneliness updated: Recent research on loneliness and how it affects our lives* (1. issued in paperback, pp. 88–107). Routledge.

Victor, C., Grenade, L., & Boldy, D. (2005). Measuring loneliness in later life: A comparison of differing measures. *Reviews in Clinical Gerontology, 15*(1), 63–70. https://doi.org/10.1017/S0959259805001723

Von Soest, T., Luhmann, M., & Gerstorf, D. (2020). The development of loneliness through adolescence and young adulthood: Its nature, correlates, and midlife outcomes. *Developmental Psychology, 56*(10), 1919–1934. https://doi.org/10.1037/dev0001102

Walsh, K., Scharf, T., & Keating, N. (2017). Social exclusion of older persons: A scoping review and conceptual framework. *European Journal of Ageing, 14*(1), 81–98. https://doi.org/10.1007/s10433-016-0398-8

Weiss, R. S. (1973). *Loneliness: The experience of emotional and social isolation*. MIT Press.

Yang, K., & Victor, C. (2011). Age and loneliness in 25 European nations. *Ageing and Society, 31*(8), 1368–1388. https://doi.org/10.1017/S0144686X1000139X

Marian Vasile, PhD, is currently associate professor at the Department of Sociology, Faculty of Sociology and Social Work, at the University of Bucharest in Romania and studies how social relationships affect people's quality of life, using a predominantly quantitative research approach. He is a member of the Romanian Group for the Study of Social Values, which implements the European Values Study and World Values Survey projects in Romania. His publications address topics such as subjective well-being, inequality in access to education and the labor market, social values, and the social exclusion of older people.

Marja Aartsen, PhD, is currently research professor and social gerontologist at NOVA—Norwegian Social Research at OsloMet. She is specialized in longitudinal research on social relations, social exclusion, loneliness, and cognitive functioning in the second half of life. She is interested in social issues related to ageing in place and active or successful ageing. Recent research projects and collaborations include gendered pathways to exclusion from social relations (GENPATH), reducing old-age social exclusion (ROSENET) and a multidimensional approach to social exclusion and its health consequences (AMASE). She was editor of the European Journal of Ageing from 2017 until summer 2022.

Open Access This chapter is licensed under the terms of the Creative Commons Attribution 4.0 International License (http://creativecommons.org/licenses/by/4.0/), which permits use, sharing, adaptation, distribution and reproduction in any medium or format, as long as you give appropriate credit to the original author(s) and the source, provide a link to the Creative Commons license and indicate if changes were made.

The images or other third party material in this chapter are included in the chapter's Creative Commons license, unless indicated otherwise in a credit line to the material. If material is not included in the chapter's Creative Commons license and your intended use is not permitted by statutory regulation or exceeds the permitted use, you will need to obtain permission directly from the copyright holder.

Chapter 6
Understanding Late-Life Loneliness: Micro and Meso-Level Determinants

Sunwoo Lee

6.1 Introduction

Loneliness is a mundane experience. However, in older age, it is closely associated with various ageing adversities and challenges. Over decades, extensive research has documented its prevalence and consequences, advancing our understanding of loneliness in older adults. These efforts are based on multiple theoretical frameworks, each emphasizing different aspects, including cognitive process/disparities, social relationships, and broader sociocultural relevance (e.g., Akhter-Khan et al., 2022; Heu et al., 2021; Perlman & Peplau, 1981; Rapolienė & Aartsen, 2022; Weiss, 1973; Wenger, 1996). However, the complex interplay of factors that shape loneliness remains unresolved. Given that multiple factors in different contexts contribute to older adults' loneliness as a more unique personal experience, this chapter aims to provide a nuanced perspective by examining both micro- and meso-level determinants.

To frame this discussion, two existing models are particularly relevant. Lim et al. (2020) proposed a conceptual model of loneliness that categorized risk factors into three domains: *demographic, health-related*, and *socio-environmental*. In this framework, they identified a separate domain, termed *triggers*, which refers to either a significant life event or life-stage transition that precedes and initiates the development of loneliness in an individual. Their model underscores the reciprocal relationships among these factors, highlighting how loneliness itself can be both a consequence and a mutually reinforcing risk factor. Burholt et al. (2019) developed a conceptual model of exclusion from social relations for older adults, emphasizing the necessity to integrate the human ecological approach into understanding how loneliness emerges and is experienced. This model identifies varying individual risk

S. Lee (✉)
Faculty of Physical Culture, Palacký University Olomouc, Olomouc, Czech Republic
e-mail: sunwoo.lee@upol.cz

© The Author(s) 2025

M. Aartsen et al. (eds.), *Macro Social Influences on Loneliness in Later Life*, International Perspectives on Aging 47,
https://doi.org/10.1007/978-3-031-94565-6_6

factors (e.g., socio-demographics, bio-neurological, retirement, and migration) and articulates how these factors influence an individual's evaluation of social relationships (fulfilled or unmet social needs) and social-emotional processes, resulting in different outcomes, including loneliness. Burholt et al. (2019) also highlighted that the integration of individual risk factors into social relationships and processes is greatly informed by socio-cultural, structural, and environmental contexts such as norms, values, and policy.

Building on the two frameworks and in conjunction with recent review studies, the most prevalent factors for which sufficient evidence was available were selected for inclusion. Figure 6.1 maps the most relevant factors for loneliness in older age, which are examined further in this chapter. At the micro level, it examines the role of individual characteristics and experiences, including demographics, socioeconomic status, living arrangements, health status, and psychological attributes, such as personality traits that influence how an individual processes and responds to loneliness. Micro-level factors also extend to interpersonal factors such as marital trajectories and social networks. Given the subjective nature of loneliness, involving individual awareness or cognitive process, this chapter classifies social networks and relationships as personal-level experience and thus defines it under micro-level factors. At the meso level, the focus shifts to community dynamics such as neighbourhood social cohesion and physical disorders, and the urban versus rural context. Importantly, there may be a complex relationship between factors across the micro- and meso-levels. However, these relationships are not explicitly presented in the framework for reasons of parsimony.

While there are factors frequently addressed in the literature that have a strong association with loneliness, the current body of research has yet to reach a definitive consensus on the risk factors and antecedents of loneliness. Therefore, rather than attempting to establish conclusive determinants, this chapter focuses on their varying roles contingent upon the context. Furthermore, to better understand the

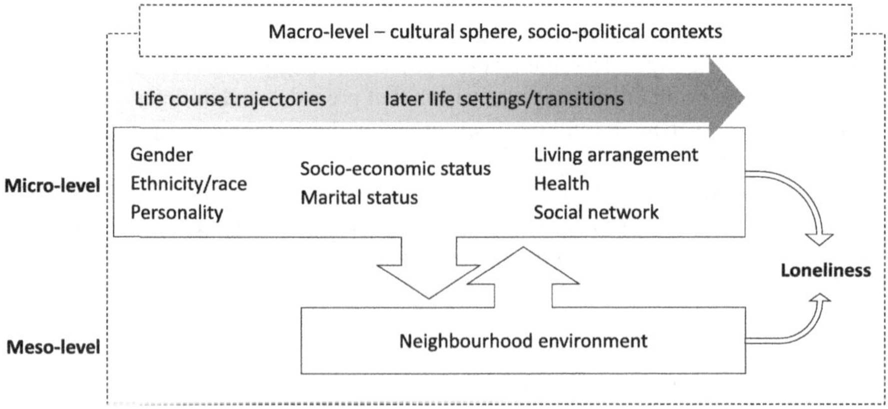

Fig. 6.1 A working framework of antecedents of loneliness in older age; adopted and modified based two conceptual models (Burholt et al., 2019; Lim et al., 2020)

influence of each factor and bridge individual experiences with broader community and environmental dynamics, the chapter integrates theoretical perspectives from multiple disciplines, such as social networks typologies and cognitive discrepancy theory, which are addressed where relevant.

6.2 Micro-level Factors

Research consistently identifies old age, female gender, widowhood, living alone, low socioeconomic status, lack of social networks and support, poor self-reported health, and depression as risk factors for loneliness. Review studies, even those published two decades apart, continue to support these findings (see Cohen-Mansfield et al., 2016; Dahlberg et al., 2022; Hajek et al., 2023b; Pinquart & Sorensen, 2001). However, more recent reviews (e.g., Barjaková et al., 2023; Susanty et al., 2024) point to inconsistencies in empirical studies, suggesting that the significance of these factors and the pathways to loneliness may vary depending on contextual differences. The chapter elaborates on each factor as follows.

6.2.1 Older Age

Loneliness tends to increase with age, suggesting that the oldest old are at greater risk for loneliness (Cohen-Mansfield et al., 2016; Dykstra et al., 2005; Fierloos et al., 2021; Niedzwiedz et al., 2016; Pagan & Malo, 2024; Vozikaki et al., 2018; Yang & Victor, 2011). A recent meta-analysis by Susanty et al. (2024) found that the prevalence of loneliness varies significantly across different age groups of older adults, showing an increasing trend with age: 21% for those aged 60–74 years, 34% for those aged 75–84, and 42% for those aged 85 and older. Sundström et al., (2009) showed that in Sweden, older adults aged 81 and over were nearly three times more likely to report loneliness than those aged 65–70 years. According to Dykstra et al. (2005), loneliness among Dutch adults aged 55 and older generally grew over a seven-year period, with the increase being more pronounced among the oldest participants; of the study respondents, 10.5%, 18%, and 17.3% experienced an increase at three respective follow-up points.

However, the relationship between age and loneliness becomes rather complicated when including younger age groups. According to Barreto et al. (2021), loneliness tends to decrease with age among a study sample that ranged from 16 to 99 years. In contrast, Nicolaisen and Thorsen (2014), using a sample aged 18 to 81 years, found that loneliness tends to increase across age groups (18–29, 30–49, 50–64, and 65–81), with prevalence rates of 21.2%, 22.3%, 23.8%, 30.2%, respectively. The percentage of individuals reporting the maximum score on loneliness (often feeling lonely) also increased across these age groups, indicating rates of 2.1%, 2.2%, 3.2% and 3.7%, respectively. When examining the frequency of loneliness (feeling lonely sometimes or often), however, the pattern showed an uneven U-shape: the prevalence was high in the 18–29 group (22.9%), lowest in the 30–49 group (18.7%), and then increased with age, reaching 20.0% for those aged 50–64, and 25.6% for those aged 65–81. Barjaková et al. (2023) suggested a U-shaped relationship between age and loneliness, with loneliness being higher in younger and older age groups. Similarly, Pinquart and Sorensen (2001) found that among three subgroups of older adults, loneliness tended to increase with age in the oldest subgroup (mean age > 80 years), while it rather tended to decrease with age in the youngest subgroup (mean age ≤ 60 years). No significant relationship was observed in the subgroup with a mean age between 60 and 80 years, resulting in a U-shaped pattern. In addition, a few studies have noted that loneliness remains relatively stable across the lifespan (Barjaková et al., 2023; Mund et al., 2020). According to Dykstra et al. (2005), in their seven-year longitudinal observations, many older adults did not necessarily experience increased loneliness (70%); some even reported a decrease in loneliness.

These findings suggest that the use of chronological age as a predictive variable can obscure significant variations or true trajectories of loneliness across the life course. Rughiniș and Humă (2015) posit that the oversimplification of socio-demographic variables, including age, in quantitative survey research should be reconsidered, notwithstanding its benefits for inferential power. Moreover, the common practice of categorizing older adults into broad age groups, such as 50+ or 60+ years, risks overlooking substantive distinctions within this population. Additionally, varying definitions of old age or older adulthood across different cultural contexts further complicates cross-cultural comparisons. As the majority of existing evidence is derived from cross-sectional studies that compare different age cohorts, longitudinal observations that follow the same age cohorts over time would provide a more precise estimation of the role of age and ageing in loneliness.

6.2.2 Gender

Older women tend to report higher levels of loneliness compared to their male counterparts (e.g., Carrasco et al., 2024; Domenech-Abella et al., 2020; Nicolaisen & Thorsen, 2024; Pagan & Malo, 2024). According to Pagan and Malo (2024), over a six-year follow-up period using data from the Survey of Health, Ageing, and Retirement in Europe (waves 4, 5, and 6), 68% of men reported *never feeling lonely*, compared to 56% of women. Additionally, women were more likely to report *always feeling lonely* (9%) than men (5%). However, some studies report no evidence of this relationship across different European countries (e.g., Fierloos et al., 2021; Lee, 2020; Myck et al., 2021; Tapia-Muñoz et al., 2022; van den Broek et al., 2024). While previous review studies have provided evidence for gender disparities in loneliness (see Cohen-Mansfield et al., 2016; Pinquart & Sorensen, 2001), more recent reviews, particularly those focusing on multivariate analyses and longitudinal observations, rarely support this hypothesis (Barjaková et al., 2023; Dahlberg et al., 2022), pointing out that the significant association between gender and loneliness is largely found in cross-sectional and bivariate analyses.

Gender differences in loneliness can be attributed to varying levels of emotional expressiveness among men and women. Compared to men, women are more prone to articulate and share their feelings, whereas men are socialized to suppress emotional expressions (Girgus et al., 2017; Thomsen et al., 2005). Jutengren and Ståhl (2024) showed that men are significantly less likely to manifest both positive and negative emotions. If men are more inclined to repress or underreport their feelings of loneliness, this gender stereotype may contribute to the observed gender gap in the loneliness measures. Unbalanced socio-demographic structures in the ageing population may also have contributed to the observed disparity. Given their longer life expectancy, women are more likely to experience widowhood and spend a longer portion of their later years living alone (Beal, 2006; Aartsen & Jylhä, 2011; Niino et al., 2025). Thus, when comparing loneliness between older men and women, gender differences may be influenced not only by gender itself, but also partially by the higher prevalence of widowhood or living alone among older women. Additionally, women's greater emotional expressivity may render them more susceptible to loneliness during life transitions, such as empty nest syndrome or bereavement.

Barjaková et al. (2023) noted that inconsistent findings on gender differences in loneliness are largely due to variations in how loneliness is measured—the use of single-item questions, frequency or intensity measures, and distinctions between emotional and social loneliness. According to Nicolaisen and Thorsen (2014), when using a direct measure (i.e., "Do you feel lonely?"), loneliness was more prevalent among women across all age groups (18–29, 30–49, 50–64 and 65–81). However, when using De Jong Gierveld Scale, which indirectly assesses loneliness through two forms—social and emotional, the prevalence of loneliness differed between men and women and across different age groups. The study added that men experience greater social loneliness, while women are more prone to emotional loneliness, particularly in the older age groups (50–64 and 65–81). Similarly, Fierloos et al. (2021) revealed that, among those older adults living with a partner, women were more likely to experience emotional loneliness than men. Another study (Jutengren & Ståhl, 2024) reported that older Swedish men were more likely to score high on social loneliness compared to their female peers. In addition, Dahlberg et al. (2015) suggested that the main predictors of loneliness differ for women and men in Sweden; for women, factors such as widowhood, depression, and reduced mobility were distinct, while for men, decreased or low levels of social contact appeared to be more relevant. Hajek and König (2021) revealed that, in older German women, the onset of obesity was significantly related to loneliness, while in men, the opposite effect was observed. These findings suggest that men and women can be equally vulnerable to loneliness, but the semantic meaning of loneliness, as well as how they experience and express it, may differ.

Gendered loneliness requires a more culturally nuanced framework. According to Sundström et al. (2009), women are significantly more likely to experience loneliness than men in countries including Spain, France, and Greece, while in other countries, there was no significant association between gender and loneliness. Pagan and Malo (2024) showed that the status and severity of disability are significantly related to the loneliness persistence, especially among women aged 50 years or older in Europe. They further noted that its negative impact on loneliness was more evident among women in Mediterranean and Eastern European countries than those in Northern countries. These findings suggest that older women, especially those living in countries with higher gender inequality, where opportunities to develop personal resources (e.g., education) are limited, can be more vulnerable to loneliness. However, the relationship between gender equality and loneliness is not straightforward. For instance, Sheftel et al. (2024) revealed that, while there was no significant relationship between female gender and chronic loneliness in counties where the gender gap is relatively small, such as Germany, Spain, England, Denmark, the Netherlands, and Poland (with gender equality index rankings of 7, 10, 14, 15, 28, and 51, respectively; World Economic Forum, 2024), in some European countries such as Switzerland, Austria, and Czech Republic (with varied gender equality rankings of 20, 49, and 104, respectively), female gender increased the likelihood of chronic loneliness. Shifting gender norms and coping strategies that evolve over time may influence how women perceive and experience loneliness, further making it challenging to discern consistent patterns in their experiences. Therefore, gendered pathways to loneliness should be examined in relation to the social and cultural contexts in which individuals have lived, together with their specific personal contexts, considering how gendered practices are integrated throughout life.

6.2.3 Living Alone

According to Eurostat (2024), in 2023, approximately 32% of individuals aged 65 and older in Europe live alone, with this percentage varying across different countries, ranging from 11% in Slovakia to 54% in Estonia. Notably, 70% of the individuals in this demographic are women (ranged 62% in Ireland to 78% in Latvia), highlighting a significant gender disparity (source: Eurostat; data code: lfst_hhindws).

Additionally, there has been an increase in the number of men aged 55–64 years who live alone, compared to that of women living alone (European Commission, Eurostat, 2020). Recent literature highlights the growing demographic of *elder orphans*—older adults who live alone (single household), are socially and/or physically isolated, and lack family caregivers (Carney et al., 2016; Kervin et al., 2022; Roofeh et al., 2020). Carney et al. (2016) emphasized the need for advocacy, awareness, and proactive strategies to improve healthcare and support systems to adequately address the unique challenges faced by this vulnerable group. While explicit statistics for Europe are unavailable, according to Roofeh et al. (2020), for example, in the United States, 2.6% of older adults qualify as elder orphans, with 21.3% at risk of becoming one. Despite ongoing debates regarding the term, elder orphan, which lacks consensus among various stakeholders, including older adults themselves (Kervin et al., 2022), this reminds us of the urgent need for preparations in Europe, particularly in countries where existing social structures and policy frameworks may be insufficient to support the growing number of older adults in this category.

According to Jutengren and Ståhl (2024), living alone is strongly associated with social loneliness that is absence of a sense of belonging and involuntary disconnection from one's social network. Similarly, de Jong Gierveld et al. (2012) found that older adults living alone are most lonely compared to older adults living with a partner or those (either single or partnered) living with one or more children. Routasalo et al. (2006) showed that older Finns aged 75 and older who live alone are about three times more likely to report frequent loneliness (feeling lonely sometimes, often, or always) compared to their counterpart who do not live alone. According to Barbosa et al. (2019), while living alone was not directly related to health, older adults living alone are more likely to experience declines in physical and mental health due to developing loneliness. Living alone—maintaining a single-person household—is often closely linked to marital trajectories, such as never having married, being widowed, or divorced/separated, all of which are considered risk factors for loneliness. This suggests that, beyond the absence of social support and informal care within the household, living alone may also reflect a person's experience of negative life transitions.

Furthermore, Sheftel et al. (2024) found that, with the degree of risk varying by country, living alone in older age is significantly associated with a higher likelihood of chronic loneliness; the negative impact of living alone was most pronounced in Switzerland, Denmark, Greece, and France, the risk is less severe but still present in Poland, Belgium, and Italy, while no relationship observed in Austria, Czech Republic, Israel, and the Netherlands. Although the study did not extend to examine commonalities among these country clusters, the findings suggest that cultural (age stereotype), structural and broader social policy-related factors (e.g., pension systems, social services) may significantly contribute to older adults' ability to live independently and maintain a sense of wellbeing, thus preventing them from translating living alone into loneliness.

In this respect, two additional considerations are worth discussing. First, we are cautious about labelling solo-living older adults as inherently vulnerable or at greater risk of loneliness. Klinenberg (2016) pointed out that living alone, social isolation, and loneliness may be correlated, but they are distinctive; living alone does not necessarily imply social isolation or feeling lonely. Living alone, when voluntarily chosen or well-adapted to, can empower various aspects of older adults' lives, allowing them to maintain independence, pursue individual interests, and engage in selective social interactions (Djundeva et al., 2019; Lee, 2022; Mair, 2019; Versey & Gibbons, 2024). If they are adequately equipped with protective factors, such as good health, sufficient household income, or strong social networks outside the home (e.g., friends or neighbours), living alone itself does not necessarily lead to social isolation and loneliness.

On the other hand, if living alone is considered a risk factor for loneliness, this raises the question of whether living with others or a larger household size protects older adults from loneliness. However, household size is not always linearly or inversely associated with loneliness. According to Lee (2020), the relationship between household size and loneliness follows a U-shaped pattern in which loneliness tends to decrease when living with two to four people, but then increases again in larger households. This suggests that living with others can reduce satisfaction with housing conditions and increase family responsibilities, potentially leading to social distress rather than satisfaction. Therefore, when examining the relationship between living alone and loneliness, it is crucial to consider the access to and availability of compensatory factors that support older adults in maintaining social well-being regardless of their living arrangements.

6.2.4 Socioeconomic Status (SES)

Literature indicates that low socioeconomic status (SES) is strongly related to higher levels of loneliness among older adults (Cohen-Mansfield et al., 2016; Hansen & Slagsvold, 2016; Myck et al., 2021; Vozikaki et al., 2018; Wang et al., 2024). Older adults with low SES are more likely to cope with material deprivation, unstable income, housing insecurity, poor living environments, and limited access to health and social services, which further compounds their isolation. Consequently, these individuals are more vulnerable to loneliness.

Hansen et al. (2021) found that financial adversities are significantly related to lower levels of social participation and higher levels of loneliness among European adults aged 60 and older. Similarly, Niedzwiedz et al. (2016) reported that older adults in the least wealthy group experienced the highest levels of loneliness, with a significant increase in risk for men when formal social activities were absent. So, structured social engagement may help buffer the negative impact of economic disadvantages on loneliness. However, older adults' ability to participate in social and community activities is also greatly influenced by their socioeconomic status; thus, material deprivation makes them more vulnerable to social isolation and loneliness, limiting social opportunities. Furthermore, Routasalo et al. (2006) reported that poverty (low income) is more prevalent among *lonely* older adults aged 75 years and over in Finland (8% of lonely individuals vs. 1.7% of the non-lonely group). According to Sheftel et al. (2024), among older adults aged 50 and over, those who were unemployed over the course of the observation period were more likely to experience chronic loneliness (Belgium, Denmark, England, France, and Spain). Employment not only provides material support but also fosters social identity, opportunities for social interaction, and a sense of purpose—resources that serve to prevent loneliness in old age.

Beyond individual disparities in socioeconomic status, income inequality across countries plays a significant role in shaping loneliness. The meta-analysis by Susanty et al. (2024) reveals a clear gradient pattern in loneliness prevalence, indicating that higher rates of loneliness were observed in lower-income countries (46%), followed by 39% in lower-middle-income countries, 33% in upper-middle-income countries, and 23% in high-income countries. Tapia-Muñoz et al. (2022) showed that older adults in countries with higher income inequality, such as Israel, Spain, and Italy, tend to experience higher levels of loneliness. In contrast, Nordic countries like Sweden and Denmark, and the Netherlands, which are generally categorized as having the least income inequality, report a lower prevalence of loneliness among older populations. High inequality driven by structural challenges such as weaker social welfare systems, greater economic insecurity, and limited access to mental health and social support services, can contribute to a sense of relative deprivation, which negatively affects social integration, community trust, and overall well-being. In this way, income inequality creates pathways that exacerbate loneliness, particularly in societies where people perceive and experience large gaps in wealth and opportunity.

A systematic review by Dahlberg et al. (2022) noted that while low income and financial difficulties, and low social status increased the risk of loneliness in older adults, the evidence for the education is weak. However, educational attainment often correlates with employment and financial security in adulthood that can help prevent material deprivation in later life. Furthermore, education helps older adults better maintain cognitive function, self-esteem and efficacy, equipping them with the skills and knowledge needed to access information and services (Balki et al., 2023; Bishop & Martin, 2007). According to Bishop and Martin (2007), although unmarried older adults might be disadvantaged due to a lack of partner support in coping with ageing adversities, those with higher education tend to engage more in social and community activities, build support networks, and access helpful resources, thereby mitigating the emotional challenges of loneliness. This highlights the role of education in enhancing protective factors against loneliness in later life.

Some studies indicate that higher educational attainment may benefit older women more (Fernández-Carro & Gumà Lao, 2022; Niedzwiedz et al., 2016). Niedzwiedz et al. (2016), for instance, showed that women with medium level education were 21% less likely, and those with high education were 16% less likely, to experience loneliness compared to women with low education. For men, although medium education was significantly associated with reduced loneliness, the impact was meagre, with only a 3% lower likelihood of loneliness compared to men with low education. Fernández-Carro and Gumà Lao (2022) pointed out that while family trajectories (e.g., having a partner or children) tend to have a stronger and more persistent impact on loneliness in older women, education attainment can provide women with opportunities to build social networks beyond traditional family roles (e.g., through careers or community involvement), thereby reducing their risk of loneliness. These findings suggest that the relationship between education and loneliness may be less straightforward, with higher educational attainment potentially acting as a buffer against other factors that more directly impact loneliness.

Hajek et al. (2024a, b) provide further insights into the role of education. Among older adults aged 80 years and above in Germany, low education was significantly associated with higher levels of loneliness, but this association was significant only in men (Hajek et al., 2024a). Interestingly, however, when examining specifically the sample of institutionalized older adults, higher education was significantly associated with greater loneliness (Hajek et al., 2024b). Due to more structured routines and confined physical spaces, institutionalization may diminish older adults' sense of autonomy and capacity to select social interactions compared with community living. Consequently, even for highly educated individuals, loneliness can become a challenge if psychological and behavioural adaptations are insufficient during major life transitions and when lifestyle changes are unavoidable.

6.2.5 Minority Status: Migration and Race/Ethnicity

In addition to common ageing adversities, older ethnic minorities and/or those with immigrant backgrounds encounter unique challenges, including migration-related stressors, language barriers, and experiences of discrimination or racism based on ethnicity or migrant status (Djundeva & Ellwardt, 2020; Fokkema, 2023; Joshi et al., 2024; Ruan & Cheung, 2024). Moreover, their minority status often results in limited opportunities for social and civic participation, which, in turn, exacerbates social isolation and loneliness. Furthermore, differences in cultural norms regarding ageing and formal or informal social support can influence the experience of loneliness for those ageing in a foreign country. For instance, for older adults who immigrated, with background cultures that place a strong emphasis on family support, the absence of such support in the host country can significantly heighten feelings of loneliness.

De Witte and Van Regenmortel (2022) showed that older immigrants in Belgium, whether first or second-generation, experience higher levels of loneliness than their native counterparts, and poor health status accelerates this disparity. Similarly, van Tilburg and Fokkema (2021) reported a higher prevalence of loneliness among older migrants—Moroccans and Turks living in urban areas in the Netherlands—compared to their Dutch counterparts, which is attributed to their relatively low socioeconomic status, belonging to a minority, and fewer opportunities for social participation in a foreign (host) country. The study further identified some protective factors, such as marriage, contact with children, and better health, although these factors played out differently between Moroccan and Turkish older migrants. This suggests that, while developing loneliness as a migrant and cultural minority, the way immigrants experience loneliness varies based on their unique cultural backgrounds. According to Dolberg et al. (2016), former Soviet Union (FSU) immigrants in Israel were disadvantaged across various life aspects—income, access to healthcare, education—and initially were lonelier than veteran Israelis. However, over time, FSU immigrants developed psychological adaptation and strong community support among FSU immigrants, which helped diminish loneliness. Cotterell et al. (2025) highlight the structural disadvantages older adults from ethnic minority backgrounds endure over the life course including living in neighbourhoods lacking in community resources or those with prevalent racial discrimination, and how its accumulated disadvantages exacerbate social exclusion and loneliness in later life; for them, ageing in place feel like being at home yet not truly belonging. Collectively, these studies underscore the importance of addressing both health and social support systems to alleviate loneliness among ageing ethnic minority and immigrant populations.

While this chapter considers migration status and race/ethnicity as individual demographic factors, it is also valuable to examine the relationship between migration or minority status and loneliness from the perspectives of multiple stakeholders. On the one hand, EU policies promoting mobility, along with conflicts, such as Russia's invasion of Ukraine, have accelerated migration flows, particularly in advanced Western European countries. As a result, an increasing number of older adults are ageing in foreign countries, navigating challenges associated with minority status. On the other hand, migration significantly reshapes the demographic structure of host countries, influencing policies and societal responses that impact both older immigrant and non-immigrant populations. Cohen-Mansfield et al. (2016) found that older Israeli adults perceived a decline in neighbourhood quality due to high levels of migration in their local communities. This led to increased feelings of isolation, driven by concerns such as neighbourhood deterioration, fear of crime, lack of social trust, and limited resources for socializing, thereby contributing to loneliness. Moreover, the high prevalence of migration from Eastern and Central European countries to Western European countries has broader societal implications. In Eastern and Central Europe, older adults, particularly those left behind by migrating children, often face a lack of informal social support in later life. This, combined with higher levels of socio-economic disadvantage compared to Western or Nordic regions, places them at a greater risk of loneliness. These aspects remain significantly underexplored in the current body of literature. Joshi et al. (2024) point to this gap, including the underrepresentation of non-Western contexts and the limited use of qualitative methodologies in existing studies. Therefore, understanding late-life loneliness in relation to migration requires a comprehensive perspective that considers the experiences of both migrants and non-migrants, as well as the role of social policies and broader structural factors.

6.2.6 Health Status

Poor health status, particularly physical and cognitive decline, is one of the most significant triggers for thc onsct of or chronic loneliness. According to Guthmuller (2022), health factors—having more than one chronic disease, activity limitations, and depression—were the strongest predictors of loneliness among older Europeans, surpassing the effects of social support and socio-demographic variables. The literature highlights various health conditions linked to loneliness, including poor self-rated health (e.g., Jutengren & Ståhl, 2024; Nyqvist et al., 2023; Yang, 2018), chronic illness and multimorbidity (e.g., Burholt & Scharf, 2014; Sheftel et al.,

2024; Stickley & Koyanagi, 2018), functional limitations and disability (e.g., Dahlberg et al., 2015; Dykstra et al., 2005; Pagan & Malo, 2024; Ye et al., 2024), pain (e.g., Loeffler & Steptoe, 2021), obesity and sedentary life style (e.g., Hajek & König, 2021; Hajek et al., 2021), cognitive impairments (e.g., Hajek & König, 2020; Susanty et al., 2024), and depression (Aartsen & Jylhä, 2011; Carrasco et al. 2024; Schmitz, 2021; Tapia-Muñoz et al., 2022). A recent meta-analysis (Susanty et al., 2024) provided a more comprehensive overview of the role of health status in predicting loneliness prevalence, indicating that cognitive impairment, poor self-rated health, depression, and frailty are significantly associated with increased odds of loneliness. Specifically, these factors increase the likelihood of loneliness, nearly threefold (cognitive impairment), more than double the odds (poor health and frailty), and by 74% for depression, with cognitive impairment appearing to have particularly strong effects. Except for institutionalization, which may be closely linked to functional disabilities resulting from health decline, the impact of health factors was generally higher than that of other variables, such as sex, marital status, and place of residence.

Studies explain the relationship between poor health and loneliness by revealing that declined health significantly impedes participation in social activities and diminishes social resources, thereby exacerbating loneliness (Burholt & Scharf, 2014; Loeffler & Steptoe, 2021; Pagan & Malo, 2024; Ye et al., 2024). Loeffler and Steptoe (2021) showed that declining health increases dependency on medical and social care, which leads to psychological distress, negatively impacting social competence and self-efficacy, further contributing to social withdrawal. Ye et al. (2024) identified a longitudinal association between physical frailty (e.g., difficulties in walking, hand strength, hearing impairments) and social frailty (i.e., living alone, lack of social relationships, and lack of social support) among older adults in the UK, Greece, Croatia, the Netherlands, and Spain. Stickley and Koyanagi (2018) reported that multimorbidity significantly increased the odds of loneliness among English older adults by 78% for those with four diseases and 94% for those with five or more, suggesting that multimorbidity not only poses a physical health burden but also leads to emotional and psychological challenges. Additionally, Aartsen and Jylhä (2011) found that among older Finns aged 60 and above who did not report loneliness at baseline, one third developed loneliness over a 28-year follow-up period. Those experiencing increased low mood or depression, feelings of uselessness, and tensions or nervousness were four times, 3.5 times, and nearly twice as likely to experience loneliness at follow-ups, respectively.

However, the relationship between health and loneliness is hardly clear-cut as these two aspects are mutually reinforcing. Studies often report reverse pathways, where chronic loneliness can serve as a risk factor for declining health, increase risky health behaviours (e.g., smoking, drinking), and contribute to the onset of depression and cognitive impairments (see Boss et al., 2015; Ong et al., 2015). The theory of social networks and health highlights the important role of social integration in maintaining physical health and psychological well-being (Berkman, 1995; Berkman & Glass, 2000). In other words, individuals with limited social networks and weak social ties, whether with family, friends, or their broader community, face an increased risk of chronic loneliness, which in turn heightens their vulnerability to mental health issues and physical decline over time. This suggests that older adults who are socially anchored, engage in various social activities, and receive positive social support are better equipped to cope with adversities, including loneliness, thereby preserving their overall health. These findings emphasize the need to integrate loneliness interventions with other health initiatives to disrupt this vicious cycle.

6.2.7 Personality

Studies suggest that personality traits may influence the likelihood of experiencing loneliness, as they affect an individual's social behaviour and interpretation of social experiences. Tapia-Munoz et al. (2024) found that all Big Five personality traits—extroversion, agreeableness, conscientiousness, openness (negatively), and neuroticism (positively)—were associated with baseline loneliness. Over an eight-year follow-up period, extroversion was significantly related to decline in loneliness after controlling for sociodemographic and economic factors, social isolation, health variables, depression, and the genetic risk factors for loneliness. Schutter et al. (2020) observed that lower agreeableness was significantly linked to loneliness among institutionalized older adults in the Netherlands, irrespective of gender, and women with lower extraversion and higher neuroticism were more prone to loneliness. Similarly, Guthmuller (2022) showed that the more extraverted individuals become, the less likely they are to experience loneliness: every 0.5-point increase in extraversion score was associated with a 25% reduction in loneliness, whereas individuals with higher neurotic tendencies were 20% more likely to feel lonely compared to those with lower levels of neuroticism. Guthmuller further noted that personality traits were stronger predictors of loneliness than demographic and socioeconomic factors among older Europeans. Extraversion—characterized by greater sociability, active social engagement, and diverse networks—may contribute to decreasing loneliness. In contrast, high neuroticism increases vulnerability to loneliness due to sensitivity to negative emotions and insecure attachment styles, which can often lead to strained social relationships, social withdrawal, and smaller social networks (Buecker et al., 2020). This suggests that neuroticism is a key risk factor for loneliness, emphasizing the importance of emotional regulation and social coping mechanisms, particularly as individuals age.

6.2.8 Marital Status

Marriage is one of the most important life transitions as it leads to the extension of the social networks including spouse and (grand) children, that serve as an important resource for social support in older age.

Most prior studies reinforce that older adults with non-married status including those who experience negative transitions such as separation, divorce, or widowhood or those who never married (remained as single in later life) are at greater risk for loneliness (e.g., Fokkema et al., 2012; Niino et al., 2025; Susanty et al., 2024; Tapia-Munoz et al., 2024). For instance, Arpino et al. (2022) showed that that older adults who were 'not-partnered, but having child' or 'partnered, but childless' were at greater risk of loneliness before the COVID-19 pandemic; however, during the pandemic, those 'not-partnered childless' reported the highest levels of loneliness, experiencing some transitioning from not lonely (before pandemic) to lonely (during/since pandemic). Similarly, according to Fernández-Carro and Gumà Lao (2022), women who followed traditional family paths (marriage and having children) are less lonely in old age, while older women who remained single and childless typically experience greater loneliness. Van Tilburg et al. (2015) reported that both divorcees and remarried divorcees were more likely to score high on social loneliness compared to their counterparts who were still in their first marriage.

Widowhood or bereavement has the most profound impact on the onset or worsening of loneliness in older adults across European countries. This includes Germany (Hajek et al., 2024a), Czech Republic (Štípková, 2021), the Netherlands (Dykstra et al., 2005), and Nordic regions (Aartsen & Jylhä, 2011; Dahlberg et al., 2015; Nyqvist et al., 2023). Widowhood represents the end of a long-term relationship due to death, which can result in grief and a significant disruption to one's social network. Susanty et al. (2024) showed that widowed individuals were 67% more likely to report loneliness and single individuals had a 51% increased risk. According to Fawaz and Mira (2019), older adults who had lost a spouse or close confidant reported significantly lower satisfaction with their social networks, and significantly increased loneliness and depression. Similarly, Myck et al. (2021) reported that the loss of partner led to a significant increase in loneliness, from mild to severe. Schmitz (2021) highlighted that loneliness significantly mediate the relationship between widowhood and depression, while being married appeared to offer protective benefits, reducing the likelihood of loneliness by nearly half. These findings emphasize the important role of marital status in affecting social and emotional well-being, with those lacking a close partner in old age being more vulnerable to loneliness.

However, studies suggest that the negative impact of marital transition on loneliness does not necessarily last, and it can be mitigated through psychosocial adaptation over time. A recent review (Niino et al., 2025) showed varying trajectories of loneliness after the death of a spouse, with some studies reporting linear increases, others showing decreases, and some indicating curvilinear trends. The study noted that the adverse effects of widowhood on loneliness can be attenuated by factors such as volunteering, military histories, higher income, and age. Van Tilburg et al. (2015) pointed to shifting societal attitudes towards divorce over recent decades, increased social acceptance of diverse family structures, and improved legal support, thus younger cohorts are less likely to be negatively affected by divorce compared to older cohorts. Štípková (2021) also posits that although divorce leads to social isolation and loneliness, this life transition may contribute to mitigating loneliness associated with marital strains and provide opportunities to rebuild social ties or remarry.

Importantly, whilst being married and living with a spouse or partner function as protective factors against late-life loneliness, extant marital strains, low marital satisfaction, household dysfunction related to late-life poverty, and lack of emotional support from a spouse can significantly increase older adults' vulnerability to loneliness. For instance, older caregivers providing intensive care to their spouses are particularly prone to experiencing increased physical burdens and emotional distress, including loneliness (Wagner & Brandt, 2015, 2018). Van Tilburg et al. (2015) found that among older Dutch adults, those who reported receiving emotional and instrumental support from their partner had an 8% probability of experiencing the highest levels of emotional and social loneliness, while for those without partnership support, the chance of scoring highest on loneliness jumps to 13%. Hansen et al. (2021) showed that older adults (both men and women) who *often* perceived constraints due to high family responsibilities were significantly more likely to experience loneliness; for women, *occasional* feelings of constraints were also linked to loneliness. These findings align with the cognitive discrepancy theory in explaining loneliness (e.g., Burholt et al., 2017; Perlman & Peplau, 1981), suggesting that loneliness arises when individuals experience psychological distress due to a perceived disparity or an unmet need for emotional or practical support in social relationships.

6.2.9 Social Networks and Support

Individuals develop various forms of social relationships throughout their lives, each shaping different levels of engagement, expectations, and experiences. Older adults may exhibit varying capabilities to maintain and redefine social roles, needs, and activities within their familial and community contexts. Wenger's seminal studies on social network typology (1996, 1997) identified five forms of informal social support systems based on local relationships, family, friends, neighbours, and community group engagement). These typologies, labelled 'locally integrated', 'community-focused', 'local self-contained', 'private-restricted', and 'friend- and family dependent', are distinguished by their accessibility to family, frequency of interactions, and community engagement. Indicating that each typology has its own benefits and limitations, Wenger noted that older adults within a private restricted support network—those without local family or informal support—are at greater risk. Furthermore, she emphasized that having a balanced combination of these social networks is most beneficial in protecting against adversities, such as loneliness and depression, rather than relying on a single resource. Similarly, Fiori et al. (2006) proposed five distinct social network types—nonfamily-restricted, nonfriends, family, diverse, and friends—reflecting available social networks (i.e., married, number of children, contact with children, religious services attendance, contact with friends, meetings attendance), and showed that these network types vary depending on factors, such as age, education, income, and functional health. This section elaborates how various forms and typologies of social networks are linked to loneliness.

A deficit in social relationships and support—both quantity and quality—significantly increases the risk for loneliness and vice versa (Carrasco et al., 2024; Fokkema et al., 2012; Pinquart & Sorensen, 2001; Guthmuller, 2022; Santini et al., 2016). Vasile et al. (2024) found that low-frequency contact with family/relatives living outside the household, friends, and neighbours is significantly associated with loneliness among older Europeans aged 65 and above. Santini et al. (2016) highlighted that lower social integration, lack of emotional support from social networks, and increased social strains significantly contribute to loneliness among older Irish adults aged 50 years or older. While the size of social networks continues to influence loneliness, there is a growing emphasis on the quality of these networks over mere size or status (Abramowska-Kmon & Timoszuk, 2020; Štípková, 2021; Yang, 2018). Yang (2018) suggested that a strong sense of feeling close to their spouse or partner, rather than being in a relationship (married), plays a more critical role in determining the likelihood of feeling—never or only occasionally—lonely. Moreover, although women are more likely to become widowed, research indicates that widowers tend to experience greater loneliness than their widow counterparts (Niino et al., 2025; Štípková, 2021). Fierloos et al. (2021) reported that men living without a partner are almost twice as likely to experience social loneliness compared to those living with a partner, and the association between poor relationship quality with spouse or partner and loneliness is more pronounced in men, suggesting thus gender differences in emotional needs among married couples in older age.

Beyond the impact of spousal relationships in later life, intergenerational relations significantly affect older adults' loneliness. However, the relationship with adult children and/or grandchildren and its potential role in loneliness is rather complex. According to de Jong Gierveld et al. (2012), among older adults (whether single or partnered) living with one or more children aged 25 or older, there is a greater likelihood of providing support to their adult children than receiving support from them. Although there is a protective effect of co-residence (living with children) on loneliness, the impact is smaller than living solely with a spouse or partner (couple-only household). The study further noted that in both Eastern and Western European countries (France, Germany, Russia, Bulgaria, and Georgia), older adults who are primarily on the receiving side are most lonely. Abramowska-Kmon and Timoszuk (2020) reported that having at least one child in the social network is significantly related to higher levels of loneliness among older women aged 65 years and over in Poland. Santini et al. (2016) found that, for women, social strain from children—feeling unsupported or stressed in the parent-child relationship—significantly contributes to feelings of loneliness, which in turn influence depression. Furthermore, Hajek and König (2022) noted that in Southern Europe (Spain, Italy and Slovenia), as older women start caring for their grandchildren, their loneliness tends to increase, while no significant change in loneliness is observed among men in those countries. This might suggest that men tend to be less involved in caregiving roles or perceive these responsibilities differently. These findings, together with previous studies (e.g., Fierloos et al., 2021; Niino et al., 2025; Štípková, 2021) suggest that partnership and spousal support are more important for older men's emotional well-being, while women are more likely to be affected by broadened social engagement derived from parenthood and relationships with their children.

Wenger (1997) stressed that, while family networks are important, they are not as protective in isolation if community or friend involvement is lacking. As traditional family structures and roles weaken, older adults may increasingly need to seek social support from diverse sources beyond their families. Mair (2019) found that older adults without kin or whose relatives are unavailable tend to report having more friends in their networks, based on data from individuals aged 50 and older across 17 EU countries. Djundeva et al. (2019) showed that older adults living alone in Eastern and Southern European countries are more likely to have *restricted, child-based* networks, whereas in Western and Northern European countries, *friend-oriented* networks are more prevalent and friendships are highly valued among those living alone. According to Routasalo et al. (2006), unmet expectations of the contact with friends and feeling poorly understood by close people nearly doubled the likelihood of feeling lonely, while the frequency of contact was not significantly related to loneliness among older Finns. Neighbours, due to their physical proximity, often become essential social resources for older adults, frequently forming friendship, particularly for those living alone or without children (Seifert & König, 2019; Pinquart & Sorensen, 2001). According to Seifert and König (2019), 6–8% of older adults aged 50 to their early 70 s reported providing help to their neighbours, but this rate declined with age, with only 2% of those aged 80 and older serving as help providers. Conversely, the proportion of older adults receiving help from their neighbours more than doubled among those aged 80 and above compared to those in their 50 s. The proportion of older adults who receiving neighbourly help was particularly higher among those in poor health, those without children or whose children not living in a same community, and people who were widowed or divorced. Hajek et al. (2023a) showed that changes in close contact with neighbours during the pandemic significantly affected loneliness among older German adults; specifically, decreased closeness and increased loneliness among men, while decreased involvement in neighbourhood activities and increased loneliness among women.

6.3 Meso-level Factors

Neighbourhood dynamics—comprising its physical and material assets, as well as how individuals integrate these into their needs and expectations—can significantly contribute to loneliness. A recent scoping review categorized neighbourhood factors associated with loneliness and social isolation among older populations (see Meehan et al., 2023). Factors that increased loneliness included neighbourhood disadvantage, rurality, lack of social security, and higher proportion of migrated populations, while factors that help diminish loneliness included open green spaces, accessible services, neighbourhood satisfaction, social cohesion and neighbourhood belonging, walkability, transport access, neighbourhood safety, and housing diversity. Based on this review, the relevant literature addressing the meso-level factors for loneliness narrows down into two domains: (1) perceived neighbourhood environments—built environment and social cohesion, and (2) urban versus rural contexts.

6.3.1 Perceived Neighbourhood Environments

According to Shiovitz-Ezra (2015), perceived physical environment (service availability), and social capital and cohesion in neighbourhood—sense of belonging to the local area, having people to rely on in times of need—are significantly associated with loneliness in older adults; these impacts are particularly pronounced in the "oldest-old" group of older Europeans (aged 75 years or older). Domenech-Abella et al. (2020) found that higher usability (available facilities, access to third places, transportation) and walkability of neighbourhoods were significantly associated with lower levels of loneliness among older adults aged 50 years old and over living in Finland, Poland, and Spain. Similarly, Gibney et al. (2020) reported that higher levels of age-friendliness (i.e., perceived safety, access to services, and walkability) was significantly related to lower levels of loneliness among older Irish adults. Favourable neighbourhood conditions, such as safe and walkable environments and easy access to daily amenities, allow older adults to more engage in out-of-home activities, thereby helping them maintain social connectedness and a sense of belonging to their local community.

Kemperman et al. (2019) explored how perceived neighbourhood environments (i.e., neighbourhood attachment, safety, and satisfaction with amenities) and objective physical characteristics (i.e., distances to public green spaces and daily shopping amenities) influence loneliness among older Dutch adults. The study found that neighbourhood safety appeared to contribute to neighbourhood attachment, while satisfaction with amenities was related to loneliness by increasing satisfaction with social networks. In other words, neighbourhood safety and access to facilities promote social engagement and participation, thereby contributing to lower levels of loneliness. In a similar context, a recent review by Bower et al. (2023) suggested that the built environment itself is not directly associated with loneliness but rather plays a supportive role through providing opportunities to promote social connectedness and a sense of belonging.

Conversely, neighbourhood disorder and deprivation can hinder social integration and neighbourhood cohesion, leading to increased isolation and loneliness among older adults (see also Chap. 4; Van Regenmortel et al., 2025). Vandalism, high crime rates, and poorly maintained housing may create anxiety and fear, causing older adults to withdraw from activities outside of their homes. Scharf and de Jong Gierveld (2008) showed significantly higher prevalence rates of loneliness among older adults living in deprived neighbourhoods in England—that representing higher prevalence of low income, unemployment, poor access to health care and public transportation, higher prevalence of illness, low education, and poor housing and homelessness. Similarly, Victor and Pikhartova (2020), reported that 25% of English older adults experienced area-based loneliness (often felt lonely within the area of residence), compared to 18% who reported individual-based loneliness; 9% experienced both types of loneliness. In particular, area-based loneliness was significantly related to deprivation score, with higher deprivation scores correlating with a higher prevalence of loneliness.

6.3.2 Urban versus Rural Contexts

Urban and rural contexts differ significantly in demographic, social, economic, cultural, and environmental features, each presenting unique challenges and opportunities that affect how older adults experience loneliness. Urban areas are typically characterized by high population density, diverse populations and cultures, and higher levels of industrialization, offering greater opportunities for job, access to services, available technology and transportation, and resources for education, social participation, and leisure. Rural areas, on the other hand, represent less populated, more homogeneous, often older, and have limited health and social services and infrastructure. Therefore, compared to those living in urban areas, older adults living in rural areas seem to be more disadvantaged and vulnerable to loneliness (Hussain et al., 2023; Susanty et al. 2024). In their recent meta-analysis, Susanty et al. (2024) reported that living in rural areas significantly increased the likelihood of loneliness, indicating an 18% higher risk of loneliness for rural residents compared to those in different settings.

Conversely, Myck et al. (2021) found that living in a rural area did not impact on either severe loneliness or the likelihood of becoming lonely over a two-year follow-up period among individuals aged 50 and older across 13 European countries. Similarly, Kemperman et al. (2019) reported that the degree of urbanization was not significantly related to loneliness among Dutch older adults aged 65 years and over, suggesting that loneliness is shaped by multiple factors beyond mere geography. Additionally, Burholt and Scharf (2014) observed no significant relationship between rurality and loneliness among older Irish adults. While rurality was related to lower participation in social leisure activities (e.g., attending films, plays, concerts; sports/exercise, traveling for pleasure), it was positively related with social resources. Burholt and Scharf (2014) further noted that poor health was inversely related to social resources, and the association was considerably stronger in rural areas than urban areas. Lee (2020) found that older adults in rural areas or small villages experienced less loneliness than those in cities or large towns in the Czech Republic. Despite various disadvantages of rural living in later life, older adults in rural areas may benefit from socially tighter local communities, that can provide stronger social bonds and support networks, thereby protecting them against loneliness.

The inconsistent findings suggest that the rural-urban divide in loneliness should be examined in light of the diverse underlying factors within each context and their different influence in forming social networks and experiences that collectively contribute to loneliness. For instance, in urban settings, higher levels of mental health issues are related to stress, social isolation and anonymity, pollution, noise, and crime, whereas older adults in rural regions can develop poor mental health because of limited access to health and social services (Alcañiz et al., 2020; Kovess-Masfety et al., 2005). Relatedly, policy definitions and public perceptions of rurality and urbanity are country-specific, and thus vary across Europe; for instance, rural areas in the UK may differ from those in other European countries. Some rural areas may benefit from active local organizations, whereas others may experience population decline and weakened social cohesion. Certain cultural factors, such as higher levels of civic participation and cycling culture, prevalent in the Netherlands, for example, may play a significant role in protecting older adults in rural areas from social isolation and loneliness. Furthermore, these cultural norms influence the development of regional policies and infrastructure, thereby promoting the age-friendliness of rural environments. To advance the understanding of loneliness among older adults, it is imperative to better integrate geographical and cultural variability across Europe, moving beyond the simplistic view of rurality as merely a disadvantage or vulnerability.

6.4 Intersectionality of Risk Factors

Each of the aforementioned factors plays a distinct role. However, they do not act in isolation and their influence varies across different contexts, resulting in older adults experiencing loneliness in more nuanced ways. Moreover, these factors extend beyond the micro- and meso-levels to include macro-level influence. Research reflects this complexity.

According to Liu (2021), among regular Internet users, Caucasian women and those with higher social status reported lower levels of loneliness, while women from Black and minority ethnic backgrounds had significantly higher levels of loneliness; in contrast, both Caucasian and black/minority ethnic men reported lower loneliness levels. Arnoso et al. (2023) highlighted the complex and intersecting factors contributing to loneliness among Spanish women, expounding on how their lived experiences as women, such as limited opportunity, socioeconomic disparities, family responsibilities, and (for some) minority backgrounds, exacerbated exclusion and stigma, thereby intensifying loneliness. Furthermore, Merodio et al. (2024) substantiated that gendered ageism, abuse, and discrimination based on minority backgrounds (e.g., sexuality, disabilities) create intersectional inequalities that impede older women's social participation. These findings suggest that female sex, low socioeconomic status, and minority backgrounds constitute multilayered constraints for women, resulting in a specific subgroup of older adults being more vulnerable to loneliness. This also potentially explains the inconsistent reporting in its prevalence and correlates when simply using the gender as a binary variable in research.

Li and Spini (2022), examined how multiple identities are associated with loneliness among adults aged 18 or older residing in a Swiss municipality; the sample consisted of approximately 39% people aged 18–40, 39% aged 41–64, and 21% aged 65 or older. The study classified participants into 36 intersectional strata based on nationality (foreign vs. Swiss), gender (male vs. female), age (18–40, 41–64, 65+), and education (primary, secondary, tertiary), and analysed how these strata were related to loneliness. The findings indicated that nationality and education were the strongest predictors of loneliness, with certain social clusters, particularly those involving older age, lower socioeconomic status, and migrant backgrounds, being at higher risk of loneliness. An individual develops and embodies multiple social identities throughout life; some, such as gender and nationality, remain relatively stable, while others, such as marital status and employment, may change over time due to key life transitions. Grills and Prus (2008) stressed the need to move beyond a conventional approach, using social categories as static, as this approach risks oversimplifying the complex and interactive mechanisms underlying human experiences. This reinforces the importance of examining how individuals navigate and are influenced by multiple (social) identities, constructing different meanings through their everyday practices and interaction in relation to experiencing loneliness.

Beyond the intricate interplay of multiple social identities, vulnerable situations or conditions in older age are also highly correlated and contribute to loneliness in combination. Sundström et al. (2009) revealed that older adults living alone with poor health had significantly higher odds of loneliness compared to those living alone with good health, or those not living alone but with poor health; in particular, there was a tenfold increase in the likelihood of loneliness compared to those living with others and in good health. Similarly, Carrasco et al. (2024) showed that among older Spanish adults living alone with poor mental health (presence of depression and anxiety) and low quality of life, about 73% reported loneliness, while less than 1% reported loneliness among those living with others and being in good mental health and with a high quality of life. Likewise, as older adults with low socioeconomic status are more likely to reside in disadvantaged neighbourhoods, the combined effects of these individual- and neighbourhood-level factors can place them at greater risk for severe and chronic loneliness. Importantly, the effects of individual and meso-level factors while interacting are largely governed by the societal, historical, and cultural contexts in which individuals have lived. According to Nyqvist et al. (2019), both individual resources (e.g., self-rated health, household size, marital status) and welfare regimes influence the absence of loneliness among older Europeans. The study emphasised that in Nordic countries, older adults are less reliant on personal resources to avoid loneliness, whereas in other regimes, such as Southern and Eastern European countries, they are more reliant on family and social ties. Furthermore, Langenkamp et al. (2024) found that social cohesion had a relatively small impact on reducing loneliness in countries where cultural pluralism—the acceptance and celebration of diverse cultures—is highly valued, such as

Germany, Denmark, Finland, and Sweden. However, the impact of social cohesion on loneliness is considerably stronger in countries with lower cultural pluralism.

For older adults, the interaction between multiple identities and life transitions within a given societal and environmental context can expose them to increased risk factors (see also Chap. 2 of this book; Nyqvist et al., 2025). Acknowledging the diverse and multifaceted experiences of loneliness, this intersectional approach provides a framework for a better understanding of why some older adults are more resilient to loneliness, while others are more susceptible, moving beyond the notion of older adults as a homogeneous group.

6.5 Childhood Experiences and Loneliness in Old Age

The intersectionality approach reminds us that loneliness in older age is accounted for by considering individual attributes within the social, economic, and cultural contexts that shape unique intersectional characteristics. Factors such as sex, race/ethnicity, and chronological age are typically determined at birth, and factors such as education, job experience, and family trajectories are largely set in early adulthood, both of which are barely modifiable in old age. However, these factors contribute to the development of various identities and roles that evolve, interact, and accumulate throughout life, often exerting cumulative advantages or disadvantages that influence how one experiences loneliness in later life.

According to Dannefer (2003, 2020), ageing is not merely biological but a process deeply intertwined with social stratification and the life-long accumulation of advantages and disadvantages. That is, the systemic accumulation of any advantages or disadvantages across the life course is significantly related to widening disparities in health and socioeconomic status and social integration in later life. Early life conditions (e.g., education and family background) shape trajectories that either reinforce privileges or disadvantages, and these processes are further informed by societal-structural systems, such as labour markets, institutional discrimination, and policy, leading to increasing divergence in living standards and well-being in later life. For instance, Nurius et al. (2019) found that adverse childhood experiences are significantly related to lower income, the development of unhealthy behaviours (i.e., tobacco use, sedentary lifestyle), and poor physical health (e.g., obesity) in adulthood, all of which collectively contribute to poor health in older age. Similarly, Ferraro et al. (2016) showed that socioeconomic disadvantage and frequent parental abuse hinder the development of positive social resources and increase the likelihood of risky behaviours (smoking and obesity) and additional health problems (heart disease and cancer). These findings suggest that the impact of early life adversities intensifies inequality and chronic stressors, creating a chain of risks that makes individuals with such disadvantages more vulnerable to physical and mental health challenges. However, there remains a gap in understanding how early life experiences, particularly those in childhood and youth, influence loneliness in older age.

According to Guthmuller (2022), early life circumstances (e.g., relationship with parents and peers, childhood socioeconomic status, physical abuse) account for 7% of the factors contributing to loneliness in later life, compared to other demographic and socioeconomic factors (6%) or country-level characteristics (5%). The results indicated that experiences of physical harm, poor health as a child, and low household wealth during childhood all increased the odds of loneliness in old age. The study further highlighted the important role of the mother–child relationship, noting that those who reported having a fair or poor relationship with their mother during childhood were 34% more likely to experience loneliness compared to those who had an excellent relationship. Similarly, Liu and Liu (2023) found that a higher number of early life adversities, such as household dysfunction, parental mental health issues, and substance abuse, was significantly related to loneliness in later life. While the negative effects of childhood adversities seem to be mitigated by active social participation in older age, lifetime discrimination based on political beliefs, religion, ethnicity, nationality, or sexual orientation significantly undermines the protective benefits of social engagement, thereby increasing loneliness. Tiilikainen et al. (2024) showed that Finnish older adults who experienced greater adversities in childhood or youth (fear of a family member, emotionally cold upbringing, or the loss of a parent) were more likely to follow a severe loneliness trajectory, reinforcing the important role of early social environments and its lifelong influence on social and emotional well-being. Additionally, Finkel et al. (2025) found that financial difficulties experienced in both childhood and adulthood were significantly associated with emotional well-being (anxiety, depression, and loneliness) over a 25-year follow-up period in a Swedish sample of participants aged 45–88 years at baseline. The study revealed that individuals experiencing high financial strain in both childhood and adulthood tended to show a gradual, linear increase in anxiety, depression, and loneliness over time and that the combined effect of childhood and adult financial strain was significantly linked to loneliness, not to anxiety or depression.

Early life environments and experiences influence not only sequential adulthood conditions, such as education and employment, but also play a pivotal role in the development of personality, attachment styles, social intelligence, and coping strategies, all of which have enduring effects on resilience or vulnerability to adversities in later life. Although childhood and youth circumstances may not be as strongly predictive of loneliness as more straightforward factors, such as widowhood or poor health in old age, they represent important life course risk factors that unfold over time. Understanding the longitudinal associations between early life experiences and loneliness in older adults will provide an opportunity to identify risk factors, potentially early on, and implement adequate interventions and preventive measures to mitigate social exclusion and loneliness in later life.

6.6 Diversity in Ageing Populations and Emerging (Risk) Factors

Population ageing has become increasingly heterogeneous, leading to more diverse family structure and living environments in later life. However, the potential impact of these changes on loneliness among older adults requires further investigation. Here, we elaborate on several aspects that merit additional research.

Minority statuses extend beyond major determinants such as migration history or racial/ethnic backgrounds. For instance, as individuals more openly define their unique gender, sexual, and social identities, the number of older adults identifying as LGBTQ+ is rapidly growing. This demographic faces a greater risk of loneliness compared to their heterosexual peers, experiencing lifelong experiences of discrimination, stigma, social isolation, and a lack of community support, particularly in countries where cultural norms predominantly adhere to traditional gender roles and familial structures (Buczak-Stec et al., 2023; Elmer et al., 2024; Ribeiro-Gonçalves et al., 2024; Willis et al., 2022). Yet, this group remains significantly underrepresented in ageing research. It is important to provide a better understanding of how older adults navigate non-traditional life (family) pathways in their ageing trajectories, including those from minority backgrounds, and how they develop adaptive strategies to protect against loneliness in old age.

While living alone is often linked to loneliness, other living arrangements among older adults may deserve greater attention. For instance, many older adults transition into institutional settings such as retirement communities, assisted living facilities, nursing homes, or palliative care. These shifts may leave older adults more vulnerable, as their independent living diminishes. However, the availability of prompt medical and social services, as well as increased opportunities for interaction with peers and leisure activities within these institutions, can make institutionalization beneficial for preventing loneliness. According to Dykstra et al. (2005), admissions to residential care did not significantly affect loneliness among older Dutch adults. In contrast, Susanty et al. (2024) reported that institutionalization was strongly associated with a higher risk of loneliness, with individuals in institutional settings nearly three times more likely to experience loneliness compared to those living independently. It is essential to address the emotional and social challenges arising from these transitions that contribute to the development of loneliness.

It is also worth noting that older cohorts face global challenges including digitalization (see Chap. 8 of this book; Seifert, 2025), climate change (see Chap. 9 of this book; Ayalon, 2025), and pandemics which require them to adapt their lifestyles and behaviours. For instance, use of advanced digital technologies such as the Internet and smartphones can potentially mitigate loneliness by fostering social connections and developing new social networks and activities (Petersen et al., 2023; Rennoch et al., 2023; Silva et al., 2022). The increasing integration of AI-powered social robots into social and healthcare services demonstrates potential in caregiving and providing emotional support, particularly for older adults living alone (Pu et al., 2018). However, older adults who are less equipped with or unable to afford necessary services or who have poor digital literacy, often associated with low socioeconomic status, are more vulnerable to social isolation and loneliness. These digital disparities were further exacerbated during the COVID-19 pandemic as the adoption of digital technology became essential for accessing health and social services (Balki et al., 2023; Lee, 2021; Seifert et al., 2021). Moreover, rapid societal changes including digitalization may leave some older adults experiencing more alienation or marginalization. If they lack sufficient support and cognitive resources to assess misinformation, they may be more susceptible to conspiracy theories (Ford et al., 2013; Zwar et al., 2022). This mistrust of emerging technologies can further deepen distrust in medical care systems, institutions, and governments, exacerbating social isolation and feelings of loneliness. These challenges are not only relevant for older adults today but will also significantly impact younger cohorts as they age, when encountering these challenges early in life.

6.7 Conclusion

This chapter addressed both the most salient and subtle yet important risk factors that contribute to loneliness in later life. Six key findings are highlighted.

1. While older age, female sex, and living alone are commonly associated with loneliness, their effects are context-specific and mixed and should be interpreted with greater nuance rather than assumed as universal risk factors.
2. The relationship between health and loneliness is still ambiguous as they appear to be mutually reinforcing.
3. Marital status and experience, family trajectories, and social relationships serve as key mechanisms underlying loneliness; greater attention should be directed towards the quality of relationships (e.g., marital strain, perceived support, and satisfaction) and how older adults reconcile discrepancies in role expectations and experiences in both the development and alleviation of loneliness.
4. Given the complex interplay of multiple factors, studies should integrate an intersectional approach when examining the potential risk factors of loneliness.
5. Loneliness is shaped not only by contemporary conditions but also by early life experiences, including childhood living conditions and the family environment. Understanding these early experiences can explain how prevalent risk factors evolve over the course of life.
6. Societal-historical and cultural variations in their influence on loneliness have emerged as significant factors, yet largely underexplored areas.

While providing an in-depth discussion of the various risk factors, several delimitations were set to maintain a focused scope. The majority of the evidence presented is derived from empirical studies conducted on European populations, and the impact of the COVID-19 pandemic is considered only where relevant. Importantly, the narrative literature review approach has limitations in terms of providing conclusive evidence. The inclusion criteria for the discussed factors were primarily based on systematic reviews and key quantitative studies, which, while rigorous, may have excluded important factors such as biology and genetics, owing to the limited available evidence.

These limitations encourage future research to adopt a more inclusive approach and develop clearer insights into potential areas for intervention and policy provisions. To clarify the underlying mechanism, future studies should (1) provide more robust evidence of causality between loneliness and its risk factors, (2) examine the cumulative impact of these risk factors over time, considering early life experiences, and (3) differentiate between modifiable and non-modifiable factors while exploring how certain factors mediate or moderate the experience of loneliness. To further advance our understanding of loneliness in older age, future research should develop methodologies and theoretical frameworks that incorporate an intersectionality and life course approach (see also Chaps. 11 and 14 of this book; Precupetu et al., 2025; Suanet & Aartsen, 2025). By integrating these perspectives, researchers and policymakers can design and implement targeted interventions to address the specific needs of different subgroups within an ageing population. Finally, research on loneliness, particularly in European contexts, requires an expanded understanding of the varying cultural and historical influences that have shaped older cohorts' life trajectories, material living, and societal attitudes toward ageing in myriad ways.

Competing Interests The author has no conflict of interest to declare that are relevant to the content of this chapter.

References

Aartsen, M., & Jylhä, M. (2011). Onset of loneliness in older adults: Results of a 28 year prospective study. *European Journal of Ageing, 8*, 31–38. https://doi.org/10.1007/s10433-011-0175-7

Abramowska-Kmon, A., & Timoszuk, S. (2020). Family and social networks, subjective well-being and loneliness among older adults in Poland. *Studia Demograficzne, 177*(1), 9–36. https://doi.org/10.33119/SD.2020.1.1

Akhter-Khan, S. C., Li, L., Prina, M., Wong, G. H.-Y., & Mayston, R. (2022). Understanding and addressing older adults' loneliness: The social relationship expectations framework. *Perspectives on Psychological Science, 18*(4), 762–777. https://doi.org/10.1177/17456916221127218

Alcañiz, M., Riera-Prunera, M. C., & Solé-Auró, A. (2020). "When I retire, I'll move out of the city": Mental well-being of the elderly in rural vs. urban settings. *International Journal of Environmental Research and Public Health, 17*(7), 2442. https://doi.org/10.3390/ijerph17072442

Arnoso, A., Arnoso, M., Elgorriaga, E., Asla, N., Aiertza, M., Bengoetxea, A., & Pizarro, M. (2023). Meanings of loneliness for women using social services in Spain: An intersectional analysis. *Affilia, 38*(1), 91–110. https://doi.org/10.1177/088610992211087

Arpino, B., Mair, C. A., Quashie, N. T., & Antczak, R. (2022). Loneliness before and during the COVID-19 pandemic—are unpartnered and childless older adults at higher risk? *European Journal of Ageing, 19*(4), 1327–1338. https://doi.org/10.1007/s10433-022-00695-1

Ayalon, L. (2025). Climate change and the risk of loneliness. In M. Aartsen, I. Precupetu, & B. Suanet (Eds.), *Macro social influences on loneliness in later life: Towards a better understanding of the loneliness paradox in later life*. Springer.

Balki, E., Hayes, N., & Holland, C. (2023). The indirect impact of educational attainment as a distal resource for older adults on loneliness, social isolation, psychological resilience, and technology use during the COVID-19 pandemic: Cross-sectional quantitative study. *JMIR Aging, 6*, e47729. https://doi.org/10.2196/47729

Barbosa, F., Cunha, C., Voss, G., & Matos, A. D. (2019). 25 The impact of living alone on physical and mental health: Does loneliness matter?. *Health and Socio–economic Status Over the Life Course, 243*. https://doi.org/10.1515/9783110617245-025

Barjaková, M., Garnero, A., & d'Hombres, B. (2023). Risk factors for loneliness: A literature review. *Social Science & Medicine, 334*, 116163. https://doi.org/10.1016/j.socscimed.2023.116163

Barreto, M., Victor, C., Hammond, C., Eccles, A., Richins, M. T., & Qualter, P. (2021). Loneliness around the world: Age, gender, and cultural differences in loneliness. *Personality and Individual Differences, 169*, 110066. https://doi.org/10.1016/j.paid.2020.110066

Beal, C. (2006). Loneliness in older women: A review of the literature. *Issues in Mental Health Nursing, 27*(7), 795–813. https://doi.org/10.1080/01612840600781196

Berkman, L. F. (1995). The role of social relations in health promotion. *Psychosomatic Medicine, 57*(3), 245–254. https://doi.org/10.1097/00006842-199505000-00006

Berkman, L. F., & Glass, T. (2000). Social integration, social networks, social support, and health. In L. F. Berkman & I. Kawachi (Eds.), *Social epidemiology* (Online ed.). Oxford Academic. https://doi.org/10.1093/oso/9780195083316.003.0007

Bishop, A. J., & Martin, P. (2007). The indirect influence of educational attainment on loneliness among unmarried older adults. *Educational Gerontology, 33*(10), 897–917. https://doi.org/10.1080/03601270701569275

Boss, L., Kang, D., & Branson, S. (2015). Loneliness and cognitive function in the older adult: A systematic review. *International Psychogeriatrics, 27*, 541–553. https://doi.org/10.1017/S1041610214002749

Bower, M., Kent, J., Patulny, R., Green, O., McGrath, L., Teesson, L., et al. (2023). The impact of the built environment on loneliness: A systematic review and narrative synthesis. *Health & Place, 79*, 102962. https://doi.org/10.1016/j.healthplace.2022.102962

van den Broek, T., Lam, J., & Potente, C. (2024). Do middle-aged and older people underreport loneliness? Experimental evidence from the Netherlands. *European Journal of Ageing, 21*(1), 29. https://doi.org/10.1007/s10433-023-00772-0

Buczak-Stec, E., König, H. H., & Hajek, A. (2023). Sexual orientation and psychosocial factors in terms of loneliness and subjective well-being in later life. *The Gerontologist, 63*(2), 338–349. https://doi.org/10.1093/geront/gnac116

Buecker, S., Maes, M., Denissen, J. J., & Luhmann, M. (2020). Loneliness and the Big Five personality traits: A meta–analysis. *European Journal of Personality, 34*(1), 8–28. https://doi.org/10.1002/per.2229

Burholt, V., & Scharf, T. (2014). Poor health and loneliness in later life: The role of depressive symptoms, social resources, and rural environments. *Journals of Gerontology: Series B, 69*(2), 311–324. https://doi.org/10.1093/geronb/gbt121

Burholt, V., Windle, G., Morgan, D. J., & CFAS Wales team. (2017). A social model of loneliness: The roles of disability, social resources, and cognitive impairment. *The Gerontologist, 57*(6), 1020–1030. https://doi.org/10.1093/geront/gnw125

Burholt, V., Winter, B., Aartsen, M., Constantinou, C., Dahlberg, L., Feliciano, V., De Jong Gierveld, J., Van Regenmortel, S., Waldegrave, C., & Working Group on Exclusion from Social Relations, part of the COST-financed Research Network 'Reducing Old-Age Exclusion: Collaborations in Research and Policy' (ROSENet). (2019). A critical review and development of a conceptual model of exclusion from social relations for older people. *European Journal of Ageing, 17*(1), 3–19. https://doi.org/10.1007/s10433-019-00506-0

Carney, M., Fujiwara, J., Emmert, B., Liberman, T., & Paris, B. (2016). Elder orphans hiding in plain sight: A growing vulnerable population. *Current Gerontology and Geriatrics Research*, 2016. https://doi.org/10.1155/2016/4723250

Carrasco, P. M., Crespo, D. P., García, A. I. R., Ibáñez, M. L., Rubio, B. M., & Montenegro-Peña, M. (2024). Predictive factors and risk and protection groups for loneliness in older adults: A population-based study. *BMC Psychology, 12*(1), 238. https://doi.org/10.1186/s40359-024-01114-2

Cohen-Mansfield, J., Hazan, H., Lerman, Y., & Shalom, V. (2016). Correlates and predictors of loneliness in older-adults: A review of quantitative results informed by qualitative insights. *International Psychogeriatrics, 28*(4), 557–576. https://doi.org/10.1017/S1041610215001532

Cotterell, N., Buffel, T., Nazroo, J., & Qualter, P. (2025). Loneliness among older ethnic minority people: Exploring the role of structural disadvantage and place using a co-research methodology. *Ethnic and Racial Studies, 48*(1), 206–228. https://doi.org/10.1080/01419870.2024.2311833

Dahlberg, L., Andersson, L., McKee, K. J., & Lennartsson, C. (2015). Predictors of loneliness among older women and men in Sweden: A national longitudinal study. *Aging & Mental Health, 19*(5), 409–417. https://doi.org/10.1080/13607863.2014.944091

Dahlberg, L., McKee, K. J., Frank, A., & Naseer, M. (2022). A systematic review of longitudinal risk factors for loneliness in older adults. *Aging & Mental Health, 26*(2), 225–249. https://doi.org/10.1080/13607863.2021.1876638

Dannefer, D. (2003). Cumulative advantage/disadvantage and the life course: Cross-fertilizing age and social science theory. *The Journals of Gerontology: Series B, 58*(6), S327–S337. https://doi.org/10.1093/geronb/58.6.s327

Dannefer, D. (2020). Systemic and reflexive: Foundations of cumulative dis/advantage and life-course processes. *The Journals of Gerontology: Series B, 75*(6), 1249–1263. https://doi.org/10.1093/geronb/gby118

De Jong Gierveld, J., Dykstra, P. A., & Schenk, N. (2012). Living arrangements, intergenerational support types and older adult loneliness in Eastern and Western Europe. *Demographic Research, 27*, 167–200. https://doi.org/10.4054/DemRes.2012.27.7

De Witte, J., & Van Regenmortel, T. (2022). The relationship between loneliness and migration among Belgian older adults. *Ageing International, 47*(4), 672–694. https://doi.org/10.1007/s12126-022-09484-0

Djundeva, M., & Ellwardt, L. (2020). Social support networks and loneliness of Polish migrants in the Netherlands. *Journal of Ethnic and Migration Studies, 46*(7), 1281–1300. https://doi.org/10.1080/1369183X.2019.1620416

Djundeva, M., Dykstra, P. A., & Fokkema, T. (2019). Is living alone "aging alone"? Solitary living, network types, and well-being. *The Journals of Gerontology: Series B, 74*(8), 1406–1415. https://doi.org/10.1093/geronb/gby119

Dolberg, P., Shiovitz-Ezra, S., & Ayalon, L. (2016). Migration and changes in loneliness over a 4-year period: The case of older former Soviet Union immigrants in Israel. *European Journal of Ageing, 13*, 287–297. https://doi.org/10.1007/s10433-016-0370-5

Domenech-Abella, J., Mundo, J., Leonardi, M., Chatterji, S., Tobiasz-Adamczyk, B., Koskinen, S., et al. (2020). Loneliness and depression among older European adults: The role of perceived neighborhood built environment. *Health & Place, 62*, 102280. https://doi.org/10.1016/j.healthplace.2020.102280

Dykstra, P. A., van Tilburg, T. G., & Gierveld, J. D. J. (2005). Changes in older adult loneliness: Results from a seven-year longitudinal study. *Research on Aging, 27*(6), 725–747. https://doi.org/10.1177/0164027505279712

Elmer, E. M., van Tilburg, T. G., & Fokkema, T. (2024). Age and gender identity in the relationship between minority stress and loneliness: A global sample of sexual and gender minority adults. *The Journal of Sex Research*, 1–20. https://doi.org/10.1080/00224499.2024.1985285

European Commission, Eurostat. (2020). *Ageing Europe: Looking at the lives of older people in the EU: 2020 edition*. Publication Office of the European Union. https://data.europa.eu/doi/10.2785/628105

Eurostat. (2024). *Number of persons by sex, age groups, household composition and working status* (lfst_hhindws). Publications Office of the European Union. https://data.europa.eu/doi/10.2908/LFST_HHINDWS. Accessed August 20, 2024.

Fawaz, Y., & Mira, P. (2019). 27 Bereavement, loneliness and health. *Health and Socio-economic Status Over the Life Course*, 259. https://doi.org/10.1515/9783110617245-027

Fernández-Carro, C., & Gumà Lao, J. (2022). A life-course approach to the relationship between education, family trajectory and late-life loneliness among older women in Europe. *Social Indicators Research, 162*(3), 1345–1363. https://doi.org/10.1007/s11205-022-02894-4

Ferraro, K. F., Schafer, M. H., & Wilkinson, L. R. (2016). Childhood disadvantage and health problems in middle and later life: Early imprints on physical health? *American Sociological Review, 81*(1), 107–133. https://doi.org/10.1177/0003122415619617

Fierloos, I. N., Tan, S. S., Williams, G., Alhambra-Borrás, T., Koppelaar, E., Bilajac, L., et al. (2021). Socio-demographic characteristics associated with emotional and social loneliness among older adults. *BMC Geriatrics, 21*, 1–10. https://doi.org/10.1186/s12877-021-02170-5

Finkel, D., Hyde, M., Hasselgren, C., Sacco, L., Sindi, S., & Nilsen, C. (2025). Both childhood and adult perceived financial strain impact age trajectories of change in emotional health in late adulthood. *Aging & Mental Health*, 1–8. https://doi.org/10.1080/13607863.2025.2464709

Fiori, K., Antonucci, T., & Cortina, K. (2006). Social network typologies and mental health among older adults. *The Journals of Gerontology: Series B, 61*(1), 25–32. https://doi.org/10.1093/GERONB/61.1.P25

Fokkema, T. (2023). Loneliness among older migrants. In *Handbook on migration and ageing* (pp. 290–300). Edward Elgar Publishing. https://doi.org/10.4337/9781800886116.00028

Fokkema, T., De Jong Gierveld, J., & Dykstra, P. A. (2012). Cross-national differences in older adult loneliness. *The Journal of Psychology, 146*(1-2), 201–228. https://doi.org/10.1080/00223980.2011.631612

Ford, C., Wallace, S., Newman, P., Lee, S., & Cunningham, W. (2013). Belief in AIDS-related conspiracy theories and mistrust in the government: Relationship with HIV testing among at-risk older adults. *The Gerontologist, 53*(6), 973–984. https://doi.org/10.1093/geront/gns192

Gibney, S., Zhang, M., & Brennan, C. (2020). Age-friendly environments and psychosocial wellbeing: A study of older urban residents in Ireland. *Aging & Mental Health, 24*(12), 2022–2033. https://doi.org/10.1080/13607863.2019.1652245

Girgus, J. S., Yang, K., & Ferri, C. V. (2017). The gender difference in depression: Are elderly women at greater risk for depression than elderly men? *Geriatrics, 2*(4), 35. https://doi.org/10.3390/geriatrics2040035

Grills, S., & Prus, R. (2008). The myth of the independent variable: Reconceptualizing class, gender, race, and age as subcultural processes. *The American Sociologist, 39*(1), 19–37. http://www.jstor.org/stable/41217765

Guthmuller, S. (2022). Loneliness among older adults in Europe: The relative importance of early and later life conditions. *PLoS One, 17*(5), e0267562. https://doi.org/10.1371/journal.pone.0267562

Hajek, A., & König, H. H. (2020). Which factors contribute to loneliness among older Europeans? Findings from the survey of health, ageing and retirement in Europe: determinants of loneliness. *Archives of Gerontology and Geriatrics, 89*, 104080. https://doi.org/10.1016/j.archger.2020.104080

Hajek, A., & König, H. H. (2021). Does obesity lead to loneliness and perceived social isolation in the second half of life? Findings from a nationally representative study in Germany. *Geriatrics & Gerontology International, 21*(9), 836–841. https://doi.org/10.1111/ggi.14264

Hajek, A., & König, H. H. (2022). Grandchild care and loneliness among older Europeans: Longitudinal evidence from the Survey of Health, Ageing and Retirement in Europe. *International Journal of Geriatric Psychiatry, 37*(8), 1–8. https://doi.org/10.1002/gps.5713

Hajek, A., Kretzler, B., & König, H. H. (2021). The association between obesity and social isolation as well as loneliness in the adult population: A systematic review. *Diabetes, Metabolic Syndrome and Obesity*, 2765–2773. https://doi.org/10.2147/DMSO.S320806

Hajek, A., Kretzler, B., Walther, C., Aarabi, G., Zwar, L., & König, H. H. (2023a). Neighbourhood cohesion, loneliness and perceived social isolation prior and during the COVID-19 pandemic. Longitudinal evidence from the German Ageing Survey. *Social Psychiatry and Psychiatric Epidemiology, 58*(9), 1411–1420. https://doi.org/10.1007/s00127-023-02448-w

Hajek, A., Volkmar, A., & König, H. H. (2023b). Prevalence and correlates of loneliness and social isolation in the oldest old: A systematic review, meta-analysis and meta-regression. *Social Psychiatry and Psychiatric Epidemiology*, 1–23. https://doi.org/10.1007/s00127-023-02428-0

Hajek, A., Gyasi, R. M., & König, H. H. (2024a). Factors associated with loneliness among individuals aged 80 years and over: Findings derived from the nationally representative "Old Age in Germany (D80+)" study. https://doi.org/10.1016/j.archger.2024.105443

Hajek, A., Zwar, L., Gyasi, R. M., et al. (2024b). Prevalence and determinants of loneliness among the oldest old living in institutionalized settings. *Zeitschrift für Gerontologie und Geriatrie, 57*(3), 214–219. https://doi.org/10.1007/s00391-023-02196-x

Hansen, T., & Slagsvold, B. (2016). Late-life loneliness in 11 European countries: Results from the generations and gender survey. *Social Indicators Research, 129*(1), 445–464. https://doi.org/10.1007/s11205-015-1111-6

Hansen, T., Kafková, M. P., Katz, R., Lowenstein, A., Naim, S., Pavlidis, G., et al. (2021). Exclusion from social relations in later life: micro-and macro-level patterns and correlations in a European perspective. *International Journal of Environmental Research and Public Health, 18*(23), 12418. https://doi.org/10.3390/ijerph182312418

Heu, L. C., van Zomeren, M., & Hansen, N. (2021). Does loneliness thrive in relational freedom or restriction? The culture-loneliness framework. *Review of General Psychology, 25*(1), 60–72. https://doi.org/10.1177/1089268020959033

Hussain, B., Mirza, M., Baines, R., Burns, L., Stevens, S., Asthana, S., & Chatterjee, A. (2023). Loneliness and social networks of older adults in rural communities: A narrative synthesis systematic review. *Frontiers in Public Health, 11*, 1113864. https://doi.org/10.3389/fpubh.2023.1113864

Joshi, M., Finney, N., & Hale, J. M. (2024). Loneliness and social isolation of ethnic minority/immigrant older adults: A scoping review. *Ageing & Society*, 1–31. https://doi.org/10.1017/S0144686X23000835

Jutengren, G., & Ståhl, F. (2024). Determinants of social loneliness among older adults in job retirement and the role of emotional expressivity. *Aging & Mental Health*, 1–9. https://doi.org/10.1080/13607863.2023.2277001

Kemperman, A., van den Berg, P., Weijs-Perrée, M., & Uijtdewillegen, K. (2019). Loneliness of older adults: Social network and the living environment. *International Journal of Environmental Research and Public Health, 16*(3), 406. https://doi.org/10.3390/ijerph16030406

Kervin, L. M., Chamberlain, S. A., Wister, A. V., & Cosco, T. D. (2022). (Older) Adults without advocates: Support for alternative terminology to "elder orphan" in research and clinical contexts. *Journal of the American Geriatrics Society, 70*(11), 3329–3333. https://doi.org/10.1111/jgs.17960

Klinenberg, E. (2016). Social isolation, loneliness, and living alone: Identifying the risks for public health. *American Journal of Public Health, 106*(5), 786–787. https://doi.org/10.2105/AJPH.2016.303166

Kovess-Masfety, V., Alonso, J., Graaf, R., & Demyttenaere, K. (2005). A European approach to rural—urban differences in mental health: The ESEMeD 2000 comparative study. *The Canadian Journal of Psychiatry, 50*, 926–936. https://doi.org/10.1177/070674370505001407

Langenkamp, A., Mund, M., & Hawkley, L. (2024). The role of country-level characteristics for the association between loneliness and neighborhood cohesion–A multi-level analysis. *Journal of Social and Personal Relationships*, 02654075241262321. https://doi.org/10.1177/02654075241262321

Lee, S. (2020). Loneliness among older adults in the Czech Republic: A socio demographic, health, and psychosocial profile. *Archives of Gerontology and Geriatrics, 90*, 104068. https://doi.org/10.1016/j.archger.2020.104068

Lee, S. (2021). Urgent call for health education to promote eHealth literacy in aging populations: A brief note. *Educational Gerontology, 47*(5), 193–195. https://doi.org/10.1080/03601277.2021.1899796

Lee, S. (2022). Does living alone affect self-perceptions of aging? Findings from two waves of the Health and Retirement Study. *Gerontology & Geriatric Medicine, 8*, 23337214221077798. https://doi.org/10.1177/23337214221077798

Li, Y., & Spini, D. (2022). Intersectional social identities and loneliness: Evidence from a municipality in Switzerland. *Journal of Community Psychology, 50*(8), 3560–3573. https://doi.org/10.1002/jcop.22855

Lim, M. H., Eres, R., & Vasan, S. (2020). Understanding loneliness in the twenty-first century: An update on correlates, risk factors, and potential solutions. *Social Psychiatry and Psychiatric Epidemiology, 55*(7), 793–810. https://doi.org/10.1007/s00127-020-01889-7

Liu, B. C. P. (2021). The impact of intersectionality of multiple identities on the digital health divide, quality of life and loneliness amongst older adults in the UK. *The British Journal of Social Work, 51*(8), 3077–3097. https://doi.org/10.1093/bjsw/bcaa149

Liu, B. C. P., & Liu, R. H. L. (2023). Early life adversities and discrimination, social activity, and loneliness among older adults in Europe: A moderated mediation analysis. *Aging & Mental Health, 27*(8), 1627–1635. https://doi.org/10.1080/13607863.2022.2144355

Loeffler, A., & Steptoe, A. (2021). Bidirectional longitudinal associations between loneliness and pain, and the role of inflammation. *Pain, 162*(3), 930–937. https://doi.org/10.1097/j.pain.0000000000002103

Mair, C. A. (2019). Alternatives to aging alone?: "Kinlessness" and the importance of friends across European contexts. *The Journals of Gerontology: Series B, 74*(8), 1416–1428. https://doi.org/10.1093/geronb/gbz029

Meehan, D. E., Grunseit, A., Condie, J., HaGani, N., & Merom, D. (2023). Social-ecological factors influencing loneliness and social isolation in older people: A scoping review. *BMC Geriatrics, 23*(1), 726. https://doi.org/10.1186/s12877-023-04208-6

Merodio, G., De Zárate, A., Zhu, F., & Morentin-Encina, J. (2024). The impact of gendered ageism and related intersectional inequalities on the health and well-being of older women. *Research on Ageing and Social Policy*. https://doi.org/10.17583/rasp.15017

Mund, M., Freuding, M. M., Möbius, K., Horn, N., & Neyer, F. J. (2020). The stability and change of loneliness across the life span: A meta-analysis of longitudinal studies. *Personality and Social Psychology Review, 24*(1), 24–52. https://doi.org/10.1177/1088868319850738

Myck, M., Waldegrave, C., & Dahlberg, L. (2021). Two dimensions of social exclusion: Economic deprivation and dynamics of loneliness during later life in Europe. In K. Walsh, T. Scharf, S. Van Regenmortel, & A. Wanka (Eds.), *Social exclusion in later life* (Vol. 28, pp. 311–326). Springer. https://doi.org/10.1007/978-3-030-51406-8_24

Nicolaisen, M., & Thorsen, K. (2014). Who are lonely? Loneliness in different age groups (18–81 years old), using two measures of loneliness. *The International Journal of Aging and Human Development, 78*(3), 229–257. https://doi.org/10.2190/AG.78.3.b

Nicolaisen, M., & Thorsen, K. (2024). Gender differences in loneliness over time: A 15-year longitudinal study of men and women in the second part of life. *The International Journal of Aging and Human Development, 98*(1), 103–132. https://doi.org/10.1177/00914150231172280

Niedzwiedz, C. L., Richardson, E. A., Tunstall, H., Shortt, N. K., Mitchell, R. J., & Pearce, J. R. (2016). The relationship between wealth and loneliness among older people across Europe: Is social participation protective? *Preventive Medicine, 91*, 24–31. https://doi.org/10.1016/j.ypmed.2016.07.016

Niino, K., Patapoff, M. A., Mausbach, B. T., Liu, H., Moore, A. A., Han, B. H., Palmer, B. W., & Jester, D. J. (2025). Development of loneliness and social isolation after spousal loss: A systematic review of longitudinal studies on widowhood. *Journal of the American Geriatrics Society, 73*(1), 253–265. https://doi.org/10.1111/jgs.19156

Nurius, P. S., Fleming, C. M., & Brindle, E. (2019). Life course pathways from adverse childhood experiences to adult physical health: A structural equation model. *Journal of Aging and Health, 31*(2), 211–230. https://doi.org/10.1177/0898264317726448

Nyqvist, F., Nygård, M., & Scharf, T. (2019). Loneliness amongst older people in Europe: A comparative study of welfare regimes. *European Journal of Ageing, 16*, 133–143. https://doi.org/10.1007/s10433-018-0487-y

Nyqvist, F., Näsman, M., Hemberg, J., & Nygård, M. (2023). Risk factors for loneliness among older people in a Nordic regional context–a longitudinal study. *Ageing & Society, 43*(10), 2372–2393. https://doi.org/10.1017/S0144686X22000345

Nyqvist, F., McHugh Power, J., & Coll-Planas, L. (2025). Theorizing loneliness in later life: Micro, meso, and macro perspectives. In M. Aartsen, I. Precupetu, & B. Suanet (Eds.), *Macro social influences on loneliness in later life: Towards a better understanding of the loneliness paradox in later life*. Springer.

Ong, A., Uchino, B., & Wethington, E. (2015). Loneliness and health in older adults: A mini-review and synthesis. *Gerontology, 62*, 443–449. https://doi.org/10.1159/000441651

Pagan, R., & Malo, M. A. (2024). Dynamic analysis of loneliness at older ages in Europe by gender. *Applied Research in Quality of Life*, 1–30. https://doi.org/10.1007/s11482-023-10110-w

Perlman, D., & Peplau, L. A. (1981). Toward a social psychology of loneliness. In S. W. Duck & R. Gilmour (Eds.), *Personal relationships in disorder* (pp. 31–56). Academic.

Petersen, B., Khalili-Mahani, N., Murphy, C., Sawchuk, K., Phillips, N., Li, K., & Hebblethwaite, S. (2023). The association between information and communication technologies, loneliness and social connectedness: A scoping review. *Frontiers in Psychology*, 14. https://doi.org/10.3389/fpsyg.2023.1063146

Pinquart, M., & Sorensen, S. (2001). Influences on loneliness in older adults: A meta-analysis. *Basic and Applied Social Psychology, 23*(4), 245–266. https://doi.org/10.1207/S15324834BASP2304_2

Precupetu, I., Pop, C., & Aartsen, M. (2025). Macro-level influences on loneliness in later life: An fsQCA analysis. In M. Aartsen, I. Precupetu, & B. Suanet (Eds.), *Macro social influences on loneliness in later life: Towards a better understanding of the loneliness paradox in later life*. Springer.

Pu, L., Moyle, W., Jones, C., & Todorovic, M. (2018). The effectiveness of social robots for older adults: A systematic review and meta-analysis of randomized controlled studies. *The Gerontologist, 59*, e37–e51. https://doi.org/10.1093/geront/gny046

Rapolienė, G., & Aartsen, M. (2022). Lonely societies: low trust societies? Further explanations for national variations in loneliness among older Europeans. *European Journal of Ageing, 19*(3), 485–494. https://doi.org/10.1007/s10433-021-00649-z

Rennoch, G., Schlomann, A., & Zank, S. (2023). The relationship between internet use for social purposes, loneliness, and depressive symptoms among the oldest old. *Research on Aging, 45*, 630–642. https://doi.org/10.1177/01640275221150017

Ribeiro-Gonçalves, J. A., Jesus, J. C., Costa, P. A., & Leal, I. (2024). Sexual stigma and mental health of LGB older adults: A Systematic scoping review. *Sexuality Research and Social Policy*, 1–23. doi:https://doi.org/10.1007/s13178-023-00741-z.

Roofeh, R., Smith, D. M., & Clouston, S. A. P. (2020). Estimated prevalence of elder orphans using National Health and Aging Trends Study. *Journal of Aging and Health, 32*(10), 1443–1449. https://doi.org/10.1177/0898264320932382

Routasalo, P. E., Savikko, N., Tilvis, R. S., Strandberg, T. E., & Pitkälä, K. H. (2006). Social contacts and their relationship to loneliness among aged people – A population-based study. *Gerontology, 52*(3), 181–187. https://doi.org/10.1159/000091828

Ruan, Y. X., & Cheung, M. C. (2024). Systematic review of factors influencing loneliness in older-adult migrants. *Aging & Mental Health*, 1–13. https://doi.org/10.1080/13607863.2023.2277151

Rughiniş, C., & Humă, B. (2015). Who theorizes age? The "socio-demographic variables" device and age–period–cohort analysis in the rhetoric of survey research. *Journal of Aging Studies, 35*, 144–159. https://doi.org/10.1016/j.jaging.2015.07.005

Santini, Z. I., Fiori, K. L., Feeney, J., Tyrovolas, S., Haro, J. M., & Koyanagi, A. (2016). Social relationships, loneliness, and mental health among older men and women in Ireland: A prospective community-based study. *Journal of Affective Disorders, 204*, 59–69. https://doi.org/10.1016/j.jad.2016.06.032

Scharf, T., & de Jong Gierveld, J. (2008). Loneliness in urban neighbourhoods: an Anglo-Dutch comparison. *European Journal of Ageing, 5*, 103–115. https://doi.org/10.1007/s10433-008-0080-x

Schmitz, A. (2021). Gendered experiences of widowhood and depression across Europe: The role of loneliness and financial resources from a longitudinal perspective. *Journal of Affective Disorders, 280*, 114–120. https://doi.org/10.1016/j.jad.2020.11.070

Schutter, N., Koorevaar, L., Holwerda, T. J., Stek, M. L., Dekker, J., & Comijs, H. C. (2020). 'Big Five' personality characteristics are associated with loneliness but not with social network size in older adults, irrespective of depression. *International Psychogeriatrics, 32*(1), 53–63. https://doi.org/10.1017/S1041610219000215

Seifert, A. (2025). Information and communication technologies and the risk of loneliness. In M. Aartsen, I. Precupetu, & B. Suanet (Eds.), *Macro social influences on loneliness in later life: Towards a better understanding of the loneliness paradox in later life*. Springer.

Seifert, A., & König, R. (2019). Help from and help to neighbors among older adults in Europe. *Frontiers in Sociology, 4*. https://doi.org/10.3389/fsoc.2019.00046

Seifert, A., Cotten, S. R., Xie, B., & Carr, D. (2021). A double burden of exclusion? Digital and social exclusion of older adults in times of COVID-19. *The Journals of Gerontology: Series B, 76*(3), e99–e103. https://doi.org/10.1093/geronb/gbaa098

Sheftel, M. G., Margolis, R., & Verdery, A. M. (2024). Loneliness trajectories and chronic loneliness around the world. *The Journals of Gerontology: Series B, 79*(8). https://doi.org/10.1093/geronb/gbac158

Shiovitz-Ezra, S. (2015). 15 Loneliness in Europe: Do perceived neighbourhood characteristics matter?. *Ageing in Europe: Supporting Policies for an Inclusive Society*, 169–182. doi:https://doi.org/10.1332/policypress/9781447310727.003.0015.

Silva, P., Matos, A. D., & Martinez-Pecino, R. (2022). Can the internet reduce the loneliness of 50+ living alone? *Information, Communication & Society, 25*(1), 17–33. https://doi.org/10.1080/1369118X.2020.1736128

Stickley, A., & Koyanagi, A. (2018). Physical multimorbidity and loneliness: A population-based study. *PLoS One, 13*(1), e0191651. https://doi.org/10.1371/journal.pone.0191651

Štípková, M. (2021). The impact of marital status transitions on loneliness in later life: Divorce versus widowhood. *Journal of Gerontology: Social Sciences, 76*(3), 587–599. https://doi.org/10.1093/geronb/gbaa180

Suanet, B., & Aartsen, M. (2025). Linking life course theory to multi-level explanations of loneliness: Towards a sociology of loneliness. In M. Aartsen, I. Precupetu, & B. Suanet (Eds.), *Macro social influences on loneliness in later life: Towards a better understanding of the loneliness paradox in later life*. Springer.

Sundström, G., Fransson, E., Malmberg, B., & Davey, A. (2009). Loneliness among older Europeans. *European Journal of Ageing, 6*, 267–275. https://doi.org/10.1007/s10433-009-0134-8

Susanty, S., Nadirawati, N., Setiawan, A., Haroen, H., Pebrianti, S., Harun, H., … & Banda, K. J. (2024). Overview of the prevalence of loneliness and associated risk factors among older adults across six continents: A meta-analysis. *Archives of Gerontology and Geriatrics*, 105627. https://doi.org/10.1016/j.archger.2023.105627

Tapia-Muñoz, T., Staudinger, U. M., Allel, K., Steptoe, A., Miranda-Castillo, C., Medina, J. T., & Calvo, E. (2022). Income inequality and its relationship with loneliness prevalence: A cross-sectional study among older adults in the US and 16 European countries. *PLoS One, 17*(12), e0274518. https://doi.org/10.1371/journal.pone.0274518

Tapia-Munoz, T., Ajnakina, O., Fancourt, D., & Steptoe, A. (2024). Personality traits and loneliness among older people in the UK: Cross-sectional and longitudinal analysis from the English Longitudinal Study of Ageing. *European Journal of Personality, 38*(4), 599–614. https://doi.org/10.1002/per.2447

Thomsen, D. K., Mehlsen, M. Y., Viidik, A., Sommerlund, B., & Zachariae, R. (2005). Age and gender differences in negative affect—Is there a role for emotion regulation? *Personality and Individual Differences, 38*(8), 1935–1946. https://doi.org/10.1016/j.paid.2004.12.001

Tiilikainen, E., Aartsen, M., & Kraav, S. L. (2024). Early-life circumstances and late life loneliness trajectories among Finnish older adults. *BMC Geriatrics, 24*(1), 459. https://doi.org/10.1186/s12877-024-04967-6

van Tilburg, T. G., & Fokkema, T. (2021). Stronger feelings of loneliness among Moroccan and Turkish older adults in the Netherlands: In search for an explanation. *European Journal of Ageing, 18*(3), 311–322. https://doi.org/10.1007/s10433-020-00591-2

van Tilburg, T. G., Aartsen, M. J., & van der Pas, S. (2015). Loneliness after divorce: A cohort comparison among Dutch young-old adults. *European Sociological Review, 31*(3), 243–252. https://doi.org/10.1093/esr/jcu086

Van Regenmortel, S., Tiilikainen, E., Ristolainen, H., Burholt, V., & Dahlberg, L. (2025). Social exclusion perspective on loneliness in later life. In M. Aartsen, I. Precupetu, & B. Suanet (Eds.), *Macro social influences on loneliness in later life: Towards a better understanding of the loneliness paradox in later life*. Springer.

Vasile, M., Aartsen, M., Precupetu, I., Tufă, L., Dumitrescu, D. A., & Radogna, R. M. (2024). Association between social isolation and mental well-being in later life. What is the role of loneliness? *Applied Research in Quality of Life, 19*(1), 245–267. https://doi.org/10.1007/s11482-023-10115-5

Versey, H.S., & Gibbons, J. (2024). Aging alone (while Black): Living alone, loneliness, and health among older Black women. *The Gerontologist*. https://doi.org/10.1093/geront/gnae175

Victor, C. R., & Pikhartova, J. (2020). Lonely places or lonely people? Investigating the relationship between loneliness and place of residence. *BMC Public Health, 20*, 1–12. https://doi.org/10.1186/s12889-020-08923-y

Vozikaki, M., Papadaki, A., Linardakis, M., & Philalithis, A. (2018). Loneliness among older European adults: Results from the survey of health, aging and retirement in Europe. *Journal of Public Health, 26*, 613–624. https://doi.org/10.1007/s10389-018-0896-2

Wagner, M., & Brandt, M. (2015). 16 Loneliness among informal caregivers aged 50+ in Europe. *Ageing in Europe-Supporting Policies for an Inclusive Society*, 9783110444414-018. https://doi.org/10.1515/9783110444414-018

Wagner, M., & Brandt, M. (2018). Long-term care provision and the well-being of spousal caregivers: An analysis of 138 European regions. *The Journals of Gerontology: Series B, 73*(4), e24–e34. https://doi.org/10.1093/geronb/gbx133

Wang, Y., Liu, M., Yang, F., Chen, H., Wang, Y., & Liu, J. (2024). The associations of socioeconomic status, social activities, and loneliness with depressive symptoms in adults aged 50 years and older across 24 countries: Findings from five prospective cohort studies. *The Lancet Healthy Longevity, 5*(9). https://doi.org/10.1016/S2666-7568(23)00182-5

Weiss, R. S. (1973). *Loneliness: The experience of emotional and social isolation*. MIT Press.

Wenger, G. C. (1996). Social networks and gerontology. *Reviews in Clinical Gerontology, 6*(3), 285–293. https://doi.org/10.1017/S0959259800004780

Wenger, G. C. (1997). Social networks and the prediction of elderly people at risk. *Aging & Mental Health, 1*(4), 311–320. https://doi.org/10.1080/13607869757001

Willis, P., Vickery, A., & Jessiman, T. (2022). Loneliness, social dislocation and invisibility experienced by older men who are single or living alone: Accounting for differences across sexual identity and social context. *Ageing & Society, 42*(2), 409–431. https://doi.org/10.1017/S0144686X20000803

World Economic Forum. (2024). *Global Gender Gap Report 2024*. https://www.weforum.org/publications/gender-gap-report-2024

Yang, K. (2018). Longitudinal loneliness and its risk factors among older people in England. *Canadian Journal on Aging, 37*, 12–21. https://doi.org/10.1017/S0714980817000624

Yang, K., & Victor, C. (2011). Age and loneliness in 25 European nations. *Ageing & Society, 31*(8), 1368–1388. https://doi.org/10.1017/S0144686X1000139X

Ye, L., van Grieken, A., Alhambra-Borrás, T., Zhou, S., Clough, G., Markaki, A., et al. (2024). Interplay of physical, psychological, and social frailty among community-dwelling older adults in five European countries: A longitudinal study. *Journal of Urban Health, 101*(4), 730–739. https://doi.org/10.1007/s11524-023-00707-7

Zwar, L., König, H., & Hajek, A. (2022). Are informal caregivers more likely to believe in conspiracy theories during the COVID-19 pandemic?: Findings of a representative study from Germany. *Aging & Mental Health, 27*, 588–594. https://doi.org/10.1080/13607863.2022.2102141

Sunwoo Lee, PhD, is Senior Researcher in the Faculty of Physical Culture at Palacký University Olomouc, Czech Republic. After completing her PhD from Texas A&M university in 2013, she worked as a research fellow at Charles University and Palacký University Olomouc. With over 10 years of experience in social gerontology, her research explores attitudinal and behavioral factors influencing ageing trajectories, with a focus on civic participation, sport and exercise, resilience, and positive psychology. Her current work involves developing theoretical frameworks and methodologies to apply a life-course approach to healthy ageing, aiming to better understand resilience development across life stages.

Open Access This chapter is licensed under the terms of the Creative Commons Attribution 4.0 International License (http://creativecommons.org/licenses/by/4.0/), which permits use, sharing, adaptation, distribution and reproduction in any medium or format, as long as you give appropriate credit to the original author(s) and the source, provide a link to the Creative Commons license and indicate if changes were made.

The images or other third party material in this chapter are included in the chapter's Creative Commons license, unless indicated otherwise in a credit line to the material. If material is not included in the chapter's Creative Commons license and your intended use is not permitted by statutory regulation or exceeds the permitted use, you will need to obtain permission directly from the copyright holder.

Chapter 7
The Social Infrastructure of Loneliness. A Scoping Review of Societal Influences and Their Implications

Laura Tufă

7.1 Introduction

The infrastructure of loneliness encapsulates the interplay between macro-societal factors such as social resources, economic conditions, cultural norms, technological access, urban design, and various other global phenomena, like migration, in shaping individuals' experiences of connection or isolation. Understanding this infrastructure is crucial for developing strategies aimed at alleviating loneliness within communities and at an individual level. From a theoretical perspective, adding knowledge about how macro-societal factors shape loneliness could benefit a further pool of well-designed social studies. From a policy perspective, this could beneficially impact the design of targeted policies to address interventions (Jentoft et al., 2025) that not only focus on changing behaviors, patterns, and the social interactions of individuals, but could, for example, help redesign neighborhoods and environments to deter loneliness. However, studies dealing with macro-societal influences on loneliness, while often attempting to address the importance of disentangling these effects (Fokkema et al., 2013), rarely manage to do so. That is to say, the authors try to isolate the macro-social influences, but are hindered by the limits of available data and their underlying conceptualizations. Moreover, there are sometimes varied and distinct understandings of what a macro-social factor is. For example, the understanding that some factors, generally viewed as meso-level factors (family and social connections, area and neighborhood quality, access to digital infrastructure), could, because of the way they are embedded in contextual and cultural values of a particular place at a particular time, be considered

L. Tufă (✉)
Research Institute for Quality of Life within the Romanian Academy, Bucharest, Romania

Research Institute of the University of Bucharest, Bucharest, Romania
e-mail: laura.tufa@sas.unibuc.ro

© The Author(s) 2025

M. Aartsen et al. (eds.), *Macro Social Influences on Loneliness in Later Life*, International Perspectives on Aging 47,
https://doi.org/10.1007/978-3-031-94565-6_7

macro-social level factors. Moreover, there are also "genuine macro-level factors, that is, factors that can only be conceptualized and measured at the macro-level" (Luhmann et al., 2023:19). Additionally, the use of various proxies for different aspects of the macro context limits inference on which factors are important and studying them separately can hinder the analysis of correlated factors. We also need to acknowledge that it usually takes time for loneliness to develop, which implies that studying it from a longitudinal perspective could offer greater insights into how different macro-social influences impact transitions in and out of loneliness across the life course (Ciobanu & Fokkema, 2021; Cifci, 2024) and shape particular life biographies of loneliness.

This chapter is based on a number of cross-national studies that have attempted to explain differences in the prevalence of loneliness by focusing on certain macro-level features. These attributes include a society's sociodemographic structure (Fokkema et al., 2013), social wealth and welfare regime type (Nyqvist et al., 2019), as well as generalized trust (Rapolienė & Aartsen, 2022), family (Dykstra, 2009; Luhmann et al., 2023) and social interaction norms (Jylhä & Jokela, 1990), internet availability, and a favorable opportunity structure for societal engagement (Swader & Moraru, 2023). There are also ways of gaining a comprehensive understanding of loneliness variations at the national level: either by examining the same macro-level factors in each country or by taking into account the interplay between micro and macro social factors and how they affect loneliness (Wu et al., 2022).

Expanding on this literature, the current chapter aims to comprehensively review research done on macro-social factors of loneliness and answer the following questions: (1) What are the potential macro-social influences on loneliness? (2) How are these factors empirically engaged and are there different strategies and methods employed to underline the effects of these factors? (3) What are the research gaps on macro-social factors?

7.2 Methodology

The current chapter aims to comprehensively review research on macro-social factors of loneliness through a scoping review. Scoping reviews have been used before for researching the macro-social factors that contribute to loneliness (Meehan et al., 2023), and among immigrant and older adult groups (Johnson et al., 2019). A scoping review's main goal is to map the body of research on a given subject, highlighting important ideas, knowledge gaps, and different kinds of evidence (Munn et al., 2018). The research objectives aid in narrowing down the search, even when there are varying perspectives on the existing literature. To comprehend complex issues or emerging fields where the body of existing literature may be sparse or diverse and heterogeneous, scoping reviews are intended to methodically identify and map the breadth of evidence available on a given topic (Munn et al., 2018, 2022). According to Munn et al. (2018) and Peters et al. (2021), this method enables researchers to gather a variety of data, such as primary research, reviews, giving them a thorough snapshot of the environment. This could be furthered through the selection of studies with different designs (Arksey & O'Malley, 2005).

To draw upon a wide primary range of studies, the eligibility criteria for inclusion in the current study were broad. Selected disciplines were psychology, economics, sociology, health and medical sciences, gerontology, policy, community, and urban studies. The geographical area criteria for the selected studies were that they should include European countries. While it was important that the studies address macro social influences on loneliness, there was no particular focus on a certain methodology of the eligible studies. However, it was important for loneliness to be treated as an outcome variable or in association with macro-level variables.

The search approach for this study went through several stages to make sure all pertinent reviews were included in the analysis. Web of Science, Scopus, and Google Scholar were the principal three databases through which the search was conducted. Several keywords were employed, and Boolean operators (AND, OR) were used to efficiently combine them: macro-level variables, macro-social determinants of loneliness, macro-social elements of loneliness, or macro impacts on loneliness, AND older adults/persons. The study type (original research, reviews) and language (only English) were two of the filters that were applied. The search, which was carried out between August 22, 2024, and September 2, 2024, produced a total of 6573 item-results of which 5652 items were eliminated after the titles were filtered. The remaining 921 papers in the database were additionally screened. A total of 53 publications were eliminated for select reasons, including the following: (a) they were written in a language other than English, or (b) they addressed loneliness solely as an input variable, predictor, or factor, or they focused on individual/meso-level aspects of loneliness. This left 868 studies in the database. A second search for publications was carried out between November 25, 2024, and December 13, 2024. This led to 1052 new entries into the database of which 184 were added based on the same selection criteria. Author name, title, abstract, year, key findings, and methodology were all included in the database. The domain, loneliness as a correlate or outcome, the study's conformity with the research aims, and duplicate studies that were not initially eliminated were all considered in a third screening step. After abstract screening, 866 papers were removed because they dealt with other topics. An additional search in References sections and through Connected Papers graphs for networks of citations took place between January 15, 2025, and February 16, 2025. After adding 5 more papers, the result was a total number of 191 studies. Further selection criteria focused on titles, to reflect the idea of loneliness as an outcome. Six studies that focused on interventions to alleviate loneliness, while important, didn't address the response to our questions, but rather dealt with loneliness post-hoc, so they were also removed. If loneliness was a part of collective measures of wellbeing (eight studies), but effects weren't easily identifiable, then the study was not selected. Concurrently, while many of the studies marginally mentioned loneliness as being potentially influenced by or contributing to life satisfaction, since loneliness was not the primary outcome or, in many cases, was rather a mediator or a moderator, the option was to not include them in the sample (two of such studies). A similar strategy was used in dealing with studies focused on explaining health outcomes in general, which only mentioned loneliness as a potential effect. An additional number of seven paper didn't address macro-factors.

This led to 168 studies. After removing 13 duplicates and 21 studies focused exclusively on areas outside Europe, a total of 134 studies resulted. After further screening the References section of papers considered relevant, an additional seven titles were included, resulting in a final sample of 141 papers. In-depth screening and reading of the papers using criteria related to whether macro-social factors were considered in the design led to a sample of 62 papers, after removing 79 papers (see Fig. 7.1).

7.2.1 Quality Appraisal

The methodological quality of the included research was assessed by two evaluators (the author and another trained evaluator) using the Mixed Methods Appraisal Tool (MMAT) (Hong et al., 2018) and the Critical Appraisal Skills Programme (CASP) (Long et al., 2020) for reviews as part of the quality evaluation, due to the variety of paper types (14 reviews, nine qualitative studies, 36 quantitative, and three mixed-methods).

The MMAT tool enables a more thorough review by considering important facets of study design, data collection, and analysis. The tool is a flexible and popular instrument to assess empirical studies' methodological quality critically, including mixed-methods, qualitative, and quantitative research. MMAT was used to evaluate 48 of the 62 studies and evaluated factors including the rigor of data analysis, the suitability of study design, the clarity of research questions, and the sufficiency of data collection techniques. Among the factors assessed were sample representativeness, the presence of controls for confounding variables, and measurement reliability in quantitative research. Additionally, for the sample of qualitative studies (N = 9), the suitability of the sampling plan, the techniques used for data collection, and the comprehensiveness of data analysis were evaluated. For mixed-methods studies (N = 3), the integration of qualitative and quantitative components was assessed to ensure both were appropriately addressed and integrated. As a result, one qualitative paper was eliminated from the sample.

The Critical Appraisal Skills Programme (CASP) checklist for systematic reviews evaluates important areas of the methodology of the reviews, and 14 papers were assessed using the CASP checklist. Clarity of the review's goals, the effectiveness of the search strategy, the suitability of the research selection and data extraction procedures, and the comprehensiveness of findings synthesis are the evaluation factors. Additionally, it was assessed whether the reviews sufficiently addressed potential biases and limitations and whether the data presented supported the conclusions reached. The reviews were also evaluated according to whether they sufficiently addressed potential biases and limitations and if the data presented supported the findings reached. CASP can specifically determine if research topics are well-articulated, whether thorough search techniques are employed to find pertinent

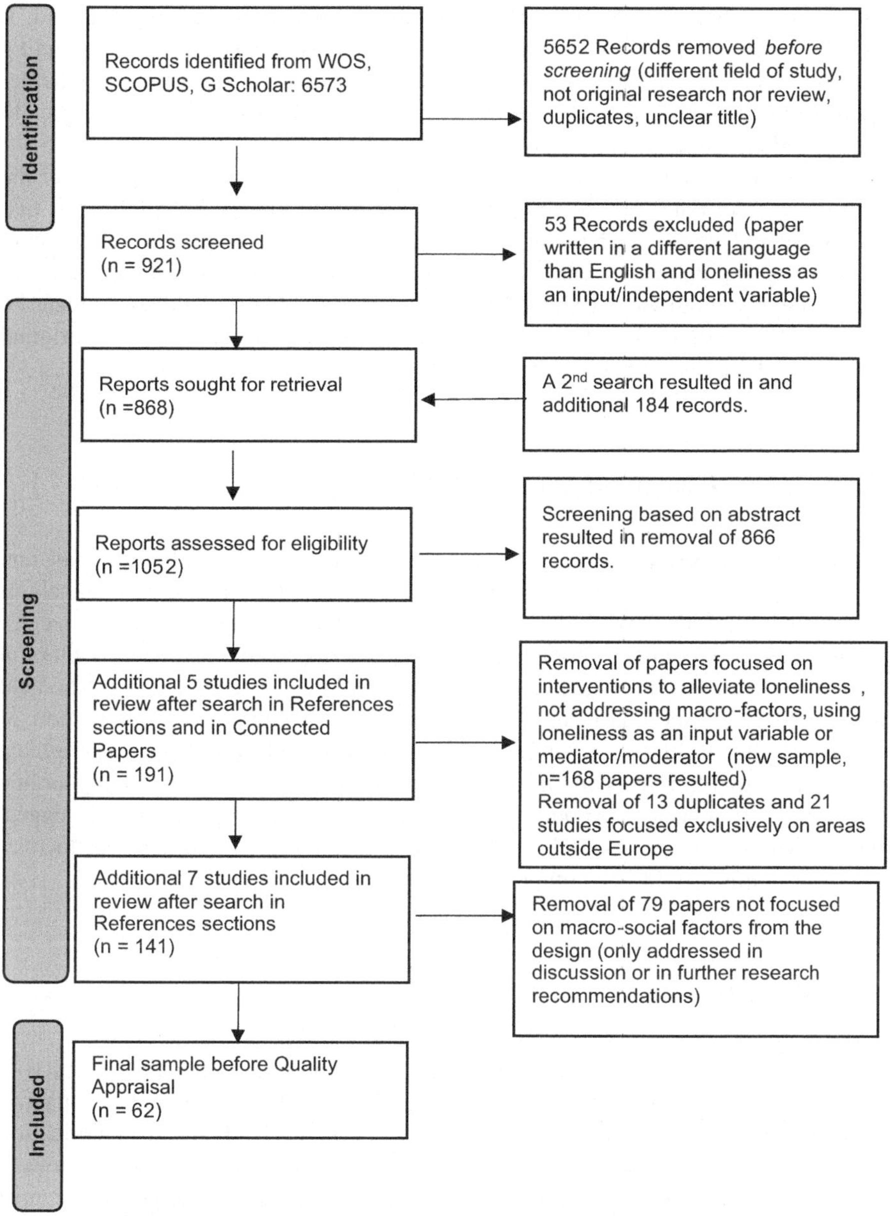

Fig. 7.1 Flowchart of search, exclusion criteria, and selection (PRISMA)

papers, and whether suitable inclusion and exclusion criteria are implemented. It can also establish if the reviews offered a clear summary of the findings, including any meta-analyses carried out. Using CASP was also useful for assessing whether the reviews considered the consequences of any methodological flaws and critically considered the implications of any limitations.

During the evaluation process, disagreements occurred for nine papers over the interpretation of data and the application of the tools' criteria. To resolve this disagreement, debates to reach consensus among reviewers were organized to compare evidence. Disagreements were logged, and each reviewer was given the chance to convey their point of view, followed by a collective analysis of the relevant material in accordance with each of the assessment tool criteria and a review of the original articles' techniques to ensure clarity.

7.2.2 Data Extraction and Analysis

The following information was collected from the studies: the author(s), goals and objectives, duration, dataset, overall design, the participants, and represented countries (see Table 7.1). Data for participants included age group and sample size. To put the results in context, a broad summary of the distribution of macro-factors in the sample was also recorded. These components were arranged in a methodical manner to enable comparisons between studies and pinpoint the distribution of influences. For instance, research conducted in different periods or geographical areas showed differences in the distribution of macro-factors, including policy effects or differences in resource access. To identify research gaps and suggest frameworks for future research that addresses understudied macro-social factors, the study synthesized these components.

7.3 Results

The following macro-social factors associated with loneliness were identified across 62 studies (Table 7.2), with their prevalence reflecting their documented impact in shaping loneliness patterns. These categorizations were based on self-identification done by cited authors, but also by own categorization, to ensure fewer categories.

Cultural values, norms, and social expectations (28 studies) emerged as the most frequently cited factor. These factors act as societal standards for social relationships that directly influence perceptions of loneliness. For example, individualistic cultures often prioritize self-reliance over communal bonds, raising expectations for personal achievement that can exacerbate feelings of inadequacy when unmet (Barrett & Mosca, 2013; Lykes & Kemmelmeier, 2014). Conversely, collectivist societies may foster stronger communal ties but also create pressures to conform to group norms, potentially isolating those who deviate (Dykstra, 2009; Rokach,

Table 7.1 Studies' characteristics (data extracted)

Author(S)	Aim(s)/Objectives	Period of the study	Dataset	Design	Participants (Sample size, age group)	Countries
Albert, I	Family Cohesion and Cultural Attachment impact on loneliness	2013–2015	IRMA	Quantitative	131 Portuguese immigrants in Luxembourg	Luxembourg
Barreto, M., Doyle, D. M., & Qualter, P.	Loneliness as a social justice issue, focus on structural conditions.	2021	Literature	State-of-the-art review	n/a	n/a
Barreto, M., Victor, C., Hammond, C., Eccles, A., Richins, M. T., & Qualter, P.	Examine the effects of culture, age, and gender on loneliness.	2018	BBC Loneliness survey	Quantitative	46,054	237 Countries & territories (UK mostly)
Barrett, A; Mosca, I	Loneliness among return migrants vs. Baseline	2009–2011	Tilda wave 1	Longitudinal Quantitative	8500+	Ireland
Buecker, S., Ebert, T., Götz, F. M., Entringer, T. M., & Luhmann, M.	Loneliness across regions in Germany.	2013	SOEP	Longitudinal Quantitative	17,602	Germany
Burholt, V.	Effects of culture on loneliness and SI in later life.	n/a	Literature	State-of-the-art review	n/a	worldwide (with a focus on Wales)

(continued)

Table 7.1 (continued)

Author(S)	Aim(s)/Objectives	Period of the study	Dataset	Design	Participants (Sample size, age group)	Countries
Cifci, F.	A conceptual framework for intergenerational loneliness trajectories	n/a	Literature	State-of-the-art review	n/a	n/a
Ciobanu, RO; Fokkema, T	Investigate role of religion on loneliness mitigation among migrants.	2013–2014	established Romanian migrants	Qualitative	27 older Romanian migrants	Switzerland
Ciobanu, RO; Fokkema, T	A life course analysis on "what protects Romanian migrants from loneliness"	2013–2014	established Romanian migrants	Qualitative	21 older Romanian migrants	Switzerland
Cohen-Mansfield, J., Hazan, H., Lerman, Y., & Shalom, V.	Identify predictors & correlates of loneliness through review & panels	n/a + 2012	Literature	Mixed methods	2 panels, 25 participants total	Israel (panels)
Cotterell, N., Buffel, T., Nazroo, J., & Qualter, P.	Loneliness and life course disadvantage in older ethnic minorities	2019	structured Interviews	Qualitative	17	UK
Dahlberg, L.	A critique of studies on older adult loneliness during the COVID-19 pandemic	2021	n/a	State-of-the-art review	n/a	n/a
de Jong Gierveld, J., & Tesch-Römer, C.	An integrated theoretical framework for east/west European old age loneliness differences	n/a	Literature	Theoretical Framework (review)	n/a	n/a

de Jong Gierveld, J., Dykstra, P. A., & Schenk, N.	Differentiating support types in east/west European intergenerational living	2004–2012	GGS-I wave 1	Quantitative		
Delaruelle, K	Migration-related inequalities in loneliness in Europe	2010–2014	ESS waves 5,6,7	Quantitative	121,835	26 countries
Doblas, J. L., Palomares-Linares, I., & Martínez, M. S.	How the prevalence of loneliness (and its correlates) varies between four South European countries	2015	SHARE	Quantitative		Spain, Italy, Greece, Portugal
Doyle, D. M., Qualter, P., Victor, C., & Barreto, M.	Social stigma against older/younger LGB persons and how it correlates to loneliness	n/a	Sample of LGB persons	Quantitative	7000	113 Countries
Dykstra, P. A.	A systematic analysis on several "myths" ad realities about older adult loneliness	2009	Literature	State-of-the-art review	n/a	n/a
Fernández-Carro, C; Lao, JG	A longitudinal analysis of the factors leading to late life loneliness, with a focus on older women	2009–2013, 2017	SHARE	Longitudinal Quantitative	10,615	EU
Fokkema, T; Naderi, R	Loneliness among Turkish migrants in Germany vs. Natives	2005–2008	GGS	Quantitative	3248 Germans,494 Turks	Germany

(continued)

Table 7.1 (continued)

Author(S)	Aim(s)/Objectives	Period of the study	Dataset	Design	Participants (Sample size, age group)	Countries
Fokkema, T., Gierveld, J. D. J., & Dykstra, P. A.	A cross-national analysis of differences in older adult loneliness	2008	SHARE Wave 2	Quantitative	12,248 50+ adults	EU
Goldman, N., Khanna, D., El Asmar, M. L., Qualter, P., & El-Osta, A.	A scoping review of national policies for addressing loneliness and social isolation		Policy Documents	Qualitative	23 policy documents	52 Countries
Hansen, T; Slagsvold, B	identify sources of country differences in late-life loneliness in west/north and eastern Europe	2004–2011	GGS	Quantitative	33,832	11 countries
Hansen, T., Kafková, M. P., Katz, R., Lowenstein, A., Naim, S., Pavlidis, G., ... & Aartsen, M.E	Chart micro/macro-level patterns and correlations in later-life ESR across Europe	2011–2015	SHARE Wave 4, 6	Quantitative	6558 men, 9795 women	EU
Heu, L. C., Hansen, N., van Zomeren, M., Levy, A., Ivanova, T. T., Gangadhar, A., & Radwan, M.	Investigate loneliness across cultures in a qualitative approach	2017	42 semi-structured Interviews	Qualitative	42	Austria, Bulgaria, Israel, Egypt, India

Heu, L. C., van Zomeren, M., & Hansen, N.	The articles offers a novel framework between culture and loneliness and supports it with data	2006+	Literature & ESS Round 3	Mixed methods	n/a	EU
Horn, V., & Fokkema, T.	An analysis of older migrants needs with recommendations for multi-level intervention	2013–2016	IAB-BAMF-SOEP wave 1,2	Quantitative	958	Germany
Hunter, A	An analytical framework for understanding inequalities among aging among older migrants	n/a	Literature	Theoretical Framework (review)	n/a	n/a
Jentoft, E. E., Sandset, T., & Haldar, M.	An analysis of British policy documents problematizing loneliness as a public health issue	2016–2021	Policy Documents	Quantitative	20 documents	UK
Jentoft, E. E.	A discourse analysis study focused on lonely older adults and technological mitigation measures for loneliness	2017–2021	100 Documents including 13 strategies	Qualitative	n/a	UK

(continued)

Table 7.1 (continued)

Author(S)	Aim(s)/Objectives	Period of the study	Dataset	Design	Participants (Sample size, age group)	Countries
Joshi, M., Finney, N., & Hale, J. M.	A scoping review of loneliness among older adults of immigrant and minority background	2021	Literature	State-of-the-art review	73 + 3 studies	n/a
Jylhä, M., & Jokela, J.	A classic study charting loneliness in a cross-cultural manner	1986	Eleven Country Study on Health Care of the Elderly	Quantitative	6 regions, varied no of respondents per region	Finland, West Berlin, Greece, Yugoslavia, Italy
King, R; Cela, E; Fokkema, T; Vullnetari, J	Loneliness and trans-generational care among older Albanians	2002–2013	Interviews	Qualitative	First generation-migrants and Zero generation, parents and grandparents left behind migration of younger cohorts	Albania, Greece
Klok, J; van Tilburg, TG; Suanet, B; Fokkema, T; Huisman, M	Belonging as a protective mechanism against loneliness among migrants in the Netherlands	2013–2014	Quantitative, Longitudinal Aging Study Amsterdam (LASA)	Quantitative Longitudinal	269 Turks, 202 Moroccans	Netherlands
Langenkamp, A., Mund, M., & Hawkley, L. T	An analysis of three country-level characteristics which explain cross-national disparities in loneliness	2012	ESS, EUROSTAT	Quantitative	45,042	EU and other European countries

Luhmann, M., Buecker, S., & Rüsberg, M.	An analysis of loneliness focusing on time and space differences focusing on four groups of predictors	2023	n/a	state-of-the-art review	n/a	n/a
Lykes, V. A., & Kemmelmeier, M.	Loneliness as a function of cultural values	1992, 2006	ESS, Eurobarometer	Quantitative	1992 Eurobarometer; N = 3902 and 2006 European Social Survey, N = 38,867	12 (1992) 22(2006) European societies
Meehan, D. E., Grunseit, A., Condie, J., HaGani, N., & Merom, D.	A scoping review of loneliness among older adults focused on social- ecological predictors	n/a	52 studies	Meta-analysis	n/a	n/a
Mohan, G., & Lyons, S.	A study linking comparing of life and loneliness with high-speed internet availability in Ireland	2018	TILDA	Quantitative	2674 geopositioned out of 3416 investigated	Ireland
Morgan, D., Dahlberg, L., Waldegrave, C., Mikulionienė, S., Rapolienė, G., Lamura, G., & Aartsen, M.	A study of micro and macro-level correlates for ESL	2013–2015	SHARE Wave 5, 6, Eurobarometer, ESS	Quantitative	52,562 at W5 39,628 at W6	EU

(continued)

Table 7.1 (continued)

Author(S)	Aim(s)/Objectives	Period of the study	Dataset	Design	Participants (Sample size, age group)	Countries
Neves, BB; Petersen, A	Understanding the stigma of late life loneliness	2018–2020	Two separate qualitative projects	Qualitative	22 residents of care homes (2018) 35 individuals (2020)	Australia
Newmyer, L., Verdery, A. M., Wang, H., & Margolis, R.	A complex modelling of the potential old age "tide" of loneliness coming with demographic aging	unclear	SHARE, CHARLS, ELSA, HART, HRS, TILDA, IFLS, KLoSA, MHAS	Quantitative	199,644 total	27 countries including most EU, China, US, Mexico, Korea etc.
Nyqvist, F; Nygård, M; Scharf, T	A comparative study of European welfare regimes as relating to loneliness	2014	ESS wave 7	Quantitative	11,389	20 countries
Rapolienė, G., & Aartsen. M.	An analysis of loneliness relating to low levels of trust in "post totalitarian" European countries	2012	ESS wave 6	Quantitative	12,042 of which 4827 from "post totalitarian countries"	29 countries 12 "post totalitarian"
Reine, I., Miķelsone, M., Tomsone, S., Guðmundsson, H., Ivanovs. A., Guðmundsson, H. S., & Koroļeva, I.	Post-covid study on loneliness and financial wellbeing in Nordic and Baltic countries	2020	SHARE wave 8, HL20	Quantitative	5313 participants 2377 - Sweden, Denmark, and Finland 2936 Estonia, Latvia, and Lithuania.	Iceland, Sweden, Denmark, Finland, Estonia, Latvia, Lithuania
Rokach, A.	A review of the effects of gender and culture on loneliness	n/a	Literature	state-of-the-art review	n/a	n/a

Ruan, Y. X., & Cheung, M. C.	A systematic review of articles dealing with loneliness in older adult migrants	2024	35 studies	Meta-analysis	n/a	n/a
Shiovitz-Ezra, S., Shemesh, J., & McDonnell/ Naughton, M.	An analysis of the links between ageism and loneliness	n/a	Literature	State-of-the-art review	n/a	n/a
Sundström, G; Fransson, E; Malmberg, B; Davey, A	Replication of earlier cross-cultural loneliness studies - Loneliness more prevalent in Southern Europe	2004–2006	SHARE	Quantitative	8787	Europe
Surkalim, D. L., Luo, M., Eres, R., Gebel, K., Van Buskirk, J., Bauman, A., & Ding, D.	A broad meta-analysis of loneliness prevalence		57 studies	Meta-analysis	n/a	113 Countries and territories
Swader, C. S.	This article explains perceived loneliness among people in Europe by accounting for cultural factors as well as social isolation.	2014	ESS wave 7	Quantitative	36,760	21 countries

(continued)

Table 7.1 (continued)

Author(S)	Aim(s)/Objectives	Period of the study	Dataset	Design	Participants (Sample size, age group)	Countries
Swader, C. S., & Moraru, A. V.	An analysis of the ways in which social infrastructure alleviates loneliness	2014	ESS wave 7 + others	Mixed methods	unclear due to QCA	26 countries
Taniguchi, H., & Kaufman, G.	An analysis of how "collectivism" and "individualism" affect loneliness from a cross-country perspective	2017	ISSP Social Networks and Social Resources	Quantitative	44,492	29 countries
Tapia-Muñoz, T., Staudinger, U. M., Allel, K., Steptoe, A., Miranda-Castillo, C., Medina, J. T., & Calvo, E.	A look at how the GINI coefficient relates to loneliness prevalence	2013–2014	HRS, ELSA, SHARE	Quantitative	75,891	15 EU countries, England, US
van den Broek, T., & Tosi, M.	An analysis on whether more children lead to less loneliness in eastern Europe	2004–2012	GGS-I Wave 1	Quantitative	25,479 parents aged 50–80	Bulgaria, Czechia, Estonia, Georgia, Lithuania, Poland, Romania, Russia
van Tilburg, T., Havens, B., & de Jong Gierveld, J.	A classic study on differences in the type of loneliness in different cultures	1992–1996	three studies	Quantitative	3543 (all samples)	Canada, Italy, Netherlands

Victor, C. R., Burholt, V., & Martin, W.	An exploratory study with confirmation on loneliness among ethnic minority elders in the UK	2001–2002	two studies	Quantitative	300 elderly migrants 169 elderly east-Asians	UK
Wagner, M., & Brandt, M.	Loneliness among informal caregivers aged 50+ in Europe.	2012	SHARE	Quantitative	3633/50,797	Europe
Wu, J., Zhang, J., & Fokkema, T.	A comparative study of data from Europe and China on the interplay between macro factors and micro	2012	SHARE, CHARLS	Quantitative	62,084	Europe, China
Yang, K.	An intersectional approach to loneliness	2014	ESS	Quantitative	2252	UK
Zoutewelle-Terovan, Mioara; Liefbroer, Aart Cornelis	A look at links between adulthood events and loneliness later in life	2004–2012	GGS-I Wave 1	Quantitative	61,082	12 European countries

Table 7.2 Macro-social factors

Macro factor	Number of studies
Cultural values, norms, and expectations	28
Welfare spending/state/generosity	16
Migration	15
Structural and institutional discrimination	7
Opportunity structure for societal participation/ for social networks	7
Social exclusion	7
Sociodemographic composition of society	5
Ageism	4
Digitalization and digital exclusion	4
Economic factors/Income inequality	3
Fertility and demographic change	3
Societal trust	2
Religiosity	1
COVID-19 restrictions, measures and policy changes	1

2018). Migration (15 studies) and structural discrimination (7 studies) highlight systemic barriers to social integration. Migrants often face language barriers, cultural dissonance, and exclusionary policies that limit access to social networks (Goldman et al., 2024). Discrimination—whether based on race, ethnicity, or socioeconomic status—can further affect migrants' loneliness (Horn & Fokkema, 2023). Welfare spending and state generosity (16 studies) demonstrate how institutional support buffers loneliness risks. Economic factors and income inequality (3 studies) reveal how wealth disparities might influence loneliness. Opportunity structures for societal participation (7 studies) and the sociodemographic composition of the society (5 studies) underscore how societal frameworks shape social engagement. Ageism (4 studies) and social exclusion (7 studies) reflect systemic marginalization of older adults. Digitalization (3 studies) presents a twofold influence, while at the same time changing the very nature of social interactions (Luhmann et al., 2023). Older adults are seen as being the beneficiaries of technology enabled remote connections (Jentoft, 2023), while over-reliance on digital platforms can deepen isolation for those lacking digital literacy or preferring in-person interactions. Demographic shifts (3 studies), including low fertility rates and aging populations, can alter support systems. Smaller families and increased longevity may leave older adults without immediate caregivers and social relationships in their immediate environment, heightening reliance on formal services that often lack the intimacy of familial bonds. Finally, COVID-19 restrictions (1 study) and societal trust (2 studies) illustrate acute and chronic influences. Pandemic lockdowns disrupted routines, while low societal trust—often linked to inequality or having a totalitarian past at the country-level reduces willingness to engage with others, perpetuating loneliness (Rapolienė & Aartsen, 2022).

7.3.1 Cultural Values, Norms, and Expectations

Cultural norms significantly influence loneliness across societies. The norm deviations and loneliness (NoDeL) framework suggests that individuals who deviate from social norms are at higher risk of loneliness due to factors like alienation and social rejection (Heu, 2023). The culture-loneliness framework proposes that restrictive relationship norms may protect against physical isolation but increase emotional and perceived isolation (Heu et al., 2021a). Cultural norms about individual choice in relationships also play a role, with higher relational mobility associated with lower loneliness, while lower relational stability may increase loneliness risk (Heu et al., 2021b). Loneliness is characterized by an undesired absence of reciprocal empathic understanding across cultures, with cultural meanings shaping expectations of closeness and social connectedness (Burholt, 2023). Both individualist and communal cultures can exhibit a "culture of loneliness," albeit of different kinds (van Staden & Coetzee, 2010). These findings highlight the complex interplay between cultural norms and loneliness experiences (Reine et al., 2024).

The study of how cultural norms and social expectations affect loneliness is quite disparate and spread out in the literature. Most of the studies focus on cultural norms around individualism or collectivism (Swader, 2019; Barreto et al., 2021; Taniguchi & Kaufman, 2022; Dahlberg et al., 2022). Research focusing on other cultural norms apart from cultural individualism, is scarce (Langenkamp et al., 2024), with few mentions that look also at how materialism might affect loneliness (Luhmann et al., 2023). Few studies on cultural pluralism exist (Langenkamp et al., 2024), and even fewer were found that focus on norms around ageing and intergenerational interactions (Albert, 2021). This is somewhat paradoxical, since many studies in the literature examining loneliness are concerned with older age groups (Langenkamp et al., 2024). Moreover, discussions of the limitations that stem from not considering interactions between macro-level factors stemming from the same domain (for example interactions between cultural individualism/pluralism/collectivism and cultural expectations around ageing) or from different domains (e.g. digitalization and individualistic cultures), while mentioned in several studies (Hunter, 2018; Luhmann et al., 2023; Langenkamp et al., 2024), are not routinely addressed. This individualization of research on loneliness points to larger issues related to the social reproduction of stigma in neoliberal contexts, where individualistic values thrive (Barreto et al., 2024). For a theoretical exploration of how cultural factors impact on loneliness, see also Chap. 3 of this book (van Tilburg, 2025).

7.3.2 Welfare State Generosity

Welfare state generosity is one of the most frequently investigated macro-social level influences on loneliness (Barreto et al., 2024; de Jong Gierveld & Tesch-Römer, 2012), with 15 out of 62 studies pointing to various degrees and different ways that various mechanisms embedded in welfare spending could reduce loneliness (Swader & Moraru, 2023; Barreto et al., 2024). It has been demonstrated that the generosity of the welfare state, especially through public spending on welfare and old-age pensions, considerably lowers the chance of loneliness among older people (Wu et al., 2022). In welfare systems characterized by greater generosity, such as those found in Nordic countries, older adults exhibit reduced dependence on personal resources to address loneliness, owing to their access to social services and benefits (Sundström et al., 2009; Fokkema et al., 2013; Nyqvist et al., 2019; Hansen et al., 2021). In contrast, in regions with less generous welfare provisions, such as Southern and Eastern Europe, there tends to be a higher prevalence of loneliness, as individuals often rely more significantly on familial and social connections (Fokkema et al., 2013; Nyqvist et al., 2019). Eastern European countries, despite having strong types of social integration mostly in family convoys, have higher scores on loneliness compared to Western countries (de Jong Gierveld & Tesch-Römer, 2012). This is due to the fact that substantial welfare provisions can improve social integration by giving people access to social services and benefits that enable them to build and sustain social networks without being unduly hampered by necessities like shelter, food, and medical care (Barreto et al., 2024) and without bearing the burden of mixing financial needs with family obligations (de Jong Gierveld & Tesch-Römer, 2012; Wagner & Brandt, 2015; Preoteasa et al., 2018). However, while research mostly presents homogeneity across a particular welfare regime, intra-welfare regime variability is addressed less often. According to more recent research Southern European countries exhibit distinct patterns in loneliness, while others share similarities with central and northern European trends (Doblas et al., 2020).

There are three different narratives around welfare spending influences on loneliness. First, there are studies where the main focus is on the individual and meso-level influences, while structural factors offer context for interpretation of the results (de Jong Gierveld et al., 2012; Fokkema et al., 2013; Hansen & Slagsvold, 2016). Second, the societal factors are integrated in the research design (de Jong Gierveld & Tesch-Römer, 2012; Fokkema et al., 2013; Hansen et al., 2021), using proxies like social expenditure as percentage of GDP (de Jong Gierveld & Tesch-Römer, 2012; Wu et al., 2022) and recommendations pointing cautiously to consider how individual-level factors play out in different welfare spending regimes (de Jong Gierveld & Tesch-Römer, 2012; Wu et al., 2022). Third, societal factors are presented as the most important factors, while this approach is also complemented by an underlying critique of the way most of the studies can in fact, despite good intentions, obscure the role of societal factors through a rather narrow focus in individual-level factors (Barreto et al., 2024). A newly considered focus is how loneliness can be influenced by access to welfare entitlements in more than one country (Hunter, 2018).

7.3.3 Migration

One of these principal directions of investigation is the impact of displacement and migration on loneliness, including the impact of specific integration policies. Migration can convey loneliness twofold: either for those who migrate in the destination countries (Fokkema et al., 2013; Fokkema & Naderi, 2013; Klok et al., 2017) or for those left behind, so-called "orphaned pensioners" (King et al., 2014). International migration affects opportunities and constraints for older persons to connect in their new environments (Fokkema et al., 2013; Joshi et al., 2024), but also in their origin countries, potentially leading to a transnational sense of not belonging, affecting loneliness (Klok et al., 2017). Klok et al. (2017) highlight that the concept of belonging shapes different outcomes, such as assimilation, integration, separation, or marginalization- in the context of integration policies for migrants. These outcomes evolve over time and are influenced by what other researchers use to explain cross-national differences in loneliness distribution: the cultural pluralism orientation (Langenkamp et al., 2024), or the acceptance of different lifestyles. In essence, belonging not only drives integration policy development, but also interacts with cultural pluralism to shape societal experiences of loneliness. A strong sense of belonging to one's own group (separation) is equally effective against loneliness as integration (or assimilation) (Klok et al., 2017). Additionally, the experience of displacement as a refugee often leads to increased loneliness, primarily due to insufficient preparation for both the displaced individuals and the societies or communities receiving them (Rüdel & Joly, 2024). First-generation migrants who arrived after the age of 18 report more loneliness in comparison to those who migrated earlier, while at the same time those of the second-generation report less loneliness, which could reflect the better integration policies that were introduced later and mainly impacted the later-born migrants (Delaruelle, 2023). Furthermore, migrants from cultures with greater relational mobility may feel less lonely in host societies with similar features (Heu et al., 2021b). These findings illustrate the complicated relationship between migration and loneliness. Interestingly, countries with more positive opinions toward immigrants may have wider loneliness disparities, indicating complicated societal processes (Delaruelle, 2023).

7.3.4 Structural and Institutional Discrimination

Studies focusing on older individuals with a migratory background typically emphasize structural and institutional discrimination (Horn & Fokkema, 2023). By creating obstacles to social integration and sustaining feelings of exclusion, structural and institutional discrimination is somewhat elusively identified as a macro-social latent factor by various authors (Yang, 2023; Barreto et al., 2023, 2024), a factor that strongly influences loneliness in later life. When older persons encounter institutional discrimination, such as when they are treated unjustly in the workplace, housing market, or healthcare system, they frequently feel increased stress and fewer possibilities for meaningful social engagement. Additionally, age-related difficulties frequently overlap with disadvantaged identities, exacerbating the negative impacts of discrimination on loneliness (Neves & Petersen, 2025). Ageism and racial/ethnic discrimination, for instance, can be twin burdens for older persons from minority groups, making them feel even more excluded. Such encounters may cause people to lose faith in peers and institutions, which further distances them from possible support networks. During more conservative political eras, these groups could experience higher degrees of discrimination, which might greatly raise their likelihood of loneliness (Luhmann et al., 2023). More progressive eras, on the other hand, frequently offer a more welcoming atmosphere, which lessens this possibility (Luhmann et al., 2023).

7.3.5 Opportunity Structure for Societal Participation

Research indicates that older individuals with fewer children often experience higher levels of loneliness and social isolation due to diminished familial ties and support networks (Diaz-Venegaz et al., 2017). In Southern and Eastern Europe, strong familial ties traditionally mitigate feelings of loneliness; however, when these support systems weaken, older adults may experience heightened isolation (Sandu et al., 2022). However, the effects of declining fertility differ across cohorts. For instance, younger cohorts (born after 1937) tend to benefit from lower fertility in terms of fewer depressive symptoms and better health outcomes. Conversely, older cohorts (born in 1937 or earlier) may experience negative economic impacts due to fewer children to provide support (Hansen & Slagsvold, 2016). In any case, the decline in family size correlates with increased loneliness among older adults (Cohen-Mansfield et al., 2016). In regions with high widowhood rates and fewer children, seniors often find themselves without close family members nearby, exacerbating feelings of loneliness. This is evident particularly in Eastern Europe, where socioeconomic factors further compound the issue, leading to higher vulnerability among seniors, particularly for women in Eastern Europe (van den Broek & Tosi, 2020). But older adults in Eastern Europe reported higher instances of loneliness even when co-residential arrangements were in place (de Jong Gierveld & Tesch-Römer, 2012) highlighting that proxies such as co-habitation might fail to account for cultural and contextual factors influencing social integration and emotional well-being. Proxy indicators (socio economic status, health, network size) nonetheless remain a contentious topic, studies employing proxies may inadvertently promote policy responses that are ineffective or misaligned with the actual needs of older adults.

7.3.6 Social Exclusion

Social exclusion linked to loneliness in a total of seven papers with broad methodological approaches (see also Chap. 4 of this book; Van Regenmortel et al, 2025). Barreto et al. argue for a focus away from individual predictors and towards a social-justice centric view of loneliness focused on factors such as "cultural hegemony" (Barreto et al., 2024), discriminatory practices and deprivation that signal social exclusion, the main argument being that this would also lead to better ways of tackling it. Loneliness is treated as resulting from a cumulation of disadvantages among older migrants in the UK (Cotterell et al., 2025; Victor et al., 2012). It is also tracked as an interplay between country specific stigma and young/old differences in social capital among sexual minorities across 113 countries (Doyle et al., 2022). Social exclusion is a significant result in both cases. Exclusion from social relations is the primary concern in the work of Hansen and colleagues, which chart loneliness as one of the dimensions of social exclusion across their European sample (Hansen et al., 2021). Fernández-Carro and Gumà Lao (2022) have a different approach, looking at the life-courses of older women and the predictive background factors (education, family) which correlate with loneliness and exclusion in later life, transcending the meso- or individual level. At a larger, literature corpus scale, Ruan and Cheung do a thorough and systematic review of these factors which lead to loneliness among older adult migrants (Ruan & Cheung, 2024) and list social exclusion by way of social barriers to participation among the factors. The authors are dissatisfied with the current state of the literature and call for more "longitudinal studies with a rigorous design" on migrant loneliness and a general moving away from one-item questions.

7.3.7 Sociodemographic Composition of Society

Five studies tackle the link between the sociodemographic composition of society and loneliness, with a focus on the loneliness of older adults. A study of Portuguese migrants in Luxembourg (Albert, 2021) deals heavily with acculturative stress and the issue of intergenerational belonging as impacting loneliness and highlights that experiencing challenges in balancing multiple cultural identities appears to be a key factor contributing to feelings of loneliness among migrants. Regional differences can also be predictors of loneliness (Buecker et al., 2021) especially when looking at countries with a powerful regional divide (as is the case of Germany). Demographic differences, be they across regions (Buecker et al., 2021) or different European societies (de Jong Gierveld & Tesch-Römer, 2012) can have significant impact even in cases when all other factors are equal. Loneliness here is seen as a derived outcome, one resulting from the interplay between individual level factors and macro-level demographic predictors. De Jong Gierveld and Tesch-Römer (2012) suggest that a person without children may experience greater loneliness in a society where having children is common, compared to someone living in a society where childlessness is more prevalent and accepted. This implies that the social context of childlessness can significantly influence feelings of loneliness (Zoutewelle-Terovan & Liefbroer, 2018). Demographic differences and adult child interactions make the object of another study (de Jong Gierveld et al., 2012) that investigates loneliness among coresident households. Finally, current trends of sociodemographic change are raising an alarm on the future prevalence of loneliness (Newmyer et al., 2022) as global populations and the "demographic metabolism" continues to age. Most papers in this category look at evolving societies and thus many limitations are based on the amount of sociodemographic data.

7.3.8 Ageism

Societal ageism contributes to loneliness through social rejection, self-embodiment of stereotypes, and social exclusion (Shiovitz-Ezra et al., 2018) but there are a host of other associated factors, like lack of intergenerational interactions, as well as public reproduction of ageist stereotypes against older individuals (Dykstra, 2009). Older and younger people are physically, culturally, and institutionally separated, which limits their ability to build enduring relationships with people of different ages. Negative associations were identified between perceptions of ageism and loneliness (Meehan et al., 2023), moreover since loneliness stigma is particularly more present for older individuals (Neves & Petersen, 2025). Digital barriers and ageism could particularly lead to new forms of exclusion based on sociotechnological ageism (Neeves et al., 2023) the representation of older individuals as being less technologically savvy and less flexible in acquiring digital skills, a form of ageism that goes beyond digital ageism, as it is rooted in common misconceptions about older people's capacity or willingness to engage with emerging technologies, alongside broader societal views on aging (Neeves et al., 2023).

7.3.9 Digitalization and Digital Exclusion

Digitalization (as in the degree of its spread), accessibility and the use of digital technology in everyday life influence loneliness across countries (Luhmann et al., 2023; Swader & Moraru, 2023; Langenkamp et al., 2024). Macro-level factors related to digitalization usually relate to infrastructure—the spread of digital infrastructure, the availability of broadband and expansions to digital services particularly catering to older-age users (Langenkamp et al., 2024). There is, however, little direct impact on loneliness (Mohan & Lyons, 2024). Technology can both alleviate and exacerbate loneliness, a complex phenomenon labelled in literature as *the dual role of technology* (Long et al., 2024). Technology provides the tools for maintaining social connections, but studies show it can also lead to unsatisfactory interactions and increased isolation if not balanced with in-person connections (Long et al., 2024; Jentoft, 2023). In more collectivist societies, where social relationships are highly valued, digital technologies may be used to enhance existing social connections, potentially reducing loneliness. In contrast, individualist cultures might see digital tools as a substitute for in-person interactions and therefore attract stigma, which could exacerbate loneliness (Heu et al., 2021a). The pace and distribution of digital transitions influences how individuals develop digital competencies and adopt various technologies. The shift towards digital services can exacerbate loneliness for those who lack access to or are uncomfortable using technology, leading to digital exclusion (Jentoft, 2023).

Digital exclusion, particularly among older persons, exacerbates loneliness by cutting people off from important social contacts and services (see also Chap. 8 of this book; Seifert, 2025). As technology becomes more integrated into daily life, those without access are left behind, experiencing more social isolation. Older persons frequently lack digital literacy or resources to interact with digital technology, resulting in exclusion from online communities and services that could otherwise give support and connection (Lu et al., 2024). The pivot to digital services means that physical locations where seniors used to socialize, such as markets and community centers, are closing or becoming less important, perhaps isolating them even further. If digital regulations are not carefully constructed, they may accidentally exacerbate loneliness. For example, a "digital by default" approach to service delivery may exclude those who lack digital skills thus making them dependent on others for basic needs (Moroney & Jarvis, 2020). Moreover, while digital interventions like video conferencing can reduce loneliness, they require access to technology and internet, which many individuals in late life could lack (Welch et al., 2023).

Policies often prioritize market-driven solutions over public services, which can widen the digital divide. Older adults, in particular, may face barriers to accessing digital technologies due to cost or lack of skills, further isolating them from social networks (Jentoft, 2023). This exclusion can be exacerbated by policies that rely heavily on digital solutions without addressing underlying inequalities. There are several research gaps that can be highlighted. While plenty of studies focus on individual use, individual digital competency and other individual-level factors (Xu & Köttl, 2020), as well as meso-level interventions (various technological interventions, such as ICTs, social media, telecare systems, and assistive robots, have been found to mitigate feelings of hopelessness and alienation among older groups), country-level or other macro-level factors like digital exclusion are lacking in their assessment of impact on loneliness.

7.3.10 Economic Factors/Income Inequality

Economic factors and income inequality significantly influence loneliness in old age, particularly through income inequality and welfare generosity. Because of weakened social cohesion and trust, older persons in more unequal countries are more prone to experience loneliness (Tapia-Muñoz et al., 2022; Wu et al., 2022). A lower socioeconomic status makes it more difficult to afford social interactions, which exacerbates loneliness. People with low income are systematically lonelier than other socio-economic groups (Niedzwiedz et al., 2016; Beller, 2024). Economic disparities also impact access to social activities and support networks, heightening feelings of isolation. Studies have shown that in more income-unequal societies, individual socioeconomic status has a stronger effect on late-life loneliness, while in more welfare-generous societies, this effect is weaker (Wu et al., 2022). Income inequality erodes social cohesion and trust, exacerbating feelings of loneliness among older adults with lower socioeconomic status. Income inequality specifically affects loneliness by creating a sense of relative deprivation, where individuals feel excluded and undervalued compared to their more affluent counterparts. This perception can lead to stress and social disengagement, increasing the likelihood of loneliness.

7.3.11 Fertility and Demographic Change

Research suggests a complex relationship between fertility rates and loneliness in older adults, influenced by various social, economic, and health factors. As fertility rates decline globally, particularly in developed countries, the implications for older adults' social structures and emotional well-being become increasingly significant. This is supported by findings that societal fertility rates are negatively correlated with suicide rates among the elderly, which may be linked to social integration (Shah, 2008). However, some studies indicate that reduced fertility doesn't necessarily lead to greater isolation in old age, as support networks may shift from offspring to other relatives or friends (Marcil-Gratton & Légaré, 1992). Social isolation, which can be influenced by factors such as living alone, being unmarried, and lack of participation in social activities, is significantly associated with increased loneliness in older adults (Taylor, 2020). Lower fertility rates lead to smaller family sizes, which can reduce the availability of immediate family support for older adults.

General decreases in fertility and in the number of children across the globe lead invariably to smaller cohorts of children and thus to an increase in old-age loneliness for parents and other aging family members. There are, however, contradictory models with some studies showing a shift of support networks away from family and towards friends or neighbors (Marcil-Gratton & Légaré, 1992). Loneliness is also greatly impacted by national and regional social models. Older adults in Eastern Europe were lonelier despite co-habiting more than those in the West. Family ties in Southern and Eastern Europe mitigate feelings of loneliness associated with aging. Yet broad proxy models centered around social network size or health cannot explain loneliness without oversimplifying complex social phenomena, which can in turn lead to poor interventions with little to no impact.

7.3.12 Societal Trust

The level of trust in a society was identified as a major factor in relation to loneliness in two of the studies included. Rapolienė and Aartsen focus on societal trust at a macro-level to explain the higher loneliness prevalence in Eastern Europe (Rapolienė & Aartsen, 2022). Singling out the impact of totalitarianism on interpersonal and systemic trust they control for most individual factors and find a link between higher loneliness prevalence and low trust in others through social disengagement. The authors do acknowledge that there could be alternative explanations mediating the relationship. Trust is also taken into account at a macro-social level in another landmark study from 2021, focusing on exclusion from social relations, with loneliness as one of the social exclusion dimensions (Hansen et al., 2021). The findings show that higher interpersonal trust is linked to lower loneliness and increased participation and the authors once again single out the case of Eastern Europe.

7.3.13 Religiosity

Religiosity appeared as a factor related to loneliness (or rather protection from loneliness) in two different studies from the same authors. In their study, Ciobanu and Fokkema looked at a qualitative sample of Romanian migrants to Switzerland. Despite the heterogeneity of their sample the authors find that many of the people interviewed are religious and attend church, while not reporting any feelings of loneliness. Apart from individual aspects like faith "sustaining" Romanian migrants they find that "Through its cultural and historical meaning, the church also recreates a familiar space, thus providing the participants with a feeling of belonging" (Ciobanu & Fokkema, 2020). The nature of the Romanian Orthodox Church as de-facto national proxy for "Romanian-ness" means that "the church recreates a safe and identifiable milieu" mediating this belonging. Despite this cross-national social aspect of Romanian religiosity and its impact on feelings of belonging (and thus not being lonely) the authors acknowledge their rather small sample of respondents and urge further, replicative studies, one of which they undertake themselves. Their 2020 life-course perspective approach (Ciobanu & Fokkema, 2020) is another qualitative study with a different sample, also focused on the protective factors against loneliness for Romanian migrants. This study also finds that many Romanian migrants find solace and companionship in organizations but especially in churches which "appear to have played a role in reducing loneliness, by being an important place to meet people and establish ties" (Ciobanu & Fokkema, 2020, p.327). The church has also a role as an intergenerational mediator leading younger churchgoers to visit older ones, in care homes or at home.

7.3.14 *COVID-19 Restrictions, Measures, and Policy Changes*

Dahlberg's paper, while more of a state-of-the-art study, constructs a brief snapshot not only of the evolution of loneliness during COVID but also of how various macro-social factors impact it in this extraordinary situation and the proposed loneliness mitigation methods (Dahlberg, 2021). Among the latter the author highlights the difficulties of using loneliness reduction methods during a worldwide pandemic, with a particular focus on older adults and those being poor. As the study provides a 2021 snapshot of COVID-related scholarship, the author acknowledges the broad limitations of the surveyed studies, particularly convenience sampling and online data collection, both factors limiting access to older respondents.

7.4 Discussion and Conclusions

As an increasingly solid corpus of research on loneliness takes shape it is becoming increasingly important to take a systematic snapshot of the field in order to identify areas where the literature is still sparse. Throughout this chapter we have taken a look at the primary macro-social factors impacting loneliness in the literature, at how they are operationalized and employed in order to identify the primary areas and methods of employment and the gaps in the literature. This scoping review identified 61 studies that focused on societal-level influences on loneliness, specifically loneliness of older individuals. While results indicate established interests in how cultural values and norms in a society, migration patterns, or welfare generosity influence loneliness, the review highlights a growing interest in less visible factors such as religiosity and societal trust. Finding the proper data to study these societal factors remains a challenge (Luhmann et al., 2023).

Policies and other macro-social factors form an important area that has not yet been properly addressed in understanding loneliness. There has been insufficient exploration into how different cultural contexts impact loneliness experiences among older adults. Cross-national studies reveal variations in loneliness prevalence, potentially due to differences in population composition or cultural values like individualism (Luhmann et al., 2023). There is a need for further longitudinal studies that assess the causal relationships between macro determinants and loneliness over time is also apparent (Dahlberg et al., 2022). This is especially important considering our limited understanding of how early life circumstances affect loneliness in later years, suggesting a need for more studies focusing on childhood influences (Guthmuller, 2022).

While some macro-level factors related to loneliness have been mentioned in the literature, there are two major barriers that impede this focus. First, conclusions on macro-social factors are still systematically overruled in the research design, because of the complexity of disentangling pathways through which macro-factors influence loneliness (Luhmann et al., 2023). Instead, macro-social factors are often mentioned either as a contextual hint for larger influences, or in post-hoc discussion, through recommendations for further research or as a part of limitations. However, the impact of macro-level factors on loneliness does not occur directly. Instead, it passes through many intermediate steps or factors and multiple pathways (Luhmann et al., 2023). For example, economic conditions might affect job availability, which in turn affects social connections, leading to loneliness. This influence is not always evident. When researchers look at how macro-level factors change over time and compare them to changes in loneliness, they not often find clear, direct relationships. This is because the connections are complex and involve many variables. Additionally, when analyzing trends over time, researchers might find patterns that seem to be related but are actually coincidental. This makes it hard to determine if there's a real cause-and-effect relationship between changes in macro-level factors and changes in loneliness.

A second barrier lies in distinguishing the relative effects of drivers at the micro and macro-levels, though some research indicates that individual-level influences have larger impacts on loneliness than macro-level factors (Morgan et al., 2021). Interactions between macro-social characteristics are seldomly investigated despite the importance of this interplay. Additionally, it could be challenging to determine the exact influence of macro-level causes because it might rely on individual characteristics, and macro-level circumstances could alter how individual traits affect loneliness (de Jong Gierveld & Tesch-Römer, 2012) and because of data limitations, methodological challenges, and interconnectedness of macro-level influences. These complexities point to the need for comprehensive, multi-level approaches to fully understand late-life loneliness.

Interventions that solely target proximal issues might not be enough because fundamental causes will continue to exist (Barreto et al., 2024). Therefore, while focusing on individual characteristics may be a viable route for change from an intervention standpoint, it may be extremely vulnerable to changes in societal factors, such as rapid policy changes, macro-social phenomena, or larger-scale catastrophes. With the aging of the global population and the resulting increased vulnerability to loneliness, new policy solutions will be required; these solutions must be grounded in empirical studies that consistently address macro-social factors.

Acknowledgements I would like to express my heartfelt gratitude to the editors of this book for their invaluable feedback, meticulous review, and thoughtful guidance throughout the whole process. Their expertise and dedication have been instrumental in shaping this chapter. I am also grateful to Dragoş Costache, whose unwavering support and generosity in providing space for me to articulate and refine my raw ideas have been a source of great encouragement. Your contributions have made a significant impact on my work, and I am deeply appreciative.

Competing Interests The author has no conflict of interest to declare that are relevant to the content of this chapter.

References

Albert, I. (2021). Perceived loneliness and the role of cultural and intergenerational belonging: The case of Portuguese first-generation immigrants in Luxembourg. *European Journal of Ageing, 18*(3), 299–310.

Arksey, H., & O'Malley, L. (2005). Scoping studies: Towards a methodological framework. *International Journal of Social Research Methodology, 8*(1), 19–32.

Barreto, M., Victor, C., Hammond, C., Eccles, A., Richins, M. T., & Qualter, P. (2021). Loneliness around the world: Age, gender, and cultural differences in loneliness. *Personality and Individual Differences, 169*, 110066.

Barreto, M., Doyle, D. M., & Qualter, P. (2023). *Loneliness inequalities evidence review*., https://www.wcpp.org.uk/wp-content/uploads/2023/08/WCPP-REPORT-Loneliness-Inequalities-Evidence-Review.pdf

Barreto, M., Doyle, D. M., & Qualter, P. (2024). Changing the narrative: Loneliness as a social justice issue. *Political Psychology, 45*, 157–181.

Barrett, A., & Mosca, I. (2013). Social isolation, loneliness and return migration: Evidence from older Irish adults. *Journal of Ethnic and Migration Studies, 39*(10), 1659–1677.

Beller, J. (2024). Social inequalities in loneliness: Disentangling the contributions of education, income, and occupation. *SAGE Open, 14*(3), 21582440241281408.

Buecker, S., Ebert, T., Götz, F. M., Entringer, T. M., & Luhmann, M. (2021). In a lonely place: Investigating regional differences in loneliness. *Social Psychological and Personality Science, 12*(2), 147–155.

Burholt, V. (2023). Culture, social isolation, and loneliness in later life. In A. Hajek, S. Riedel-Heller, & H. H. König (Eds.), *Loneliness and social isolation in old age* (pp. 51–60). Routledge.

Cifci, F. (2024). Life-course perspective on immigrant loneliness: A conceptual framework for intergenerational loneliness trajectories. *The Family Journal*, 10664807241235324.

Ciobanu, R. O., & Fokkema, T. (2020). The role of religion in protecting older Romanian migrants from loneliness. In *Ageing as a Migrant* (pp. 36–54). Routledge.

Ciobanu, R. O., & Fokkema, T. (2021). What protects older Romanians in Switzerland from loneliness? A life-course perspective. *European Journal of Ageing, 18*(3), 323–331.

Cohen-Mansfield, J., Hazan, H., Lerman, Y., & Shalom, V. (2016). Correlates and predictors of loneliness in older adults: A review of quantitative results informed by qualitative insights. *International Psychogeriatrics, 28*(4), 557–576.

Cotterell, N., Buffel, T., Nazroo, J., & Qualter, P. (2025). Loneliness among older ethnic minority people: Exploring the role of structural disadvantage and place using a co-research methodology. *Ethnic and Racial Studies, 48*(1), 206–228.

Dahlberg, L. (2021). Loneliness during the COVID-19 pandemic. *Aging & Mental Health, 25*(7), 1161–1164. https://doi.org/10.1080/13607863.2021.1875195

Dahlberg, L., McKee, K. J., Frank, A., & Naseer, M. (2022). A systematic review of longitudinal risk factors for loneliness in older adults. *Aging & Mental Health, 26*(2), 225–249. https://doi.org/10.1080/13607863.2021.1876638

CARLOS, DÍAZ-VENEGAS JOSEPH L., SÁENZ REBECA, WONG (2017) Family size and old-age wellbeing: *effects of the fertility transition in Mexico ABSTRACT Ageing and Society 37*(3) 495–516 https://doi.org/10.1017/S0144686X15001221.

Delaruelle, K. (2023). Migration-related inequalities in loneliness across age groups: A cross-national comparative study in Europe. *European Journal of Ageing, 20*(1), 35.

Doblas, J. L., Palomares-Linares, I., & Martínez, M. S. (2020). Loneliness in older adults: A comparative study of four southern European countries. In *Social problems in Southern Europe* (pp. 87–102). Edward Elgar Publishing.

Doyle, D. M., Qualter, P., Victor, C., & Barreto, M. (2022). The impact of country-level structural stigma on loneliness and social capital in older and younger LGB individuals in 113 countries. *European Journal of Public Health, 32*(Supplement_3), ckac129-193.

Dykstra, P. A. (2009). Older adult loneliness: Myths and realities. *European Journal of Ageing, 6*, 91–100.

Fernández-Carro, C., & Gumà Lao, J. (2022). A life-course approach to the relationship between education, family trajectory and late-life loneliness among older women in Europe. *Social Indicators Research, 162*(3), 1345–1363.

Fokkema, T., & Naderi, R. (2013). Differences in late-life loneliness: A comparison between Turkish and native-born older adults in Germany. *European Journal of Ageing, 10*, 289–300.

Fokkema, T., Gierveld, J. D. J., & Dykstra, P. A. (2013). Cross-national differences in older adult loneliness. In *Loneliness updated* (pp. 200–227). Routledge.

Goldman, N., Khanna, D., El Asmar, M. L., Qualter, P., & El-Osta, A. (2024). Addressing loneliness and social isolation in 52 countries: A scoping review of National policies. *BMC Public Health, 24*(1), 1207.

Guthmuller, S. (2022). Loneliness among older adults in Europe: The relative importance of early and later life conditions. *PLoS One, 17*(5), e0267562.

Hansen, T., & Slagsvold, B. (2016). Late-life loneliness in 11 European countries: Results from the Generations and Gender Survey. *Social Indicators Research, 124*, 1–20.

Hansen, T., Kafková, M. P., Katz, R., Lowenstein, A., Naim, S., Pavlidis, G., et al. (2021). Exclusion from social relations in later life: Micro-and macro-level patterns and correlations in a European perspective. *International Journal of Environmental Research and Public Health, 18*(23), 12418.

Harry Owen, Taylor (2020) Social Isolation's Influence on Loneliness Among Older Adults Clinical Social Work Journal 48(1) 140–151 https://doi.org/10.1007/s10615-019-00737-9.

Heu, L. C. (2023). The loneliness of the odd one out: How deviations from social norms can help explain loneliness across cultures. *Perspectives on Psychological Science*, 17456916231192485.

Heu, L. C., Hansen, N., & van Zomeren, M. (2021a). Resolving the cultural loneliness paradox of choice: The role of cultural norms about individual choice regarding relationships in explaining loneliness in four European countries. *Journal of Social and Personal Relationships, 38*(7), 2053–2072.

Heu, L. C., van Zomeren, M., & Hansen, N. (2021b). Does loneliness thrive in relational freedom or restriction? The culture-loneliness framework. *Review of General Psychology, 25*(1), 60–72.

Hong, Q. N., Fàbregues, S., Bartlett, G., Boardman, F., Cargo, M., Dagenais, P., et al. (2018). The Mixed Methods Appraisal Tool (MMAT) version 2018 for information professionals and researchers. *Education for Information, 34*(4), 285–291.

Horn, V., & Fokkema, T. (2023). Drivers of loneliness among older refugees. *Journal of Refugee Studies*, fead027.

Hunter, A. (2018). Older migrants: Inequalities of ageing from a transnational perspective. In *Ageing, diversity and equality* (pp. 194–209). Routledge.

Jentoft, E. E. (2023). Technology and older adults in British loneliness policy and political discourse. *Frontiers in Digital Health, 5*, 1168413.

Jentoft, E. E., Sandset, T., & Haldar, M. (2025). Problematizing loneliness as a public health issue: An analysis of policy in the United Kingdom. *Critical Policy Studies, 19*(1), 1–18.

Johnson, S., Bacsu, J., McIntosh, T., Jeffery, B., & Novik, N. (2019). Social isolation and loneliness among immigrant and refugee seniors in Canada: A scoping review. *International Journal of Migration, Health and Social Care, 15*(3), 177–190.

de Jong Gierveld, J., & Tesch-Römer, C. (2012). Loneliness in old age in Eastern and Western European societies: Theoretical perspectives. *European Journal of Ageing, 9*, 285–295.

de Jong Gierveld, J., Dykstra, P. A., & Schenk, N. (2012). Living arrangements, intergenerational support types and older adult loneliness in Eastern and Western Europe. *Demographic Research, 27*, 167–200.

Joshi, M., Finney, N., & Hale, J. M. (2024). Loneliness and social isolation of ethnic minority/immigrant older adults: A scoping review. *Ageing & Society*, 1–31.

Jylhä, M., & Jokela, J. (1990). Individual experiences as cultural–a cross-cultural study on loneliness among the elderly. *Ageing & Society, 10*(3), 295–315.

King, R., Cela, E., Fokkema, T., & Vullnetari, J. (2014). The migration and well-being of the zero generation: Transgenerational care, grandparenting, and loneliness amongst Albanian older people. *Population, Space and Place, 20*(8), 728–738.

Klok, J., Van Tilburg, T. G., Suanet, B., Fokkema, T., & Huisman, M. (2017). National and transnational belonging among Turkish and Moroccan older migrants in the Netherlands: protective against loneliness? *European Journal of Ageing, 14*, 341–351.

Langenkamp, A., Mund, M., & Hawkley, L. (2024). The role of country-level characteristics for the association between loneliness and neighborhood cohesion–A multi-level analysis. *Journal of Social and Personal Relationships, 41*(11), 3222–3247.

Long, H. A., French, D. P., & Brooks, J. M. (2020). Optimising the value of the critical appraisal skills programme (CASP) tool for quality appraisal in qualitative evidence synthesis. *Research Methods in Medicine & Health Sciences, 1*(1), 31–42.

Long, K. M., Casey, K., Bhar, S., Al Mahmud, A., Curran, S., Hunter, K., & Lim, M. H. (2024). Understanding perspectives of older adults on the role of technology in the wider context of their social relationships. *Ageing & Society, 44*(6), 1453–1476.

Lu, S. Y., Yoon, S., Yee, W. Q., Ngiam, N. H. W., Ng, K. Y. Y., & Low, L. L. (2024). Experiences of a community-based digital intervention among older people living in a low-income neighborhood: Qualitative study. *JMIR Aging, 7*(1), e52292.

Luhmann, M., Buecker, S., & Rüsberg, M. (2023). Loneliness across time and space. *Nature Reviews Psychology, 2*(1), 9–23.

Lykes, V. A., & Kemmelmeier, M. (2014). What predicts loneliness? Cultural difference between individualistic and collectivistic societies in Europe. *Journal of Cross-Cultural Psychology, 45*(3), 468–490.

Marcil-Gratton, N., & Légaré, J. (1992). Will reduced fertility lead to greater isolation in old age for tomorrow's elderly? *Canadian Journal on Aging/La Revue Canadienne du Vieillissement, 11*(1), 54–71.

Meehan, D. E., Grunseit, A., Condie, J., HaGani, N., & Merom, D. (2023). Social-ecological factors influencing loneliness and social isolation in older people: A scoping review. *BMC Geriatrics, 23*(1), 726.

Mohan, G., & Lyons, S. (2024). High-speed broadband availability, Internet activity among older people, quality of life and loneliness. *New Media & Society, 26*(5), 2889–2913.

Morgan, D., Dahlberg, L., Waldegrave, C., Mikulionienė, S., Rapolienė, G., Lamura, G., & Aartsen, M. (2021). Revisiting loneliness: Individual and country-level changes. In: *Social exclusion in later life: Interdisciplinary and policy perspectives,* 99–117.

Moroney, M., & Jarvis, A. (2020). Loneliness and digital inclusion: A Literature review. *Aging Better Middlesbrough.*

Munn, Z., Peters, M. D., Stern, C., Tufanaru, C., McArthur, A., & Aromataris, E. (2018). Systematic review or scoping review? Guidance for authors when choosing between a systematic or scoping review approach. *BMC Medical Research Methodology, 18*, 1–7.

Munn, Z., Pollock, D., Khalil, H., Alexander, L., Mclnerney, P., Godfrey, C. M., et al. (2022). What are scoping reviews? Providing a formal definition of scoping reviews as a type of evidence synthesis. *JBI Evidence Synthesis, 20*(4), 950–952.

Neves, B. B., & Petersen, A. (2025). The social stigma of loneliness: A sociological approach to understanding the experiences of older people. *The Sociological Review, 73*(2), 362–383.

Neeves et al. 2023: Neves, B. B., Petersen, A., Vered, M., Carter, A., & Omori, M. (2023). Artificial intelligence in long-term care: technological promise, aging anxieties, and sociotechnical ageism. *Journal of Applied Gerontology, 42*(6), 1274–1282.

Newmyer, L., Verdery, A. M., Wang, H., & Margolis, R. (2022). Population aging, demographic metabolism, and the rising tide of late middle age to older adult loneliness around the world. *Population and Development Review, 48*(3), 829–862.

Niedzwiedz, C. L., Richardson, E. A., Tunstall, H., Shortt, N. K., Mitchell, R. J., & Pearce, J. R. (2016). The relationship between wealth and loneliness among older people across Europe: Is social participation protective? *Preventive Medicine, 91*, 24–31.

Nyqvist, F., Nygård, M., & Scharf, T. (2019). Loneliness amongst older people in Europe: A comparative study of welfare regimes. *European Journal of Ageing, 16*, 133–143.
Peters, M. D., Marnie, C., Colquhoun, H., Garritty, C. M., Hempel, S., Horsley, T., et al. (2021). Scoping reviews: Reinforcing and advancing the methodology and application. *Systematic Reviews, 10*, 1–6.
Preoteasa, A. M., Vlase, I., & Tufă, L. A. (2018). Intergenerational support as a reaction to socio-economic crisis: Alteration of solidarity within precarious Romanian households. *European Societies, 20*(1), 111–130.
Rapolienė, G., & Aartsen, M. (2022). Lonely societies: Low trust societies? Further explanations for national variations in loneliness among older Europeans. *European Journal of Ageing, 19*(3), 485–494.
Reine, I., Miķelsone, M., Tomsone, S., Guðmundsson, H., Ivanovs, A., Guðmundsson, H. S., & Koroļeva, I. (2024). Unraveling the dynamics of loneliness in the Baltic-Nordic region: A comparative analysis in the wake of COVID-19. *Frontiers in Public Health, 12*, 1360285.
Rokach, A. (2018). The effect of gender and culture on loneliness: A mini review. *Emerging Science Journal, 2*(2), 59–64.
Ruan, Y. X., & Cheung, M. C. (2024). Systematic review of factors influencing loneliness in older-adult migrants. *Aging & Mental Health, 28*(8), 1129–1141.
Rüdel, J., & Joly, M. P. (2024). Perceived loneliness: Why are Syrian refugees more lonely than other newly arrived migrants in Germany? *Comparative Migration Studies, 12*(1), 37.
Sandu, V., Leichsenring, K., & Zólyomi, E. (2022). *Social isolation and loneliness among older people in Europe: Evidence, policies and interventions.* European Center for Social Welfare Policy and Research. https://www.eurocentreorg/projects/detail/4302
Seifert, A. (2025). Information and communication technologies and the risk of loneliness. In M. Aartsen, I. Precupetu, & B. Suanet (Eds.), *Macro social influences on loneliness in later life: Towards a better understanding of the loneliness paradox in later life*. Springer.
Shah, A. (2008). Association of suicide rates of elderly persons with fertility rates. *Psychological Reports, 102*(2), 369–376.
Shiovitz-Ezra, S., Shemesh, J., & McDonnell-Naughton, M. (2018). Pathways from ageism to loneliness. In Ayalon, L., & C. Tesch-Römer (Eds.). *Contemporary perspectives on ageism* (pp. 131–147).
Sundström, G., Fransson, E., Malmberg, B., & Davey, A. (2009). Loneliness among older Europeans. *European Journal of Ageing, 6*, 267–275.
Swader, C. S. (2019). Loneliness in Europe: Personal and societal individualism-collectivism and their connection to social isolation. *Social Forces, 97*(3), 1307–1336.
Swader, C. S., & Moraru, A. V. (2023). Social infrastructure and the alleviation of loneliness in Europe. *KZfSS Kölner Zeitschrift für Soziologie und Sozialpsychologie, 75*(Suppl 1), 387–414.
Taniguchi, H., & Kaufman, G. (2022). Family, collectivism, and loneliness from a cross-country perspective. *Applied Research in Quality of Life, 17*(3), 1555–1581.
Tapia-Muñoz, T., Staudinger, U. M., Allel, K., Steptoe, A., Miranda-Castillo, C., Medina, J. T., & Calvo, E. (2022). Income inequality and its relationship with loneliness prevalence: A cross-sectional study among older adults in the US and 16 European countries. *PLoS One, 17*(12), e0274518.
van den Broek, T., & Tosi, M. (2020). The more the merrier? The causal effect of high fertility on later-life loneliness in Eastern Europe. *Social Indicators Research, 149*(2), 733–748.
van Staden, W. C., & Coetzee, K. (2010). Conceptual relations between loneliness and culture. *Current Opinion in Psychiatry, 23*(6), 524–529.
van Tilburg, T. G. (2025). Unravelling the socio-cultural influence on loneliness. In M. Aartsen, I. Precupetu, & B. Suanet (Eds.), *Macro social influences on loneliness in later life: Towards a better understanding of the loneliness paradox in later life*. Springer.
Victor, C. R., Burholt, V., & Martin, W. (2012). Loneliness and ethnic minority elders in Great Britain: an exploratory study. *Journal of Cross-Cultural Gerontology, 27*, 65–78.

Wagner, M., & Brandt, M. (2015). 16 Loneliness among informal caregivers aged 50+ in Europe. In: A. Börsch-Supan, T. Kneip, H. Litwin, M. Myck & G. Weber (Eds.) *Ageing in Europe-supporting policies for an inclusive society*, 9783110444414-018.

Welch, V., Ghogomu, E. T., Barbeau, V. I., Dowling, S., Doyle, R., Beveridge, E., et al. (2023). Digital interventions to reduce social isolation and loneliness in older adults: An evidence and gap map. *Campbell Systematic Reviews, 19*(4), e1369.

Wu, J., Zhang, J., & Fokkema, T. (2022). The micro-macro interplay of economic factors in late-life loneliness: Evidence from Europe and China. *Frontiers in Public Health, 10*, 968411.

Xu, W., & Köttl, H. (2020). Internet use and loneliness among older adults: The moderating role of self-perceptions of ageing. In *Human Aspects of IT for the Aged Population. Technology and Society*: 6th International Conference, ITAP 2020, Held as Part of the 22nd HCI International Conference, HCII 2020, Copenhagen, Denmark, July 19–24, 2020, Proceedings, Part III 22 (pp. 364–381). Springer.

Yang, K. (2023). Loneliness and intersectionality: A progressive conditional approach. *Current Research in Behavioral Sciences, 5*, 100122.

Zoutewelle-Terovan, M., & Liefbroer, A. C. (2018). Swimming against the stream: Non-normative family transitions and loneliness in later life across 12 nations. *The Gerontologist, 58*(6), 1096–1108.

Dr. Laura Tufă is a sociologist and a researcher at the Research Institute for Quality of Life within the Romanian Academy, and the Research Institute of the University of Bucharest. She holds a PhD in Sociology from the University of Bucharest, focusing on the ethics of social research. Her work has been published in various journals, including *European Societies*, *European Journal of Ageing*, and *Applied Research in Quality of Life*. Her research explores topics like social exclusion, mental well-being, and housing pathways of older adults, offering valuable insights into the dynamics of an ageing population.

Open Access This chapter is licensed under the terms of the Creative Commons Attribution 4.0 International License (http://creativecommons.org/licenses/by/4.0/), which permits use, sharing, adaptation, distribution and reproduction in any medium or format, as long as you give appropriate credit to the original author(s) and the source, provide a link to the Creative Commons license and indicate if changes were made.

The images or other third party material in this chapter are included in the chapter's Creative Commons license, unless indicated otherwise in a credit line to the material. If material is not included in the chapter's Creative Commons license and your intended use is not permitted by statutory regulation or exceeds the permitted use, you will need to obtain permission directly from the copyright holder.

Part IV
Recent Developments and Loneliness

Chapter 8
Information and Communication Technologies and the Risk to Loneliness

Alexander Seifert

8.1 Introduction

Loneliness is common among older people, especially as social contact declines. Friends and partners die, causing social networks to shrink (Aarts et al., 2015). We define loneliness as "the unpleasant experience that occurs when a person's network of social relations is deficient in some important way, either quantitatively or qualitatively" (Perlman & Peplau, 1981, p. 31). Loneliness can, therefore, be considered the subjective feeling of lacking social contact. Social interaction is often maintained through digital tools—many times as a supplement to face-to-face contact. Thus, loneliness is closely linked to social contacts in real and digital life (Nowland et al., 2018).

The advent of digital technologies has significantly altered social interactions, influencing feelings of loneliness among both younger and older adults. Among younger adults, particularly those aged 15 to 24, excessive use of social media may ultimately lead to feelings of loneliness and isolation (Smith et al., 2021). Moreover, the adoption of contemporary digital instruments, such as social media applications, has been attributed to the tendency of social comparison and the perception of missing out on social events, which can intensify feelings of isolation. For older adults, digital technologies present both challenges and opportunities in regard to loneliness. While excessive internet use has been associated with anxiety and depression, moderate and purposeful engagement, such as using video calls and online communities, can enhance social connections and reduce feelings of isolation (Ruiz-Figueroa et al., 2025).

A. Seifert (✉)
School of Social Work, University of Applied Sciences and Arts Northwestern Switzerland, Olten, Switzerland
e-mail: alexander.seifert@fhnw.ch

© The Author(s) 2025

M. Aartsen et al. (eds.), *Macro Social Influences on Loneliness in Later Life*, International Perspectives on Aging 47,
https://doi.org/10.1007/978-3-031-94565-6_8

Age alone is not a valid predictor of loneliness; nevertheless, during the COVID-19 pandemic, older adults, especially, experienced reduced contact and relied on the telephone, for example, to communicate with loved ones (Brooke & Jackson, 2020). Although older adults can maintain contact through digital solutions, such as chats or video telephony, not all of them have technical skills, internet access, or requisite digital tools (e.g., social messenger smartphone apps) and thus cannot compensate for a lack of physical contact with digital solutions (Seifert et al., 2021; Xie et al., 2020). Thus, with the penetration of digital services into everyday life, contemporary technology can help maintain contact and social interaction. Nevertheless, those who are not technology-savvy risk exclusion and feel particularly lonely in digital-dominated everyday life because they cannot or do not want to use technology-enabled means of communication (Seifert, 2020). This two-sided view leads to the central question of to what extent digitalization affects feelings of loneliness among older people, either positively or negatively. Therefore, this chapter aims to provide a literature and empirically based answer to this question, by discussing current insights and by analyzing data from a recently conducted survey among people living in Switzerland aged between 18 and 98.

8.2 Use of Information and Communication Technologies Among Older Adults

Information and communication technologies (ICTs) are everyday tools used to seek information and communicate, including the internet, smartphone messaging, and news apps on a tablet. ICT use may enable older individuals to live independently for a longer time by positively impacting health and social isolation (Czaja et al., 2018; Schulz et al., 2015). Web-connected ICT, such as using the internet via smartphones or tablets, provides new communication capabilities. Compared with non-web-connected ICTs (e.g., landline telephones), web-connected ICTs (e.g., social network apps on a smartphone) facilitate broader access to digital information and services. Research has shown that web-connected ICT has substantially changed people's lives by enabling new forms of social participation and interaction and by enhancing access to information (Antonucci et al., 2017; Castellacci & Tveito, 2018).

Even though the digital transformation of everyday life offers opportunities to enable, for instance, the maintenance of social contact over long distances or quick access to news, successful participation in a digital society requires individuals to adapt to evolving technological innovations and possess the knowledge to perform activities digitally (Seifert & Cotten, 2021). However, not all populations are familiar with or have adequate access to ICTs. This digital divide is a global phenomenon that encapsulates the perceived gap between those with access and those without it (Compaine, 2001). The literature on older adults has shown that younger groups worldwide are more familiar with the latest technologies than older groups.

Individuals aged 65 years and older, especially those aged 80 years and older, use modern web-connected ICT less often than younger groups (Hunsaker & Hargittai, 2018; Schlomann et al., 2020).

Compared to younger adults, who are often familiar with the latest technologies (e.g., smartphones, apps, and social media), older persons are less familiar with and skilled at using newer ICTs (e.g., smartphones, smartwatches, and virtual reality tools). Alongside age differences, sociodemographic characteristics (e.g., gender, education, and income), personal factors (e.g., technical skills and technological anxiety) and environmental factors, such as ICT infrastructure and the wealth of one's region, shape this digital gap (Brandtzæg et al., 2011; König & Seifert, 2023). A representative survey across the European Union showed that 53% of people aged 50 years or older used the internet (König & Seifert, 2020). The same study revealed that people older than 80 years spent less time online than younger older adults (65–79 years) and that men and adults with higher educational and economic status aged 50 years and older were more likely to use the internet. Furthermore, individuals' health, prior experience with technology, social salience (i.e., internet use among the members of one's social network), and contextual factors, such as country-specific wealth and communication technology infrastructure, are predictors of older adults' internet use.

The COVID-19 pandemic has highlighted the significance and persistence of the "digital divide," fostering discussions about the positive and negative consequences of using or not using technology during periods of physical distancing. When physical distancing mandates were enacted during the COVID-19 pandemic, older adults—one of the most at-risk groups for COVID-19—could not interact with their social connections and were told to refrain from shopping, dining, and other outside activities. Older adults who could access ICTs could still maintain contact with social ties, buy food and groceries, and remain involved in organizations via a digital presence (e.g., many churches began broadcasting their services online). However, older adults on the wrong side of the digital divide with health and mobility limitations were likely to struggle with a "double burden of social exclusion" (Seifert et al., 2021). They could not compensate for their need for contact, for example, with their grandchildren, through digital solutions (e.g., modern ICT). Although ICT use may help older adults maintain social interaction and engagement, a sense of social exclusion and loneliness is likely for older adults who cannot access ICTs or lack the skills to use them (Robinson et al., 2020).

8.3 Potential for and Barriers to ICT Use Among Older Adults

ICT use has long been discussed in gerontological literature, as have the effects of technology on various aspects of life and well-being (Schulz et al., 2015; Wahl & Gerstorf, 2018). However, the results have been mixed, and the question of whether and to what extent technologies can improve older people's lives cannot be unequivocally answered. Rather, there is evidence of potential but also of barriers to use (Seifert & Cotten, 2021). In this context, considering the ambivalent effects of technology for older adults is crucial. For instance, the findings on the impact of technology use on quality of life have also been mixed. Quintana et al. (2018) reported no effects on evaluative and hedonic psychological well-being, instead identifying a positive effect on eudaimonic psychological well-being. Lam et al. (2020) noted positive effects of daily internet and other technology use on life satisfaction, even though its use for information seeking was associated with lower life satisfaction.

In a Swiss survey, Seifert and Schelling (2018) established that many respondents viewed the internet as useful for staying in contact with others and for coping with everyday situations and that 53% of those aged 65 and older agreed with the statement that "the internet allows me to stay independent longer into old age." These findings and those of other studies (Francis et al., 2019; Schlomann et al., 2020) suggest that the internet, a prime example of current ICT, could be a resource for facilitating everyday life by compensating for functional decline in old age. For example, instrumental ICT use—accessing services, information, or opportunities that may be unavailable through other means—has been associated with increased social engagement among older adults (Ihm & Hsieh, 2015).

In addition to the potential benefits of ICT, barriers to its use must be noted. For example, Swiss data (Seifert, 2022) revealed that the most common reasons for not using the internet were complexity of use (77%), security concerns (74%), and too much effort to learn (65%); however, over 60% of the respondents in each case stated that someone else was accessing information on the internet on their behalf (65%) or that they saw no personal benefit to using the internet (61%). The other reasons were less frequently cited, although a lack of support was also invoked by 37% of respondents as the reason for not using the internet. Only 20–29% of respondents cited cost and health problems (Seifert, 2022). There is also extensive research on the role of anxiety in older adults' technology use (Powell, 2013). Compared to younger adults, older adults are more likely to report being anxious about using technology, which has been considered relevant for explaining the digital divide between age groups.

8.4 The One Side of the Coin: Maintaining Social Contact via Modern ICT and Reducing Loneliness

Using current ICT, such as the internet, can be regarded as a resource for successful aging by providing older adults with an instrument to remain connected with and interact with the outside world (Hofer et al., 2019). However, research on the connection between older adults' internet use and their mental health has presented a mixed picture (Lam et al., 2020). Although some studies have shown negative associations between internet use and mental health (e.g., increases in anxiety or depression because of internet use; Hofer & Hargittai, 2021), other studies have been more positive, indicating that internet use can counteract depression and loneliness (Cotten et al., 2014).

In this context, previous studies on the implications of internet use for mental health have focused on outcomes such as depression and anxiety, social support, or life satisfaction. Yet one of the key challenges regarding older adults' mental health, their rich lives, and their integration into society is the maintenance of social inclusion and the avoidance of loneliness. Modern ICT can enable new forms of social interaction, especially among older adults (Antonucci et al., 2017). Nevertheless, empirical evidence on the relationship between loneliness and ICT use in old age has been mixed.

Some studies have found that loneliness is reduced (Cotten et al., 2013; Szabo et al., 2019; Yu et al., 2021). For example, a German study (Schlomann et al., 2020) revealed a significant relationship between the use of web-connected ICT and three domains of subjective well-being: loneliness, anomie, and autonomy. The participants using ICT reported lower levels of loneliness and anomie and higher levels of autonomy.

In contrast, other studies have determined that the internet does not significantly impact perceived loneliness among older people (Aarts et al., 2015; Chen & Schulz, 2016; Slegers et al., 2008). These mixed results could be related to the question of whether interactions via ICT replace real-life social interactions, which might lead to greater loneliness. However, a review of social relations and technology concluded that technology is more likely to expand traditional forms of social interaction than replace them (Antonucci et al., 2017).

Regarding longitudinal studies on internet use and loneliness, a randomized controlled trial of an internet-based intervention for older adults reported a significant reduction in perceived loneliness for the intervention group at six months, but this effect was not maintained at 12 months (Czaja et al., 2018). Another longitudinal study found that internet use for social purposes was associated with decreased loneliness the following year, while informational and instrumental internet use was unrelated to loneliness (Szabo et al., 2019). A more recent study (Yu et al., 2021) using the US-based Health and Retirement Study provided evidence based on longitudinal data on the mediating effects of social contact that indicated an association between internet use and loneliness. The study found that internet use could increase the amount of social contact.

8.5 The Other Side of the Coin: Digitalization and the Risk of Perpetuating Loneliness and Social Exclusion

As described above, the current state of research on ICT use and loneliness has been mixed. Some studies have shown a reduction in loneliness, whereas others have shown no effect. A recent review concluded that although research reviews have indicated that ICT can reduce loneliness and social isolation in older people, the causal confirmation has been limited, and evidence concerning innovative technologies, such as augmented reality systems, is scarce (Döring et al., 2022). Similarly, a UK study revealed weak associations between various online activities and loneliness but strong associations with social isolation (Stockwell et al., 2021), indicating that technology and technology-based interventions impact social interaction. Thus, technology can increase social interaction and reduce social isolation but cannot guarantee a direct impact on loneliness. Another review (Balki et al., 2022) on the effect of technological interventions on reducing loneliness concluded that technology improved social connectedness, but its effectiveness in lessening social isolation and loneliness depended on the study design and was improved by shorter durations and longer training periods. Notably, the relationship between technology use and loneliness depends on the technology and an individual's social situation.

Studies have also indicated that technology can negatively impact loneliness because technology use reduces face-to-face contact. Nowland et al. (2018) identified a complex relationship between loneliness and social internet use: When the internet serves as a tool to strengthen existing relationships or create new social connections, it can help reduce feelings of loneliness. However, when social technologies are used as a means of avoiding real-world social interactions, loneliness tends to increase. For older adults, there is an additional aspect: the non-use of digital tools. Not using for example, the internet (and digital tools) to maintain social contacts. People lacking technical skills or hardware cannot (a) enjoy the benefits of digital tools and (b) are likely to feel excluded from this digital social interaction.

For a long time, the nonuse or low use of digital technologies did not (or only to a limited extent) exclude individuals from satisfying their needs and interests because these could be achieved through widely available traditional means (e.g., in-person visitations). However, with digitalization becoming increasingly prevalent, people with few or no technical skills (among them mostly older adults) raise the question of whether the nonuse of modern technologies leads to social exclusion (Seifert & Rössel, 2019; Van Regenmortel et al., 2016). The link between the nonuse of digital technology and social exclusion is twofold. First, poor or nonuse may result in a lack of access to information and resources (e.g., goods and services) and, with this, the inability to participate in the normal daily activities available to most people (Walsh et al., 2017). For instance, as more service providers offer information and services on an online-only basis (or charge an additional fee for offline services), older adults who are not online may be increasingly disadvantaged in societal inclusion. Second, poor or no utilization of modern ICT can contribute to an increased risk of social exclusion and loneliness in old age (Reisdorf & Rhinesmith, 2020).

The increasing need to be digitally literate may contribute to a gradual loss of social integration among older adults with low or no technological skills who may no longer feel part of contemporary society. This phenomenon is known as perceived obsolescence (Brandtstädter & Wentura, 1994). In a representative German sample, 14% of older adults over the age of 60 had high levels of perceived obsolescence, which increased with the absence of internet access, fewer ICT skills, and lower internet self-efficacy (Jokisch et al., 2022).

ICTs can also generate and perpetuate ageism, with older technology nonusers seen as frail or outsiders (Cutler, 2005). If societal inclusion means active participation in the digital world, then older adults who do not own a smartphone or are not active on the internet risk social exclusion. In a Swiss survey by Seifert et al. (2018), 14% of the respondents aged 65 and older who did not use the internet stated that their nonuse led to social exclusion.

8.6 Findings from a Swiss National Survey

8.6.1 Background and Research Methods

To further consider the relationship between the use of modern ICT and loneliness, we accessed existing data from Switzerland to study how digital and nondigital social interaction may affect loneliness. We explored whether associations between social interactions and loneliness differ by mode of social interaction, that is, online, or in person. We also examined feelings of closeness to family and friends when using online communication and in-person communication.

A simple random sample of the permanent resident population of Switzerland aged 18 years and older was chosen from the sample frame (registry dataset) of the Swiss Federal Statistical Office. Personalized invitations and two reminders were sent by mail. There were no restrictions on upper-level age, current internet use, nationality, or type of housing. From October 29 to December 17, 2019, 1604 people aged 18 years and older in all the language regions (German, French, and Italian) of Switzerland were interviewed. A computer-assisted web interviewing technique was used, which was supplemented by computer-assisted telephone interviews with people who lacked an internet connection or who did not use the internet. A standardized questionnaire with closed-ended questions was used. The average interview duration for the two methods was 41.8 minutes. A total response rate of 30.5% was achieved. The respondents' ages ranged from 18 to 98 years, with a mean age of 51.5 years (SD = 17.86).

Loneliness was measured via a short three-item loneliness scale (Hughes et al., 2004). Response categories ranged from 1 = *never* to 5 = *very often* ($M = 1.96$ and $SD = 0.80$). The loneliness scale ($\alpha = .83$; scores were summed) included the following questions: "How often do you feel that you lack companionship," "How often do you feel left out," and "How often do you feel isolated from others?" To measure preferred forms of communication we used the following question: "How do you mainly communicate with the following groups of people (own partners, own children, other family members, friends)? (in person, by telephone, digital (online)". To measure feelings of closeness to different social groups (partners, children, other family members, and friends) via offline (in person) or digital (online) communication strategies, we added two questions measured on a 5-point scale (1 = *very distant* to 5 = *very close*): "When you communicate with the following groups of people in person, do you feel emotionally close or emotionally distant?" and "When you communicate with the following groups of people digital (online), do you feel emotionally close or emotionally distant?"

A set of control variables included the following sociodemographic variables: gender (1 = *female* and 0 = *male*), age (in years), education (1 = *primary level*, 2 = *secondary level*, and 3 = *tertiary level*), monthly household income (1 = *less than 4000 Swiss Francs [CHF]*, 2 = *CHF 4001–8000*, and 3 = *more than CHF 8000*), and living situation (1 = *living alone* and 0 = *not living alone*).

8.6.2 Forms of Communication

Descriptive analyses (see Table 8.1) showed that younger participants (18–64 years) and older participants (65–98 years) use mainly personal communication for contact to their partners, children and friends. For contact with children and other family members, older respondents use the telephone more often than younger respondents. For contact with friends, younger respondents are more likely to use digital communication tools in addition to face-to-face contact. For contact with family members (other than partner and own children) and friends, younger participants use digital communication tools more often than older participants.

8.6.3 Feelings of Closeness Through Offline Versus Digital Contacts

Descriptive analyses (see Table 8.2) showed that younger participants (18–64 years) reported higher levels of closeness when in face-to-face communication with children, family members, and friends than older participants (65–98 years). Older participants felt closer to their children, family members and friends when using digital communication tools than younger participants. However, when comparing face-to-face communication and digital communication within the 65–98 age group, older participants generally felt less close (lower feelings of closeness scores) to their children, family members, and friends when using digital communication tools (see Table 8.2).

We were also interested in the multivariate effect of closeness on loneliness when using digital communication tools. Employing linear regression models (one linear regression model for each category of social contacts; see Table 8.3) for people aged 65 years and older, controlling for age, gender, education, income, and living situation, the first model for feelings of closeness when using digital communication tools with children was not significant. The second model with other family

Table 8.1 Forms of communication (%)

Social groups	Own partners		Own children		Other family members		Friends	
Contact with mainly …	18–64 Years	65–98 Years	18–64 Years	65–98 Years	18–64 Years	65–98 Years	18–64 Years	65–98 Years
In person	86.5	89.8	83.6	48.4	40.1	28.9	42.1	41.8
By telephone	7.0	7.4	7.6	35.4	38.7	58.8	19.9	36.7
Digital (online)	6.4	2.8	8.8	16.2	21.1	12.3	38.0	21.5

Table 8.2 Feeling of closeness by offline versus digital contacts

Social groups Contact with …	Via communication in person		Via digital communications tools (online)	
	18–64 Years	65–98 Years	18–64 Years	65–98 Years
Own children	4.85** (0.46)	4.77** (0.51)	3.57*** (1.23)	3.89*** (1.10)
Other family members	4.62*** (0.70)	4.46*** (0.81)	3.52** (1.06)	3.69** (1.04)
Friends	4.53*** (0.72)	4.39*** (0.78)	3.52* (1.00)	3.65* (1.04)

Values shown are means and standard deviations (in brackets). Scale: 1 = *very distant* to 5 = *very close*. T test between age groups (*p < 0.05, **p < 0.01, and ***p < 0.001)

Table 8.3 Linear regression models to predict loneliness depending on feelings of closeness using digital communication tools stratified by type of social relation (only people aged 65 and older)

65+ years	Model 1: Children	Model 2: Other Family Members	Model 3: Friends
	Loneliness		
Predictor	*Beta*	*Beta*	*Beta*
Age	.144*	.141*	.149*
Female (ref. male)	.045	.048	.062
Education	.054	.026	.052
Income	−.013	.002	.018
Lives alone (ref. does not live alone)	.099	.120	.145*
Feeling of closeness using digital communication tools with children	−.080	–	–
Feeling of closeness using digital communication tools with other family members	–	−.168**	–
Feeling of closeness using digital communication tools with friends	–	–	−.204***
Model Fit	$F(6) = 1.600$; N = 310; $p = .147$; corrected $R^2 = .013$	$F(6) = 2.406$; N = 351; $p = .019$; corrected $R^2 = .034$	$F(6) = 3.792$; N = 356; $p < .001$; corrected $R^2 = .059$

Note: *$p < 0.05$, **$p < 0.01$, and ***$p < 0.001$

members was significant, revealing that, in addition to age, feelings of closeness were significantly associated with loneliness, whereas other independent variables were not. Thus, the older respondents who did not feel close to family members when they used digital communication tools were more likely to experience loneliness. The third model, with friends in the compared group, was significant, revealing that feelings of closeness, along with age and living alone, were significantly associated with loneliness. Thus, the older respondents who did not feel close to friends when using digital communication tools were more likely to experience loneliness. These analyses revealed that people who feel disconnected while using digital tools for communication are more lonely when in contact with family members and friends.

8.7 Conclusion

Modern ICTs help older adults stay connected to their social networks, overcome functional limitations, remain mobile as they age, and actively participate in society through socializing, purchasing products, being entertained and accessing information. Although technologies enable contact with social groups, such as friends or family members, there is a risk that the increasing dependence on digital tools, especially for older people who are less tech savvy, will lead to a certain degree of non-participation in social interactions, thus feelings of loneliness. Our study from Switzerland indicated that older adults aged 65 and older use less often digital communication tools for the contact to family members and friends than younger adults (18–64 years old). But if older people use digital communication they feel closer to their children, family members, and friends than adults aged 18–64 years using digital communication. Also, older adults who felt disconnected using digital tools for communication with family members and friends were more lonely. While these results should be interpreted with caution due to their limitations (regional focus on Switzerland; no longitudinal data; data did not allow for a comprehensive social network analysis of loneliness; no distinction between different technologies for maintaining contact), they suggest that digital social interaction tools are still used cautiously, particularly by older adults, and are not necessarily preferred to face-to-face contact. The preliminary data exploration suggests that older adults utilize new digital communication tools less frequently than younger adults. This may be indicative of a reduced familiarity with these tools, potentially leading to a lower perceived dependency on them within their everyday live (e.g., there using in-person contacts mostly). Older adults often rely on personal contacts and phone calls to satisfy their need for social interaction. However, the analysis also reveals that, despite the increased use of digital communication by older individuals, they report feeling less connected to their interlocutors during these digital interactions compared to their in-person interactions. This heightened sense of digital disconnection can potentially exacerbate feelings of loneliness, as digital communication is used less frequently, potentially leading to a reduced overall number of interpersonal contact attempts. Therefore, it can be posited that a considerable number of older adults in contemporary society may benefit from maintaining a balanced integration of both digital and non-digital communication methods.

The evidence in the literature so far pointed to the ambivalent role of digital tools of communication in social interaction. Modern communication tools, such as internet-based applications, enable older adults to maintain social contact. Thus, they may reduce loneliness if it is linked to missing social contacts. Consequently, technology can help protect older adults from the risks of social isolation. However, technology is only a tool and must be used wisely. For example, older adults must know who they can trust on the internet and what scams they may encounter. Therefore, in addition to technical hardware competence, literacy in the purposeful, responsible use of technological media is essential. Therefore, supporting older people who want to learn how to use modern technologies, for instance, by offering training courses or low-threshold peer-to-peer programs, is crucial (Cotten et al., 2016; Doh et al., 2015; Jokisch et al., 2020).

The relationship between digitalization and loneliness is complex and varies across age groups. For younger adults, while social media platforms offer avenues for connection, they can also lead to increased feelings of loneliness due to social comparison and reduced in-person interactions. Conversely, for older adults, digital tools like video calls and online communities can mitigate loneliness by facilitating social engagement, provided these technologies are used purposefully and not excessively. Addressing loneliness in the context of digitalization requires tailored approaches that consider the unique experiences of different age groups. Promoting digital literacy and encouraging meaningful online interactions can help maximize the benefits of technology while minimizing its potential drawbacks. Additionally, fostering offline social engagements remains crucial in combating loneliness across all demographics.

However, not all older adults are digitally savvy, and the resulting digital divide can promote digital inequality, resulting in the social exclusion of older adults unfamiliar with new technology. The literature review and analysis of Swiss data revealed that, along with the potential of technology use for maintaining social contact, older adults who were not technologically savvy felt excluded and, to an extent, lonely. However, the available data from Switzerland did not indicate longitudinal developments in the relationship between digital exclusion and loneliness. Thus, the question posed at the beginning of this chapter regarding the impact of ICT on loneliness cannot be answered conclusively. As is often the case, the answer is "it depends." On the one hand, digitalization can prevent social isolation for those who are particularly tech savvy. On the other hand, there are risks, especially among those who are not tech savvy or wish to avoid new technology, of feeling marginalized and sometimes even more lonely.

Competing Interests The author has no conflicts of interest to declare that are relevant to the content of this chapter.

References

Aarts, S., Peek, S. T. M., & Wouters, E. J. M. (2015). The relation between social network site usage and loneliness and mental health in community-dwelling older adults: Social network sites and loneliness and mental health. *International Journal of Geriatric Psychiatry, 30*(9), 942–949. https://doi.org/10.1002/gps.4241

Antonucci, T. C., Ajrouch, K. J., & Manalel, J. A. (2017). Social relations and technology: Continuity, context, and change. *Innovation in Aging, 1*(3), igx029. https://doi.org/10.1093/geroni/igx029

Balki, E., Hayes, N., & Holland, C. (2022). Effectiveness of technology interventions in addressing social isolation, connectedness, and loneliness in older adults: Systematic umbrella review. *JMIR Aging, 5*(4), e40125. https://doi.org/10.2196/40125

Brandtstädter, J., & Wentura, D. (1994). Veränderungen der Zeit-und Zukunftsperspektive im Übergang zum höheren Erwachsenenalter: Entwicklungspsychologische und differentielle Aspekte. *Zeitschrift Für Entwicklungspsychologie Und Pädagogische Psychologie, 26*(1), 2–21.

Brandtzæg, P. B., Heim, J., & Karahasanović, A. (2011). Understanding the new digital divide—A typology of internet users in Europe. *International Journal of Human-Computer Studies, 69*(3), 123–138. https://doi.org/10.1016/j.ijhcs.2010.11.004

Brooke, J., & Jackson, D. (2020). Older people and COVID-19: Isolation, risk and ageism. *Journal of Clinical Nursing, 29*(13–14), 2044–2046. https://doi.org/10.1111/jocn.15274

Castellacci, F., & Tveito, V. (2018). Internet use and well-being: A survey and a theoretical framework. *Research Policy, 47*(1), 308–325. https://doi.org/10.1016/j.respol.2017.11.007

Chen, Y.-R. R., & Schulz, P. J. (2016). The effect of information communication technology interventions on reducing social isolation in the elderly: A systematic review. *Journal of Medical Internet Research, 18*(1), e18. https://doi.org/10.2196/jmir.4596

Compaine, B. M. (Ed.). (2001). *The digital divide: Facing a crisis or creating a myth?* MIT Press.

Cotten, S. R., Anderson, W. A., & McCullough, B. M. (2013). Impact of internet use on loneliness and contact with others among older adults: Cross-sectional analysis. *Journal of Medical Internet Research, 15*(2), e39. https://doi.org/10.2196/jmir.2306

Cotten, S. R., Ford, G., Ford, S., & Hale, T. M. (2014). Internet use and depression among retired older adults in the United States: A longitudinal analysis. *The Journals of Gerontology Series B: Psychological Sciences and Social Sciences, 69*(5), 763–771. https://doi.org/10.1093/geronb/gbu018

Cotten, S. R., Yost, E. A., Berkowsky, R. W., Winstead, V., & Anderson, W. A. (2016). *Designing technology training for older adults in continuing care retirement communities*. CRC Press.

Cutler, S. J. (2005). Ageism and technology. *Generations, 29*(3), 67–72.

Czaja, S. J., Boot, W. R., Charness, N., Rogers, W. A., & Sharit, J. (2018). Improving social support for older adults through technology: Findings from the PRISM randomized controlled trial. *The Gerontologist, 58*(3), 467–477. https://doi.org/10.1093/geront/gnw249

Doh, M., Schmidt, L. I., Herbolsheimer, F., Jokisch, M. R., & Wahl, H. W. (2015). Patterns of modern ICT use among "senior technology experts": The role of demographic variables, subjective beliefs and attitudes. In J. Zhou & G. Salvendy (Eds.), *Human aspects of IT for the aged population. Design for aging* (Vol. 9193, pp. 177–188). Springer. https://doi.org/10.1007/978-3-319-20892-3

Döring, N., Mikhailova, V., Brandenburg, K., Broll, W., Gross, H.-M., Werner, S., & Raake, A. (2022). Digital media in intergenerational communication: Status quo and future scenarios for the grandparent–grandchild relationship. *Universal Access in the Information Society*. https://doi.org/10.1007/s10209-022-00957-w

Francis, J., Rikard, R. V., Cotten, S. R., & Kadylak, T. (2019). Does ICT use matter? How information and communication technology use affects perceived mattering among a predominantly female sample of older adults residing in retirement communities. *Information, Communication & Society, 22*(9), 1281–1294. https://doi.org/10.1080/1369118X.2017.1417459

Hofer, M., & Hargittai, E. (2021). Online social engagement, depression, and anxiety among older adults. *New Media & Society*, 146144482110543. https://doi.org/10.1177/14614448211054377

Hofer, M., Hargittai, E., Büchi, M., & Seifert, A. (2019). Older adults' online information seeking and subjective well-being: The moderating role of internet skills. *International Journal of Communication, 13*, 4426–4443. https://ijoc.org/index.php/ijoc/article/view/10981

Hughes, M. E., Waite, L. J., Hawkley, L. C., & Cacioppo, J. T. (2004). A short scale for measuring loneliness in large surveys: Results from two population-based studies. *Research on Aging, 26*(6), 655–672. https://doi.org/10.1177/0164027504268574

Hunsaker, A., & Hargittai, E. (2018). A review of internet use among older adults. *New Media & Society, 20*(10), 3937–3954. https://doi.org/10.1177/1461444818787348

Ihm, J., & Hsieh, Y. P. (2015). The implications of information and communication technology use for the social well-being of older adults. *Information, Communication & Society, 18*(10), 1123–1138. https://doi.org/10.1080/1369118X.2015.1019912

Jokisch, M. R., Scheling, L., Doh, M., & Wahl, H.-W. (2022). Contrasting internet adoption in early and advanced old age: Does internet self-efficacy matter? *The Journals of Gerontology: Series B, 77*(2), 312–320. https://doi.org/10.1093/geronb/gbab096

Jokisch, M. R., Schmidt, L. I., Doh, M., Marquard, M., & Wahl, H.-W. (2020). The role of internet self-efficacy, innovativeness, and technology avoidance in breadth of internet use: Comparing older technology experts and non-experts. *Computers in Human Behavior, 111*, 106408. https://doi.org/10.1016/j.chb.2020.106408

König, R., & Seifert, A. (2023). Internet usage, frequency, and intensity in old age during the COVID-19 pandemic—A case study for Switzerland. *Frontiers in Sociology, 8*, 1268613. https://doi.org/10.3389/fsoc.2023.1268613

Lam, S. S. M., Jivraj, S., & Scholes, S. (2020). Exploring the relationship between internet use and mental health among older adults in England: Longitudinal observational study. *Journal of Medical Internet Research, 22*(7), e15683. https://doi.org/10.2196/15683

Nowland, R., Necka, E. A., & Cacioppo, J. T. (2018). Loneliness and social internet use: Pathways to reconnection in a digital world? *Perspectives on Psychological Science, 13*(1), 70–87. https://doi.org/10.1177/1745691617713052

Perlman, D., & Peplau, L. A. (1981). Toward a social psychology of loneliness. *Personal Relationships, 3*, 31–56.

Powell, A. L. (2013). Computer anxiety: Comparison of research from the 1990s and 2000s. *Computers in Human Behavior, 29*(6), 2337–2381. https://doi.org/10.1016/j.chb.2013.05.012

Quintana, D., Cervantes, A., Sáez, Y., & Isasi, P. (2018). Internet use and psychological well-being at advanced age: Evidence from the English longitudinal study of aging. *International Journal of Environmental Research and Public Health, 15*(3), 480. https://doi.org/10.3390/ijerph15030480

Reisdorf, B., & Rhinesmith, C. (2020). Digital inclusion as a core component of social inclusion. *Social Inclusion, 8*(2), 132–137. https://doi.org/10.17645/si.v8i2.3184

Robinson, L., Schulz, J., Khilnani, A., Ono, H., Cotten, S. R., McClain, N., Levine, L., Chen, W., Huang, G., Casilli, A. A., Tubaro, P., Dodel, M., Quan-Haase, A., Ruiu, M. L., Ragnedda, M., Aikat, D., & Tolentino, N. (2020). Digital inequalities in time of pandemic: COVID-19 exposure risk profiles and new forms of vulnerability. *First Monday, 25(7).* https://doi.org/10.5210/fm.v25i7.10845

Ruiz-Figueroa, I., Minguela, M. Á., & Munuera, P. (2025). Diverse digital responses to loneliness in older adults: A systematic review from a social work perspective. *Clinical Social Work Journal*. https://doi.org/10.1007/s10615-024-00981-8

Schlomann, A., Seifert, A., Zank, S., Woopen, C., & Rietz, C. (2020). Use of information and communication technology (ICT) devices among the oldest-old: Loneliness, anomie, and autonomy. *Innovation in Aging, 4*(2), igz050. https://doi.org/10.1093/geroni/igz050

Schulz, R., Wahl, H.-W., Matthews, J. T., De Vito Dabbs, A., Beach, S. R., & Czaja, S. J. (2015). Advancing the aging and technology agenda in gerontology. *The Gerontologist, 55*(5), 724–734. https://doi.org/10.1093/geront/gnu071

Seifert, A. (2020). The digital exclusion of older adults during the COVID-19 pandemic. *Journal of Gerontological Social Work, 63*(6–7), 674–676.

Seifert, A. (2022). Digitale Transformation in den Haushalten älterer Menschen. *Zeitschrift für Gerontologie und Geriatrie, 55*(4), 305–311. https://doi.org/10.1007/s00391-021-01897-5

Seifert, A., & Cotten, S. R. (2021). Use of information and communication technologies among older adults: Usage differences, health-related impacts, and future needs. In D. A. Rohlinger & S. Sobieraj (Eds.), *The Oxford handbook of sociology and digital media* (pp. 1–27). Oxford University Press. https://doi.org/10.1093/oxfordhb/9780197510636.013.12

Seifert, A., Cotten, S. R., & Xie, B. (2021). A double burden of exclusion? Digital and social exclusion of older adults in times of COVID-19. *The Journals of Gerontology: Series B, 76*(3), e99–e103. https://doi.org/10.1093/geronb/gbaa098

Seifert, A., Hofer, M., & Rössel, J. (2018). Older adults' perceived sense of social exclusion from the digital world. *Educational Gerontology, 44*(12), 775–785. https://doi.org/10.1080/03601277.2019.1574415

Seifert, A., & Rössel, J. (2019). Digital participation. In D. Gu & M. E. Dupre (Eds.), *Encyclopedia of gerontology and population aging*. Springer. https://doi.org/10.1007/978-3-319-69892-2_1017-1

Seifert, A., & Schelling, H. R. (2018). Seniors online: Attitudes toward the internet and coping with everyday life. *Journal of Applied Gerontology, 37*(1), 99–109. https://doi.org/10.1177/0733464816669805

Slegers, K., Van Boxtel, M. P. J., & Jolles, J. (2008). Effects of computer training and internet usage on the well-being and quality of life of older adults: A randomized, controlled study. *The Journals of Gerontology Series B: Psychological Sciences and Social Sciences, 63*(3), P176–P184. https://doi.org/10.1093/geronb/63.3.P176

Smith, D., Leonis, T., & Anandavalli, S. (2021). Belonging and loneliness in cyberspace: Impacts of social media on adolescents' well-being. *Australian Journal of Psychology, 73*(1), 12–23. https://doi.org/10.1080/00049530.2021.1898914

Stockwell, S., Stubbs, B., Jackson, S. E., Fisher, A., Yang, L., & Smith, L. (2021). Internet use, social isolation and loneliness in older adults. *Aging and Society, 41*(12), 2723–2746. https://doi.org/10.1017/S0144686X20000550

Szabo, A., Allen, J., Stephens, C., & Alpass, F. (2019). Longitudinal analysis of the relationship between purposes of internet use and well-being among older adults. *The Gerontologist, 59*(1), 58–68. https://doi.org/10.1093/geront/gny036

Van Regenmortel, S., De Donder, L., Dury, S., Smetcoren, A.-S., De Witte, N., & Verté, D. (2016). Social exclusion in later life: A systematic review of the literature. *Journal of Population Aging, 9*(4), 315–344. https://doi.org/10.1007/s12062-016-9145-3

Wahl, H.-W., & Gerstorf, D. (2018). A conceptual framework for studying context dynamics in aging (CODA). *Developmental Review, 50*, 155–176. https://doi.org/10.1016/j.dr.2018.09.003

Walsh, K., Scharf, T., & Keating, N. (2017). Social exclusion of older persons: A scoping review and conceptual framework. *European Journal of Aging, 14*(1), 81–98. https://doi.org/10.1007/s10433-016-0398-8

Xie, B., Charness, N., Fingerman, K., Kaye, J., Kim, M. T., & Khurshid, A. (2020). When going digital becomes a necessity: Ensuring older adults' needs for information, services, and social inclusion during COVID-19. *Journal of Aging & Social Policy*, 1–11. https://doi.org/10.1080/08959420.2020.1771237

Yu, K., Wu, S., & Chi, I. (2021). Internet use and loneliness of older adults over time: The mediating effect of social contact. *The Journals of Gerontology: Series B, 76*(3), 541–550. https://doi.org/10.1093/geronb/gbaa004

Alexander Seifert, who holds a diploma in social work and a doctorate in sociology, is a senior researcher at the School of Social Work at the University of Applied Sciences Northwestern Switzerland. Prior to his current position, he held a research position at the Center for Gerontology at the University of Zurich (Switzerland) for 14 years, most recently serving as Head of Research. His research interests include social gerontology, technology use, and the lifestyles of older adults.

Open Access This chapter is licensed under the terms of the Creative Commons Attribution 4.0 International License (http://creativecommons.org/licenses/by/4.0/), which permits use, sharing, adaptation, distribution and reproduction in any medium or format, as long as you give appropriate credit to the original author(s) and the source, provide a link to the Creative Commons license and indicate if changes were made.

The images or other third party material in this chapter are included in the chapter's Creative Commons license, unless indicated otherwise in a credit line to the material. If material is not included in the chapter's Creative Commons license and your intended use is not permitted by statutory regulation or exceeds the permitted use, you will need to obtain permission directly from the copyright holder.

Chapter 9
Climate Change and the Risk of Loneliness

Liat Ayalon

9.1 Introduction

The past few decades have seen tremendous changes in the environment and the climate (United Nations, 2021), characterized by long-term variations in temperature and weather patterns. According to the International Panel on Climate Change (IPCC), the changing climate results in substantially more severe, extreme, and frequent weather events including droughts, flooding, and extremely hot and cold weather, which do not represent sporadic variations, but rather long-term deviations. This has resulted in extensive changes in the environment including the melting of glaciers, desertification, and the rise in sea levels. Whereas some of these changes are slow and gradual usually taking place over decades, such as global warming, glacier melting, or desertification, other changes are considered more rapid, such as typhoons, hurricanes, flooding, or wildfires. Regardless of their pace, these changes have a direct impact on plants and animals, resulting in the disappearance, unexpected migration patterns, and altered life cycles of certain species (Intergovernmental Panel on Climate Change, 2022).

Humans are highly impacted by the changing climate as well, with well-documented evidence of its growing impact on their health and wellbeing (An et al., 2019; Ayalon et al., 2021). It is possible to portray the impact of the changing climate on people across the lifespan as a U-shape, with both younger and older persons being particularly susceptible. Younger people are highly impacted by the changing climate, especially because they are likely to be exposed to more severe weather events for a longer period of their lives (Barford et al., 2021). Older persons as well are susceptible to the negative impact of the changing climate on their

L. Ayalon (✉)
The Louis and Gabi Weisfeld School of Social Work, Bar Ilan University, Ramat Gan, Israel
e-mail: liat.ayalon@biu.ac.il

© The Author(s) 2025

M. Aartsen et al. (eds.), *Macro Social Influences on Loneliness in Later Life*, International Perspectives on Aging 47,
https://doi.org/10.1007/978-3-031-94565-6_9

physical health (Ayalon et al., 2023) at least partially due to physiological changes and pre-morbid illness (Falchetta et al., 2024).

The present chapter explores possible associations between climate change and loneliness. This is because both represent negative phenomena of direct impact on older persons. Both climate change and loneliness are substantial risks to the population, and understanding their potential relationship is crucial. Like the changing climate, loneliness, defined as the subjective sense of having inadequate social ties (Perlman & Peplau, 1981), is characterized as a growing societal challenge of tremendous impact on individuals (Dennig et al., 2015; Henriksen et al., 2019; Lonergan-Cullum et al., 2022). In addition, like climate change (Tapia-Muñoz et al., 2022), the incidence and impact of loneliness are not shared equally by all individuals or geographic regions (Madsen et al., 2019; Neves et al., 2023). Moreover, similar to the changing climate (Åström et al., 2011), loneliness results in numerous negative health and mental health outcomes including a higher risk for mortality (Henriksen et al., 2019; Shiovitz-Ezra & Ayalon, 2010).

The chapter starts by summarizing existing evidence concerning the moderating role of social isolation, as an objective indicator of inadequate social ties (rather than loneliness, which represents the subjective experience), in the relationship between climate change and negative health and mental health outcomes. Next, I discuss the possibility of a spurious relationship between climate change and loneliness, given the similarity of moderators that make their effects more pronounced and the similarity in outcomes. I then explore three possible pathways from climate change to loneliness, while outlining potential macro-, meso-, and micro-level mediators which possibly account for the relationship between the two. An alternative pathway which explores the possible beneficial effects of the changing climate on loneliness via meso-level indicators is also explored. When reading this chapter, it is important to keep in mind the fact that research connecting the two phenomena is still scarce. Hence, much of the discussion is hypothetical in nature with limited concrete empirical data to support it. The chapter concludes with suggestions for future research to further explore whether and how these two phenomena are related as well as for future policy aimed at addressing both phenomena.

9.2 Social Isolation as a Moderator of the Relationship Between Climate Change and Negative Outcomes

There is plenty of research to show that social isolation, rather than loneliness can be a risk for inadequate preparedness and adaptation to climate change events especially among older persons (Klinenberg, 2015). Specifically, older persons who are socially isolated have been shown to be more likely to die during extreme heat events (Klinenberg, 2015). Older persons who rely on care assistance in long-term care settings also are more likely to die following evacuation due to extreme climate events such as wildfires, flooding, or tornadoes (Brown et al., 2012). Moreover, not having adequate policy representation may result in older persons not having their needs met (Willoughby et al., 2017). Figure 9.1 depicts social isolation as a moderator of the relationship between climate change and negative health and mental health outcomes, including mortality.

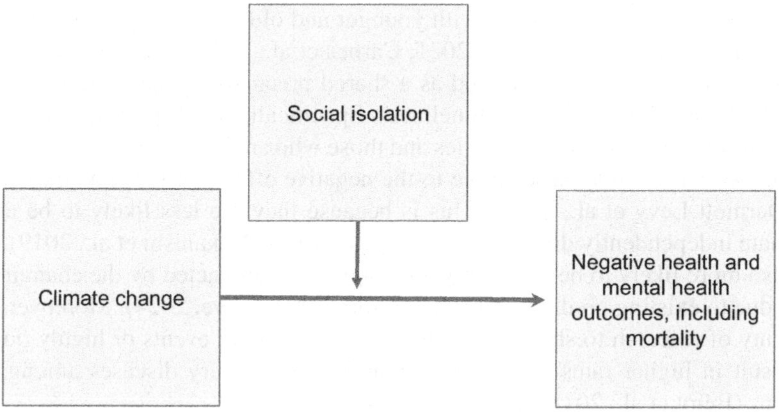

Fig. 9.1 Social isolation as moderator of the relationship between climate change and negative health and mental health outcomes including mortality

9.3 Climate Change and Loneliness May Have a Spurious Relationship

To date, only a limited number of studies have paid attention to possible links between the changing climate and loneliness (Astell-Burt et al., 2022; Bains & Turnbull, 2019; Hajek & König, 2022). Although the changing climate represents a macro-level phenomenon and loneliness is seen mainly as an individual, micro-level experience, both the changing climate and loneliness can be seen as affecting and being affected by the macro-, meso-, and micro-levels. Even though the two operate at different levels, it is possible to suggest that the effects of the changing climate and loneliness are characterized by similar moderators that make certain population groups more susceptible. However, although they may share moderators, this is by no means a causal relationship. Likewise, to a large extent, both climate change and loneliness result in similar negative outcomes. Hence, this proposed model suggests that rather than a pathway from climate change to loneliness, there is a spurious link between the two. This is due to shared moderators which make certain population groups more susceptible to both and shared negative outcomes, as detailed below.

9.3.1 Climate Change and Loneliness Have Similar Moderators Which Make Their Effects More Pronounced

Some of the same factors that make older persons particularly susceptible to the impact of the changing climate also make them susceptible to loneliness. For instance, people of different age groups are affected differently by the changing climate as well as by loneliness, with younger and older persons being particularly impacted by both (Barford et al., 2021; Carnes et al., 2014; Luhmann & Hawkley, 2016). Hence, *age* can be explored as a shared precursor to the effects of climate change as well as the effects of loneliness. Specifically, older persons who experience physical or cognitive disabilities and those who are less likely to have available care networks are more susceptible to the negative effects of the changing climate (McDermott-Levy et al., 2019). This is because they are less likely to be able to evacuate independently during climate hazard events (Nakanishi et al., 2019). They are also more likely to be physically and cognitively impacted by the changing climate due to existing predispositions (Zuelsdorff & Limaye, 2024). Moreover, there is plenty of research to show how extremely hot weather events or highly polluted air result in higher rates of cardiovascular and pulmonary diseases among older persons (Béjot et al., 2018; Kim et al., 2012).

Similar to climate change, the oldest old report high levels of loneliness, although there is no consistent evidence that the prevalence of loneliness increases with age in the older population (Chawla et al., 2021; Lee, 2025). The high levels of loneliness are partially accounted for by the fact that older persons often experience physical and cognitive impairments, which prevent them from socially interacting, thus impairing their ability to develop satisfactory social ties. Moreover, the death of close friends and family members may leave older persons socially disconnected, with limited intimate ties and heightened levels of loneliness (Ayalon et al., 2012). Retirement as well is considered a risk for loneliness as older persons often are forced to disconnect from social ties following the transition to retirement (Segel-Karpas et al., 2018).

Just like older persons, younger persons are also more likely to be impacted by the changing climate (Bunyavanich et al., 2003). Part of this is explained by their physiological susceptibility, and part is explained by the fact that the effects of the changing climate are becoming worse over time and it is younger persons who will be impacted by the changing climate throughout their remaining lifespan (Barford et al., 2021). In the case of loneliness, younger persons as well are likely to experience high levels of loneliness (Siva, 2020).

Gender also appears to have a differential association both with regard to the changing climate and with regard to the experience of loneliness (Nicolaisen & Thorsen, 2023; World Health Organization, 2014). Women in the Global South are more likely to be impacted by the changing climate (Arora-Jonsson, 2011). This has been attributed to gender norms that prevent women from accessing relief (Luna & Hilhorst, 2022). Women are also more likely to be excluded from public discourse and relevant climate policy, whereas men are the ones seen as having political power to impact climate policies. Moreover, it is men in the Global North who are more likely to pollute the environment (Arora-Jonsson, 2011). Likewise, women and especially older women are more likely to report higher levels of loneliness than men (Hajek et al., 2025). This is partially explained by the fact that older women are more likely to experience higher rates of widowhood, to live alone, and to experience cognitive or physical disabilities, which prevent them from socially interacting with others (Beal, 2006).

Belonging to a *racial or ethnic minority* group is another characteristic that makes people more susceptible to the negative impacts of the changing climate as well as to loneliness (Phuong et al., 2023; Victor et al., 2012). People of racial/ethnic minority status are more likely to experience the negative impacts of the changing climate. This is partially explained by the fact that these individuals are also more likely to experience lower levels of socioeconomic status and thus, especially in the Global South, are more likely to depend on the land for their livelihood, as many are engaged in agriculture, hunting and gathering, or animal husbandry. Under these circumstances, they are likely to experience a substantial disruption in their life and ability to make a living under severe weather events (Nguyen & Leisz, 2021; Yin et al., 2020). Moreover, individuals of racial/ethnic minority status are less likely to have adequate disaster response strategies, including adequate access to food and shelter during extreme weather events (Benevolenza & DeRigne, 2019). Loneliness as well is more likely to be reported by racial/ethnic minority groups (Joshi et al., 2024). This has been explained by the transition from traditional values to modernization, which brings with it unfulfilled expectations concerning one's social relations, by the stigma and exclusion of racial/ethnic minorities from the general society, and by lower levels of income and education of people of minority background (Cotterell et al., 2025; Taylor et al., 2024). Nevertheless, even though the changing climate and loneliness differentially impact certain population groups of similar characteristics, the exact mechanisms responsible for the effects may not be shared by the two phenomena. Rather, they may represent spurious associations.

9.3.2 Climate Change and Loneliness Have Similar Outcomes

Climate change and loneliness are related via sharing similar outcomes, which again provide no indication of a causal link between the two. Many of the negative effects of the changing climate are quite similar to the effects of loneliness, including *deteriorated health and mental health,* and even a higher *risk of mortality* (Adams et al., 2021; De Blois et al., 2015; Rico-Uribe et al., 2018). Among the most well-known risks of the changing climate are *cardiovascular diseases* which are more likely to develop in extremely hot weather events or in highly polluted environments. Cardiovascular diseases, pulmonary diseases and dementia are also associated with high levels of environmental pollution (Béjot et al., 2018; Smirnova et al., 2023). Another well-documented outcome of the changing climate is the higher *risk of death*, which primarily occurs in older persons following climate exposure (Adams et al., 2021).

Loneliness has also been shown to have a strong association with *cardiovascular conditions* (Hodgson et al., 2020). Although some have argued that it is cognitive impairment that results in higher levels of loneliness (Ayalon et al., 2016), others have shown that it is the other way around and that those who report higher levels of loneliness are more likely to develop cognitive impairment and even to be diagnosed with dementia (Sutin et al., 2018). Moreover, loneliness can also lead to other health problems such as diabetes, obesity, autoimmune diseases, and even cancer (Mushtaq et al., 2014). *Mortality* is yet another outcome commonly attributed to high levels of loneliness (Rico-Uribe et al., 2018).

The changing climate and loneliness also result in substantial *mental health outcomes* (Beutel et al., 2017; Manning & Clayton, 2018; Palinkas & Wong, 2020), which again could be similar, but do not provide any indication of a causal link between the two. Higher levels of post-traumatic stress disorder, depression, anxiety, stress, and even suicidal ideation and suicide are common mental health outcomes associated with exposure to severe weather events as well as to climate change evacuation and its aftermath (Charlson et al., 2021). Extreme heat also has been associated with high levels of anger and violence (Miles-Novelo & Anderson, 2023).

Like the changing climate, loneliness has also been shown to be a precipitator of negative *mental health outcomes* (Beutel et al., 2017). A longitudinal cross-lagged model examined the temporal associations between loneliness and depression. The study found that it is not depression that results in higher levels of loneliness, but the other way around, higher levels of loneliness at baseline result in greater depressive symptomatology at follow-up (Cacioppo et al., 2010). Likewise, research has shown that sleep problems and suicide ideation are often the products of loneliness (Ayalon & Shiovitz-Ezra, 2011; Kurina et al., 2011).

9.3.3 Conclusions

Figure 9.2 identified similar moderators which make the effects of the changing climate and of loneliness more pronounced, and outcomes associated with these effects (irrespective of each other). Whether the two are related directly, indirectly, or spuriously remains to be examined in further theoretical and empirical studies as discussed below.

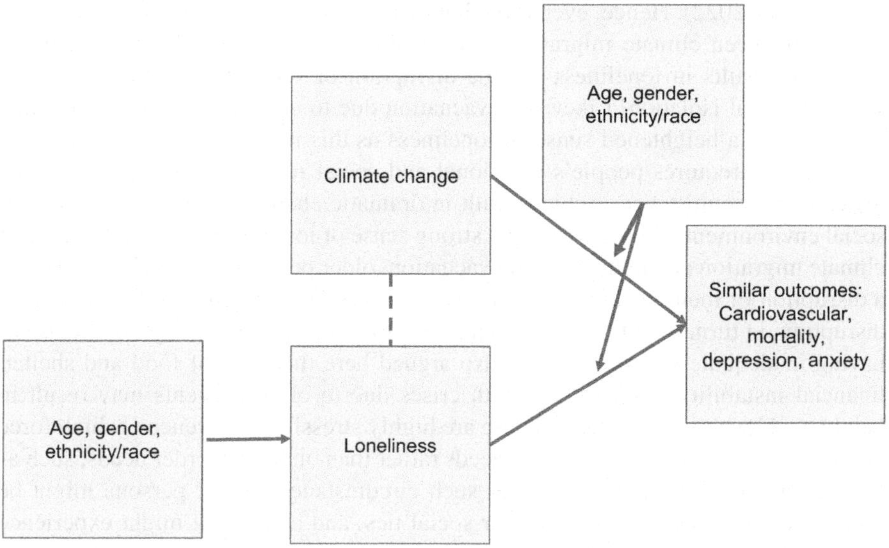

Fig. 9.2 Similar moderators and outcomes of climate change and loneliness, suggesting the possibility of a spurious relationship. *The dotted line is not discussed in the model but represents a plausible association

9.4 Climate Change Outcomes Mediate the Relationship Between Climate Change and Loneliness

9.4.1 Macro-level Mediators of the Relationship Between Climate Change and Loneliness

In addition to spurious associations mentioned above, there are possibilities of true associations between climate change and loneliness. The changing climate brings with it accompanying changes in the environment as well as changes in the entire ecosystem, including plants and animals (Intergovernmental Panel on Climate Change, 2022). Research has shown that being in a green environment has a beneficial effect on people's health and mental health, including a reduced sense of loneliness (Astell-Burt et al., 2022). Being surrounded by various animal species is yet another factor that is considered protective against loneliness. These beneficial effects are often lost once the environment, and its inhabitants, deteriorate because of the changing climate. Therefore, it is expected that under more extreme weather conditions, people will experience a greater sense of loneliness associated with environmental changes brought by the changing climate.

Another change in the social and physical environment brought by the changing climate is climate migration (Kaczan & Orgill-Meyer, 2020). Globally, there is a tendency to migrate from extremely warm areas in search of food and shelter. There is plenty of research showing that migrants experience high levels of loneliness

(Löbel et al., 2022). Hence, even though to date research has not made a direct connection between climate migration and loneliness, it is highly likely that climate migration results in loneliness via the disruption of social ties and an increased sense of social isolation. Likewise, evacuation due to extreme climate events may also result in a heightened sense of loneliness as this represents a highly stressful event, which requires people's emotional and social resources. It is possible that under such circumstances, which result in dramatic changes in one's physical and social environment, people will feel a strong sense of loneliness. Both in the case of climate migration and in the case of evacuation, older persons will likely experience a disruption of their social network due to changes in their physical location. This disruption, in turn, might result in social isolation as well as in a subjective sense of having inadequate social ties. It is also argued here that lack of food and shelter, financial instability, and public health crises due to climate events may result in heightened levels of loneliness. These are highly stressful occurrences, which force people to concentrate on their basic needs rather than on higher-order needs, such as belonging and social contact. Under such circumstances, older persons might be less geared towards investing in their social ties, and as a result might experience social isolation accompanied by an intense sense of loneliness. Figure 9.3 presents possible macro-level mediators of the relationship between climate change and loneliness.

9.4.2 *Meso-level Mediators of the Relationship Between Climate Change and Loneliness*

A substantial part of current climate change discourse reflects intergenerational divides and conflicts (Ayalon et al., 2022; Roy & Ayalon, 2022). It is younger persons who feel as if their voice and concerns are not heard. Older persons, instead, are being blamed for their (in)action and failure to protect the environment. In much of the public discourse, older persons are seen as exploiting the

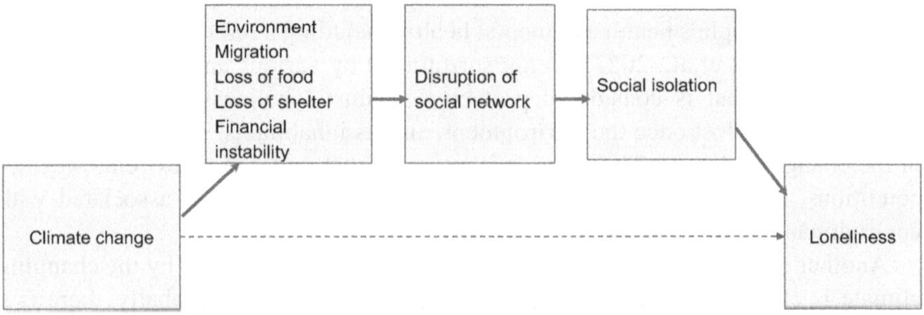

Fig. 9.3 Possible macro-level mediators of the relationship between climate change and loneliness. *The dotted line is not discussed in the model but represents a plausible association

environment for its resources and having failed to save it for the benefit of future generations. Moreover, research has shown that those who report high levels of worry and concern about the changing climate are more likely to report ageism towards older persons (Ayalon & Roy, 2023). Under such a divided environment, ageism against older persons may prevail. Moreover, older persons may internalize some of these negative messages and become increasingly more self-ageist as a result.

The link between ageism and loneliness may take several possible pathways (Shiovitz-Ezra et al., 2018). First, it is possible that more ageist individuals who feel resentment and anger toward older persons will refrain from engaging with them socially. Under such circumstances, older persons may experience a heightened sense of loneliness. In addition, heightened ageism and intergenerational conflict may also result in a sense of loneliness among younger persons, who might feel less supported and more alienated from older generations. Figure 9.4 presents possible meso-level mediators that potentially account for the relationship between climate change and loneliness via ageism, manifested in interpersonal relations, which brings with it a disruption in one's social network and social isolation as a result. It is important to note that in addition to the meso-level discussed here (e.g., ageism in interpersonal relations), ageism also manifests at the macro-level via policy and laws, which may disregard the differential impact of climate change on older persons (United Nations, 2021). The impact of ageism at the micro-level is also evident when older persons internalize negative views held towards them and as a result are less likely to engage in social interactions and report higher levels of loneliness. For instance, a study that examined the relationship between different types of care settings and loneliness, found that anxiety about aging mediated this relationship. This stresses the detrimental impact of self-directed ageism (Ayalon, 2018). Hence, self-blame and internalized ageist messages may also contribute to older persons' social isolation, which may bring with it a heightened sense of loneliness.

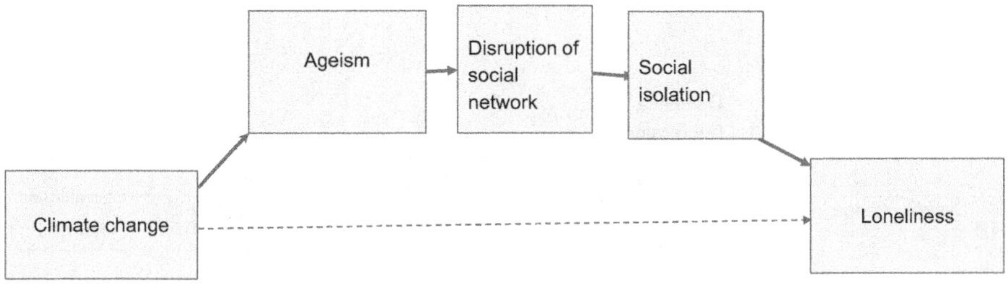

Fig. 9.4 Possible meso-level mediators of the relationship between climate change and loneliness. *The dotted line is not discussed in the model but represents a plausible association

9.4.3 *Micro-level Mediators of the Relationship Between Climate Change and Loneliness*

The changing climate and environment may also result in a reduced likelihood of engaging in various social and health behaviors, including physical activity, routine medical check-ups, or engagement in leisure time activities (Bernard et al., 2021). A reduction in one's engagement in social and health behaviors impacts not only one's health but also social life and possibly one's sense of belonging and loneliness. During extreme hot or cold periods, individuals are less likely to engage outdoors, meet people, and interact with others. This, in turn, may result in a growing sense of loneliness.

As already mentioned, the changing climate also results in a variety of negative health and mental health outcomes (Carnes et al., 2014; Ebi et al., 2021). Although similar to climate change, loneliness has been shown to be a predictor of some of these outcomes, it also could be a product of these various health and mental health outcomes (Hawkley et al., 2020). Depressed or highly anxious individuals are less likely to seek out social interactions. Instead, they may retreat to their own inner emotional struggles, invest less in social activities and, as a result, may feel a growing sense of loneliness (Franceschi et al., 2022).

Physical and cognitive impairments caused by the changing climate (Balbus & Malina, 2009; Béjot et al., 2018) may also put people at a higher risk for loneliness. People who experience physical and cognitive impairments may have fewer opportunities to engage socially because of their disability (Ayalon et al., 2012). Moreover, the stigma attached to physical and/or cognitive impairments may prevent others from socially engaging with these people (Aboseif & Woo, 2020). Mortality due to climate change (Åström et al., 2011) may also result in a heightened sense of loneliness as people may experience the loss of loved ones and as a result a lack of intimate ties. Figure 9.5 depicts micro-level mediators that possibly account for the relationship between climate change and loneliness.

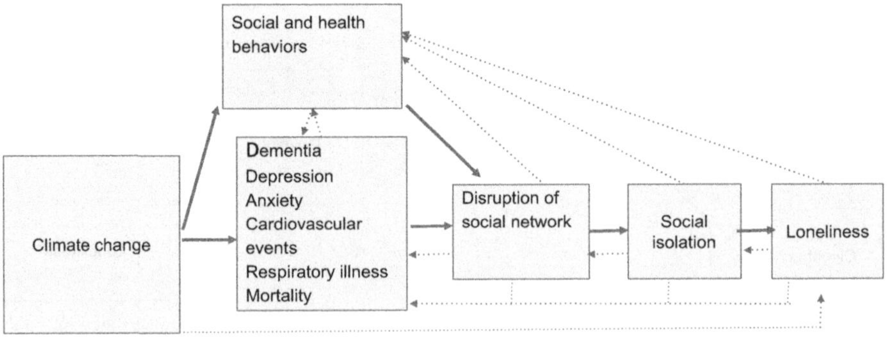

Fig. 9.5 Possible micro-level mediators of the relationship between climate change and loneliness. *Dotted lines are not discussed but reflect the cross-lagged effects of many of the variables presented in the model, as relationships are not unidirectional

9.4.4 Conclusions

This section outlines a complex model, which includes various mediators at the macro- (e.g., environmental changes), meso- (e.g., ageism), and micro- (e.g., health, mental health) levels to possibly account for an association between the changing climate and loneliness via a disruption of social relations and increased social isolation. As noted, many of the associations can be bi-directional, alluding to the complexity of the proposed model.

9.5 Engagement in the Climate Change Movement/ Pro-environmental Behaviors Alleviate Loneliness

Another possible pathway through which the link between the changing climate and loneliness can be explained is via people's engagement in the climate change movement and pro-environmental behaviors. The climate change movement is considered an informal protest movement that brings the topic of the changing climate to the forefront (Chazan & Baldwin, 2019; Ritchie, 2021). There is some research about involvement in protests in general (Okun & Ayalon, 2024) and in the climate change movement specifically as a means not only to bring certain political topics into the discourse and to create societal change, but also as a way to foster a sense of self-efficacy, improved wellbeing, increased social connectedness, and reduced loneliness (Zeigler, 2019). Related to this, Greta Thunberg, one of the most prominent climate change activists, described her own experiences as a sole and lonely activist prior to the establishment of Fridays for Future. Reportedly, her ability to establish the Fridays for Future movement and gather the support of youth worldwide has increased not only her sense of self-efficacy but also her sense of connectedness to others in the world (Olesen, 2022).

Likewise, engagement in pro-environmental behaviors can have beneficial effects by giving meaning and purpose in life (Jia et al., 2021). Engagement in pro-environmental behaviors puts one in a position of caring about the environment, taking an active stance, and contributing to society at large. Just like engaging in the climate change movement, engagement in pro-environmental behaviors helps people to group around a common cause and identify with other like-minded individuals. This may enhance one's social network, resulting in a reduced sense of loneliness. See Fig. 9.6 for details.

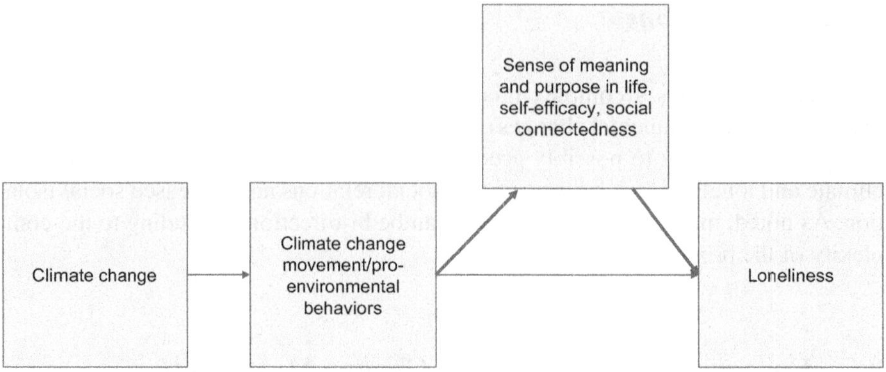

Fig. 9.6 Engagement in the climate change movement/pro-environmental behaviors possibly alleviate loneliness. *The dotted line is not discussed in the model but represents a plausible association

9.6 Conclusions

The present chapter reviewed a relatively unexplored topic, namely the association between climate change and loneliness. The chapter began by depicting the most obvious and well-explored aspect: the role of social isolation (rather than lonely) as a risk for the negative impact of climate change, especially in the case of older persons. Next, the chapter proposed a model, suggesting that climate change and loneliness may be spuriously correlated because they have similar moderators and similar outcomes. The next model examined possible mediators at the macro-, meso-, or micro- levels which potentially link the changing climate and loneliness via a disruption in one's social network and increased isolation. An alternative model also identified mediators of the link between climate change and loneliness, but this time considered the engagement in the climate change movement and pro-environmental behaviors as precipitators of an enhanced sense of social connectedness and a reduced sense of loneliness. Hence, this pathway suggests positive rather than negative effects on loneliness. When reviewing these proposed models, it is important to note the paucity of research, which makes them speculative at best. Further research is needed to better understand the possible links between the changing climate and loneliness.

Although research is scarce, the findings point to several important directions. Clearly more research is needed to explore the links between the changing climate and loneliness, which to date have largely remained under-explored. Such research should move away from cross-sectional convenience studies to experimental studies that possibly develop causal models, beyond spurious associations. Second, social justice and inequalities have received considerable attention in the context of climate change (Andrey & Jones, 2008; Antal, 2018). Far less attention has been devoted to these topics in the context of loneliness. Given the many similarities in demographics among those most susceptible to the changing climate and those susceptible to loneliness, it is important to further examine loneliness through the lens of social justice and inequalities. The effects of the changing climate on various mediators are likely moderated by various sociodemographic variables, such as age, gender, or socioeconomic status, which result in greater susceptibility of certain population groups to the effects of climate change as well as to the effect of loneliness. The moderating effects of various sociodemographic variables may explain the greater susceptibility of individuals of certain demographics, such as older persons, racial/ethnic minorities or people of lower socioeconomic status, to the changing climate (Nyahunda et al., 2021; Prina et al., 2024; Smith et al., 2022), which in turn may result in higher levels of loneliness in these population groups (Klein et al., 2020). Although this is not discussed in detail in this chapter, it is important to take into consideration the fact that climate change has a disproportionate impact on the Global South, but it is the Global North which has benefited the most from polluting and exploiting the environment for decades (Kamal Uddin, 2017). Likewise, research concerning loneliness primarily originated in the Global North, with substantially less empirical research and theoretical conceptualization concerning loneliness in the Global South (Susanty et al., 2025).

Policy-wise, it is important to acknowledge climate change as a possible precipitator of the growing phenomenon of loneliness. Such recognition can assist in targeting specific population groups as particularly susceptible to the effects of climate change as well as to the effects of loneliness. Specifically, the chapter has identified possible macro-meso-and micro-level mediators which could be improved by policy to possibly alleviate loneliness. At the macro-level, the present chapter emphasized the potential role of the environment as a factor that can enhance social engagement and alleviate f loneliness if developed adequately. Environments that are accessible to all ages, have proper shade and opportunities to interact can be established via direct policy and planning, such environments are likely to result in lower levels of loneliness (Bower et al., 2023).

Likewise, access to food, shelter and water are human rights that should be provided to all, even under extreme conditions (Levy & Patz, 2015; Nehaluddin & Lilienthal, 2021). Climate migration and immigration also deserve policy attention (Gemenne & Blocher, 2017). At the present time, even the term to describe people who are displaced due to climate events remains unclear (Berchin et al., 2017). Moreover, older persons and persons with disabilities, who represent the most susceptible population groups, often remain behind when younger and healthy generations leave due to climate events (Hauer et al., 2024). Policies that acknowledge climate migration and ensure the ability of all individuals to evacuate on time and migrate if needed are essential. Likewise, policies that support those who stay behind are also required to ensure the well-being of the most susceptible populations (Sullivan, 2017).

At the meso-level, ageism plays an important role in the lives of all of us. Both younger and older persons are particularly susceptible to the negative effects of ageism (Ayalon & Tesch-Römer, 2018; de la Fuente-Núñez et al., 2021). The World Health Organization has identified three evidence-based strategies to reduce ageism (World Health Organization, 2021). Education about ageing and about ageism can result in reduced ageism. Likewise, intergenerational contact around collaborative tasks under equal status is likely to result in reduced levels of ageism. In addition, policies that explicitly ban discrimination based on age can also be effective in reducing ageism. It is possible that these strategies can also result in the reduction of loneliness, given the varied pathways through which ageism may affect loneliness.

Micro-level mediators identified in the present chapter concern both health and mental health outcomes, as well as social and health behaviors. As the impact of the changing climate is not uniform, but rather is usually stronger and more severe in the case of the most susceptible segments of the population (Smith et al., 2022), governments and communities bear a responsibility to ensure that climate hazards do not turn into disasters. By engaging in adequate mitigation, preparation, and adaptation measures, it is possible to alleviate some of the negative health and mental health effects of the changing climate as well as its negative impact on social and health behaviors. This may also result in a reduction in loneliness among the most susceptible groups in society.

Finally, certain climate change activities, such as engagement in the climate change movement and in pro-environmental behaviors, possibly have beneficial effects (Pillemer et al., 2009) including the alleviation of loneliness. As such, it is important to encourage public engagement in the climate change movement and in pro-environmental behaviors not only to possibly tackle the growing impacts of the changing climate but also to reduce loneliness. While doing so, it is important to acknowledge the fact that certain population groups are less likely to engage in the climate change movement due to ageism (Roy & Ayalon, 2022) or other exclusionary practices and that certain population groups are less knowledgeable about the importance of engaging in pro-environmental behaviors (Liobikienė & Poškus, 2019). Hence, educational efforts are necessary.

Raising a collective awareness of climate change across all age groups has the potential to cultivate collaboration between older and younger generations. By joining forces to tackle the pressing challenges of climate change, different age groups can work toward shared objectives, creating a foundation for increased social connectedness. This collaboration can significantly reduce feelings of social isolation and loneliness, which often affect individuals across all age groups. When older people engage with younger people on environmental initiatives, they can experience a renewed sense of purpose and belonging. Mutual support and shared responsibilities in projects or community events can lead to deeper intergenerational relationships, fostering a sense of solidarity.

Moreover, the act of working together on climate-related issues encourages broader social participation. Older persons can share their life experiences and knowledge, while younger individuals can bring fresh perspectives and innovative solutions. Such exchanges can lead to greater understanding and respect between generations. Community efforts, like tree planting programs, local clean-up days, or educational workshops, not only benefit the environment but also serve as opportunities for social engagement. As people unite for a cause that impacts their futures, they build networks of support and friendship that transcend age barriers, ultimately leading to a more vibrant and connected community. By weaving together the distinct strengths of each generation, we can create a framework that reduces loneliness and encourages active involvement, reinforcing the idea that collective action on climate change is beneficial for all (Roy & Ayalon, 2023).

Acknowledgement This work received funding from the Israel Science Foundation ISF 217-20.

Competing Interests The author has no conflict of interest to declare that are relevant to the content of this chapter.

References

Aboseif, A., & Woo, B. K. P. (2020). Chapter 40 – The stigma of dementia. In C. R. Martin & V. R. Preedy (Eds.), *Genetics, neurology, behavior, and diet in dementia* (pp. 633–645). Academic. https://doi.org/10.1016/B978-0-12-815868-5.00040-2

Adams, R. M., Evans, C. M., Mathews, M. C., Wolkin, A., & Peek, L. (2021). Mortality from forces of nature among older adults by race/ethnicity and gender. *Journal of Applied Gerontology, 40*(11), 1517–1526. https://doi.org/10.1177/0733464820954676

An, R., Qiu, Y., Xiang, X., Ji, M., & Guan, C. (2019, Nov). Impact of Hurricane Katrina on mental health among US adults. *American Journal of Health Behaviours, 43*(6), 1186–1199. https://doi.org/10.5993/ajhb.43.6.15

Andrey, J., & Jones, B. (2008). The dynamic nature of social disadvantage: Implications for hazard exposure and vulnerability in Greater Vancouver. *The Canadian Geographer/Le Géographe canadien, 52*(2), 146–168. https://doi.org/10.1111/j.1541-0064.2008.00206.x

Antal, A. (2018). Climate and social justice in Eastern and Southern Europe: The social nature of climate change. *INOGOV Network: Innovations in Climate Governance*. Accessed online on March 9, 2025: chrome-extension://efaidnbmnnnibpcajpcglclefindmkaj/https://www.inogov.eu/wp-content/uploads/2018/08/Antal_WP1.pdf.

Arora-Jonsson, S. (2011, 2011/05/01/). Virtue and vulnerability: Discourses on women, gender and climate change. Global Environmental Change, 21(2), 744–751. doi:https://doi.org/10.1016/j.gloenvcha.2011.01.005.

Astell-Burt, T., Hartig, T., Eckermann, S., Nieuwenhuijsen, M., McMunn, A., Frumkin, H., & Feng, X. (2022). More green, less lonely? A longitudinal cohort study. *International Journal of Epidemiology, 51*(1), 99–110. https://doi.org/10.1093/ije/dyab089

Åström, D. O., Bertil, F., & Joacim, R. (2011). Heat wave impact on morbidity and mortality in the elderly population: A review of recent studies. *Maturitas, 69*(2), 99–105. https://doi.org/10.1016/j.maturitas.2011.03.008

Ayalon, L. (2018, Jun). Loneliness and anxiety about aging in adult day care centers and continuing care retirement communities. *Innovation in Aging, 2*(2), igy021. https://doi.org/10.1093/geroni/igy021

Ayalon, L., & Roy, S. (2023). The role of ageism in climate change worries and willingness to act. *Journal of Applied Gerontology, 42*(6), 1305–1312. https://doi.org/10.1177/07334648221130323

Ayalon, L., & Shiovitz-Ezra, S. (2011). The relationship between loneliness and passive death wishes in the second half of life. *International Psychogeriatrics, 23*(10), 1677–1685. https://doi.org/10.1017/S1041610211001384

Ayalon, L., & Tesch-Römer, C. (2018). *Contemporary perspectives on ageism*. Springer Nature.

Ayalon, L., Shiovitz-Ezra, S., & Palgi, Y. (2012). No place like home? Potential pathways to loneliness in older adults under the care of a live-in foreign home care worker. *The Journal of Psychology, 146*(1–2), 189–200. https://doi.org/10.1080/00223980.2011.574169

Ayalon, L., Shiovitz-Ezra, S., & Roziner, I. (2016). A cross-lagged model of the reciprocal associations of loneliness and memory functioning. *Psychology and Aging, 31*(3), 255. https://doi.org/10.1037/pag0000075

Ayalon, L., Keating, N., Pillemer, K., & Rabheru, K. (2021). Climate change and mental health of older persons: A human rights imperative. *The American Journal of Geriatric Psychiatry, 29*(10), 1038–1040. https://doi.org/10.1016/j.jagp.2021.06.015

Ayalon, L., Roy, S., Aloni, O., & Keating, N. (2022). A scoping review of research on older people and intergenerational relations in the context of climate change. *The Gerontologist, 63*(5), 945–958. https://doi.org/10.1093/geront/gnac028

Ayalon, L., de Mendonça Lima, C. A., Banerjee, D., Rabheru, K., & Fitzgerald, K. G. (2023). Older persons in climate change-induced hazards and building forward better. International Psychogeriatric Association, World Psychiatric Association-Section of Old Age Psychiatry, and NGO Committee on Ageing in Geneva position statement. *International Psychogeriatrics, 35*(11), 589–591. https://doi.org/10.1017/S1041610223000765

Bains, K. K., & Turnbull, T. (2019). Improving health outcomes and serving wider society: The potential role of understanding and cultivating prosocial purpose within health psychology research and practice to address climate change and social isolation and loneliness. *Frontiers in Psychology, 10*, 1787. https://doi.org/10.3389/fpsyg.2019.01787

Balbus, J. M., & Malina, C. (2009). Identifying vulnerable subpopulations for climate change health effects in the United States. *Journal of Occupational and Environmental Medicine, 51*(1), 33–37. https://doi.org/10.1097/JOM.0b013e318193e12e

Barford, A., Mugeere, A., Proefke, R., & Stocking, B. (2021). *Young people and climate change*. The British Academy. https://doi.org/10.5871/bacop26/9780856726606.001

Beal, C. (2006, 2006/01/01). Loneliness in older women: A review of the literature. Issues in Mental Health Nursing, 27(7), 795–813. doi:https://doi.org/10.1080/01612840600781196.

Béjot, Y., Reis, J., Giroud, M., & Feigin, V. (2018). A review of epidemiological research on stroke and dementia and exposure to air pollution. *International Journal of Stroke, 13*(7), 687–695. https://doi.org/10.1177/1747493018772800

Benevolenza, M. A., & DeRigne, L. (2019, 2019/02/17). The impact of climate change and natural disasters on vulnerable populations: A systematic review of literature. Journal of Human Behavior in the Social Environment, 29(2), 266–281. doi:https://doi.org/10.1080/10911359.2018.1527739.

Berchin, I. I., Valduga, I. B., Garcia, J., & De Andrade, J. B. S. O. (2017). Climate change and forced migrations: An effort towards recognizing climate refugees. *Geoforum, 84*, 147–150. https://doi.org/10.1016/j.geoforum.2017.06.022

Bernard, P., Chevance, G., Kingsbury, C., Baillot, A., Romain, A.-J., Molinier, V., Gadais, T., & Dancause, K. N. (2021, 2021/05/01). Climate change, physical activity and sport: A systematic review. *Sports Medicine, 51*(5), 1041–1059. https://doi.org/10.1007/s40279-021-01439-4

Beutel, M. E., Klein, E. M., Brähler, E., Reiner, I., Jünger, C., Michal, M., Wiltink, J., Wild, P. S., Münzel, T., & Lackner, K. J. (2017). Loneliness in the general population: prevalence, determinants and relations to mental health. *BMC Psychiatry, 17*(1), 1–7. https://doi.org/10.1186/s12888-017-1262-x

Bower, M., Kent, J., Patulny, R., Green, O., McGrath, L., Teesson, L., Jamalishahni, T., Sandison, H., & Rugel, E. (2023). The impact of the built environment on loneliness: A systematic review and narrative synthesis. *Health & Place, 79*, 102962. https://doi.org/10.1016/j.healthplace.2022.102962

Brown, L. M., Dosa, D. M., Thomas, K., Hyer, K., Feng, Z., & Mor, V. (2012). The effects of evacuation on nursing home residents with dementia. *American Journal of Alzheimer's Disease & Other Dementias®, 27*(6), 406–412. https://doi.org/10.1177/1533317512454709

Bunyavanich, S., Landrigan, C. P., McMichael, A. J., & Epstein, P. R. (2003). The impact of climate change on child health. *Ambulatory Pediatrics, 3*(1), 44–52. https://doi.org/10.1367/1539-4409(2003)003<0044:tiocco>2.0.co;2

Cacioppo, J. T., Hawkley, L. C., & Thisted, R. A. (2010). Perceived social isolation makes me sad: 5-year cross-lagged analyses of loneliness and depressive symptomatology in the Chicago Health, Aging, and Social Relations Study. *Psychology and Aging, 25*(2), 453–463. https://doi.org/10.1037/a0017216

Carnes, B. A., Staats, D., & Willcox, B. J. (2014). Impact of climate change on elder health. *Journals of Gerontology Series A: Biomedical Sciences and Medical Sciences, 69*(9), 1087–1091. https://doi.org/10.1093/gerona/glt159

Charlson, F., Ali, S., Benmarhnia, T., Pearl, M., Massazza, A., Augustinavicius, J., & Scott, J. G. (2021). Climate change and mental health: A scoping review. *International Journal of Environmental Research and Public Health, 18*(9), 4486. https://doi.org/10.3390/ijerph18094486

Chawla, K., Kunonga, T. P., Stow, D., Barker, R., Craig, D., & Hanratty, B. (2021). Prevalence of loneliness amongst older people in high-income countries: A systematic review and meta-analysis. *PLoS One, 16*(7), e0255088. https://doi.org/10.1371/journal.pone.0255088

Chazan, M., & Baldwin, M. (2019). Granny solidarity: Understanding age and generational dynamics in climate justice movements. *Studies in Social Justice, 13*(2), 244–261. https://doi.org/10.26522/ssj.v13i2.2235

Cotterell, N., Buffel, T., Nazroo, J., & Qualter, P. (2025, 2025/01/02). Loneliness among older ethnic minority people: Exploring the role of structural disadvantage and place using a co-research methodology. Ethnic and Racial Studies, 48(1), 206–228. doi:https://doi.org/10.1080/01419870.2024.2311833.

De Blois, J., Kjellstrom, T., Agewall, S., Ezekowitz, J. A., Armstrong, P. W., & Atar, D. (2015). The effects of climate change on cardiac health. *Cardiology, 131*(4), 209–217. https://doi.org/10.1159/000398787

Dennig, F., Budolfson, M. B., Fleurbaey, M., Siebert, A., & Socolow, R. H. (2015). Inequality, climate impacts on the future poor, and carbon prices. *Proceedings of the National Academy of Sciences, 112*(52), 15827–15832. https://doi.org/10.1073/pnas.1513967112

Ebi, K. L., Boyer, C., Ogden, N., Paz, S., Berry, P., Campbell-Lendrum, D., Hess, J. J., & Woodward, A. (2021). Burning embers: Synthesis of the health risks of climate change. *Environmental Research Letters, 16*(4), 044042. https://doi.org/10.1088/1748-9326/abeadd

Falchetta, G., De Cian, E., Sue Wing, I., & Carr, D. (2024, 2024/05/14). Global projections of heat exposure of older adults. *Nature Communications, 15*(1), 3678. https://doi.org/10.1038/s41467-024-47197-5

Franceschi, A., Imbimbo, E., Menesini, E., Nocentini, A., & Van As, B. A. L. (2022). The longitudinal association between loneliness and depressive symptoms in the elderly: A systematic review. *International Psychogeriatrics, 34*(7), 657–669. https://doi.org/10.1017/S1041610221000399

de la Fuente-Núñez, V., Cohn-Schwartz, E., Roy, S., & Ayalon, L. (2021). Scoping review on age-ism against younger populations. *International Journal of Environmental Research and Public Health, 18*(8), 3988. https://doi.org/10.3390/ijerph18083988

Gemenne, F., & Blocher, J. (2017). How can migration serve adaptation to climate change? Challenges to fleshing out a policy ideal. *The Geographical Journal, 183*(4), 336–347. https://doi.org/10.1111/geoj.12205

Hajek, A., & König, H.-H. (2022). Climate anxiety, loneliness and perceived social isolation. *International Journal of Environmental Research and Public Health, 19*(22), 14991. https://www.mdpi.com/1660-4601/19/22/14991

Hajek, A., Sutin, A. R., Posi, G., Stephan, Y., Peltzer, K., Terracciano, A., Luchetti, M., & König, H. H. (2025, Feb). Chronic loneliness and chronic social isolation among older adults. A systematic review, meta-analysis and meta-regression. *Aging & Mental Health, 29*(2), 185–200. https://doi.org/10.1080/13607863.2024.2385448

Hauer, M. E., Jacobs, S. A., & Kulp, S. A. (2024). Climate migration amplifies demographic change and population aging. *Proceedings of the National Academy of Sciences, 121*(3), e2206192119. https://doi.org/10.1073/pnas.2206192119

Hawkley, L. C., Buecker, S., Kaiser, T., & Luhmann, M. (2020, 2022/01/01). Loneliness from young adulthood to old age: Explaining age differences in loneliness. *International Journal of Behavioral Development, 46*(1), 39–49. https://doi.org/10.1177/0165025420971048

Henriksen, J., Larsen, E., Mattisson, C., & Andersson, N. (2019). Loneliness, health and mortality. *Epidemiology and Psychiatric Sciences, 28*(2), 234–239. https://doi.org/10.1017/S2045796017000580

Hodgson, S., Watts, I., Fraser, S., Roderick, P., & Dambha-Miller, H. (2020). Loneliness, social isolation, cardiovascular disease and mortality: A synthesis of the literature and conceptual framework. *Journal of the Royal Society of Medicine, 113*(5), 185–192. https://doi.org/10.1177/0141076820918236

Intergovernmental Panel on Climate Change. (2022). *IPCC sixth assessment report: Mitigation of climate change*. https://www.ipcc.ch/report/ar6/wg3/

Jia, F., Soucie, K., Matsuba, K., & Pratt, M. W. (2021). Meaning in life mediates the association between environmental engagement and loneliness. *International Journal of Environmental Research and Public Health, 18*(6), 2897. https://doi.org/10.3390/ijerph18062897

Joshi, M., Finney, N., & Hale, J. M. (2024). Loneliness and social isolation of ethnic minority/immigrant older adults: A scoping review. *Ageing and Society*, 1–31. https://doi.org/10.1017/S0144686X24000205

Kaczan, D. J., & Orgill-Meyer, J. (2020). The impact of climate change on migration: A synthesis of recent empirical insights. *Climatic Change, 158*(3–4), 281–300. https://doi.org/10.1007/s10584-019-02560-0

Kamal Uddin, M. (2017). Climate change and global environmental politics: North-South divide. *Environmental Policy and Law, 47*(3–4), 106–114. https://doi.org/10.3233/EPL-170022

Kim, Y.-M., Kim, S., Cheong, H.-K., Ahn, B., & Choi, K. (2012). Effects of heat wave on body temperature and blood pressure in the poor and elderly. *Environmental Health and Toxicology, 27*. https://doi.org/10.5620/eht.2012.27.e2012013

Klein, J., von dem Knesebeck, O., & Lüdecke, D. (2020). Social inequalities and loneliness as predictors of ageing well: A trend analysis using mixed models. *International Journal of Environmental Research and Public Health, 17*(15), 5314. https://doi.org/10.3390/ijerph17155314

Klinenberg, E. (2015). *Heat wave: A social autopsy of disaster in Chicago*. University of Chicago Press. https://doi.org/10.7208/chicago/9780226276212.001.0001

Kurina, L. M., Knutson, K. L., Hawkley, L. C., Cacioppo, J. T., Lauderdale, D. S., & Ober, C. (2011). Loneliness is associated with sleep fragmentation in a communal society. *Sleep, 34*(11), 1519–1526. https://doi.org/10.5665/sleep.1390

Lee, S. (2025). Understanding late-life loneliness: Micro and meso-level determinants. In M. Aartsen, I. Precupetu, & B. Suanet (Eds.), *Macro social influences on loneliness in later life: Towards a better understanding of the loneliness paradox in later life*. Springer.

Levy, B. S., & Patz, J. A. (2015, 2015/05/01/). Climate change, human rights, and social justice. *Annals of Globalization and Health, 81*(3), 310–322. https://doi.org/10.1016/j.aogh.2015.08.008

Liobikienė, G., & Poškus, M. S. (2019). The importance of environmental knowledge for private and public sphere pro-environmental behavior: Modifying the value-belief-norm theory. *Sustainability, 11*(12), 3324. https://doi.org/10.3390/su11123324

Löbel, L.-M., Kröger, H., & Tibubos, A. N. (2022). How migration status shapes susceptibility of individuals' loneliness to social isolation. *International Journal of Public Health, 67*, 1604576. https://doi.org/10.3389/ijph.2022.1604576

Lonergan-Cullum, M., Hooker, S. A., Levy, R., & Ricco, J. (2022). A new pandemic of loneliness. *The Journal of the American Board of Family Medicine, 35*(3), 593–596. https://doi.org/10.3122/jabfm.2022.03.210461

Luhmann, M., & Hawkley, L. C. (2016). Age differences in loneliness from late adolescence to oldest old age. *Developmental Psychology, 52*(6), 943–959. https://doi.org/10.1037/dev0000117

Luna, K. C., & Hilhorst, D. (2022). Gendered experience of disaster: Women's account of evacuation, relief and recovery in Nepal. *International Journal of Disaster Risk Reduction, 72*, 102840. https://doi.org/10.1016/j.ijdrr.2022.102840

Madsen, K., Holstein, B. E., Damsgaard, M. T., Rayce, S. B., Jespersen, L., & Due, P. (2019). Trends in social inequality in loneliness among adolescents 1991–2014. *Journal of Public Health, 41*(2), e133–e140. https://doi.org/10.1093/pubmed/fdy133

Manning, C., & Clayton, S. (2018). Threats to mental health and wellbeing associated with climate change. In *Psychology and climate change* (pp. 217–244). Elsevier. https://doi.org/10.1016/B978-0-12-813130-5.00009-6

McDermott-Levy, R., Kolanowski, A. M., Fick, D. M., & Mann, M. E. (2019). Addressing the health risks of climate change in older adults. *Journal of Gerontological Nursing, 45*(11), 21–29. https://doi.org/10.3928/00989134-20191011-04

Miles-Novelo, A., & Anderson, C. A. (2023). Avoiding a grim future: The climate crisis and its effects on human aggression and violence. *Advances in Environmental and Engineering Research, 4*(2), 1–25. https://doi.org/10.21926/aeer.2302034

Mushtaq, R., Shoib, S., Shah, T., & Mushtaq, S. (2014). Relationship between loneliness, psychiatric disorders and physical health? A review on the psychological aspects of loneliness. *Journal of Clinical and Diagnostic Research: JCDR, 8*(9), WE01. https://doi.org/10.7860/JCDR/2014/10077.4828

Nakanishi, H., Black, J., & Suenaga, Y. (2019). Investigating the flood evacuation behaviour of older people: A case study of a rural town in Japan. *Research in Transportation Business & Management, 30*, 100376. https://doi.org/10.1016/j.rtbm.2019.100376

Nehaluddin, A., & Lilienthal, G. (2021). Right to water as a human right: A critical overview of international instruments. *Environmental Policy and Law, 50*(4–5), 299–308. https://doi.org/10.3233/EPL-200232

Neves, B. B., Sanders, A., Warren, N., & Ko, P. C. (2023). Loneliness in later life as existential inequality. *Sociology*, 00380385231208649. https://doi.org/10.1177/00380385231208649

Nguyen, Y. T. B., & Leisz, S. J. (2021). Determinants of livelihood vulnerability to climate change: Two minority ethnic communities in the northwest mountainous region of Vietnam. *Environmental Science & Policy, 123*, 11–20. https://doi.org/10.1016/j.envsci.2021.04.007

Nicolaisen, M., & Thorsen, K. (2023). Gender differences in loneliness over time: A 15-year longitudinal study of men and women in the second part of life. *The International Journal of Aging and Human Development, 98*(1), 103–132. https://doi.org/10.1177/00914150231194243

Nyahunda, L., Makhubele, J. C., Mabvurira, V., & Matlakala, F. K. (2021). Vulnerabilities and inequalities experienced by women in the climate change discourse in South Africa's rural communities: implications for social work. *The British Journal of Social Work, 51*(7), 2536–2553. https://doi.org/10.1093/bjsw/bcaa118

Okun, S., & Ayalon, L. (2024). Political activism and wellbeing among older adults in Israel. *Aging & Mental Health, 28*(5), 801–811. https://doi.org/10.1080/13607863.2023.2299959

Olesen, T. (2022). Greta Thunberg's iconicity: Performance and co-performance in the social media ecology. *New Media & Society, 24*(6), 1325–1342. https://doi.org/10.1177/1461444820975416

Palinkas, L. A., & Wong, M. (2020). Global climate change and mental health. *Current Opinion in Psychology, 32*, 12–16. https://doi.org/10.1016/j.copsyc.2019.06.023

Perlman, D., & Peplau, L. A. (1981). Toward a social psychology of loneliness. *Personal Relationships, 3*, 31–56. Academic Press.

Phuong, T. T., Tan, N. Q., Dinh, N. C., Van Chuong, H., Ha, H. D., & Hung, H. T. (2023). Livelihood vulnerability to climate change: Indexes and insights from two ethnic minority communities in Central Vietnam. *Environmental Challenges, 10*, 100666. https://doi.org/10.1016/j.envc.2022.100666

Pillemer, K., Wagenet, L., Goldman, D., Bushway, L., & Meador, R. (2009). Environmental volunteering in later life: Benefits and barriers. *Generations, 33*(4), 58–63.

Prina, M., Khan, N., Akhter Khan, S., Caicedo, J. C., Peycheva, A., Seo, V., Xue, S., & Sadana, R. (2024, May 24). Climate change and healthy ageing: An assessment of the impact of climate hazards on older people. *Journal of Globalization and Health, 14*, 04101. https://doi.org/10.7189/jogh.14.04101

Rico-Uribe, L. A., Caballero, F. F., Martín-María, N., Cabello, M., Ayuso-Mateos, J. L., & Miret, M. (2018). Association of loneliness with all-cause mortality: A meta-analysis. *PLoS One, 13*(1), e0190033. https://doi.org/10.1371/journal.pone.0190033

Ritchie, J. (2021). Movement from the margins to global recognition: Climate change activism by young people and in particular indigenous youth. *International Studies in Sociology of Education, 30*(1–2), 53–72. https://doi.org/10.1080/09620214.2020.1854830

Roy, S., & Ayalon, L. (2022). Intergenerational relations in the climate movement: Bridging the gap toward a common goal. *International Journal of Environmental Research and Public Health, 20*(1), 233. https://doi.org/10.3390/ijerph20010233

Roy, S., & Ayalon, L. (2023). "They did not know what they were doing": Climate change and intergenerational compassion. *The Gerontologist*, gnad063. https://doi.org/10.1093/geront/gnad063

Segel-Karpas, D., Ayalon, L., & Lachman, M. E. (2018). Loneliness and depressive symptoms: the moderating role of the transition into retirement. *Aging & Mental Health, 22*(1), 135–140. https://doi.org/10.1080/13607863.2016.1226770

Shiovitz-Ezra, S., & Ayalon, L. (2010). Situational versus chronic loneliness as risk factors for all-cause mortality. *International Psychogeriatrics, 22*(3), 455–462. https://doi.org/10.1017/S1041610209991426

Shiovitz-Ezra, S., Shemesh, J., & McDonnell/Naughton, M. (2018). Pathways from ageism to loneliness. In L. Ayalon & C. Tesch-Roemer (Eds.), *Contemporary perspectives on ageism* (pp. 131–147). Springer. https://doi.org/10.1007/978-3-319-73820-8

Siva, N. (2020). Loneliness in children and young people in the UK. *Lancet Child and Adolescent Health, 22*(4), 567–568. https://doi.org/10.1016/S2352-4642(20)30213-3

Smirnova, N., Shaver, A. C., Mehta, A. J., Philipsborn, R., & Scovronick, N. (2023). Climate change, air quality, and pulmonary health disparities. *Clinics in Chest Medicine, 44*(3), 489–499. https://doi.org/10.1016/j.ccm.2023.03.005

Smith, G. S., Anjum, E., Francis, C., Deanes, L., & Acey, C. (2022). Climate change, environmental disasters, and health inequities: The underlying role of structural inequalities. *Current Environmental Health Reports, 9*(1), 80–89. https://doi.org/10.1007/s40572-022-00336-w

Sullivan, R. (2017). Setting a future direction for climate change policy. In *Corporate Responses to Climate Change* (pp. 334–338). Routledge. https://doi.org/10.4324/9781351280006-22

Susanty, S., Nadirawati, N., Setiawan, A., Haroen, H., Pebrianti, S., Harun, H., Azissah, D., Suyanto, J., Sarasmita, M. A., Chipojola, R., Khwepeya, M., & Banda, K. J. (2025). Overview of the prevalence of loneliness and associated risk factors among older adults across six continents: A meta-analysis. *Archives of Gerontology and Geriatrics, 128*, 105627. https://doi.org/10.1016/j.archger.2024.105627

Sutin, A. R., Stephan, Y., Luchetti, M., & Terracciano, A. (2018). Loneliness and risk of dementia. *The Journals of Gerontology: Series B, 75*(7), 1414–1422. https://doi.org/10.1093/geronb/gby112

Tapia-Muñoz, T., Staudinger, U. M., Allel, K., Steptoe, A., Miranda-Castillo, C., Medina, J. T., & Calvo, E. (2022). Income inequality and its relationship with loneliness prevalence: A cross-sectional study among older adults in the US and 16 European countries. *PLoS One, 17*(12), e0274518. https://doi.org/10.1371/journal.pone.0274518

Taylor, H. O., Chen, Y.-C., Tsuchiya, K., Cudjoe, T. K. M., Qin, W., Nguyen, A. W., & Roy, A. (2024). Racial/ethnic differences in loneliness among older adults: The role of income and education as mediators. *Innovation in Aging, 8*(8). https://doi.org/10.1093/geroni/igae068

United Nations. (2021). *Climate change 'biggest threat modern humans have ever faced', world-renowned naturalist tells security council, calls for greater global cooperation.* https://press.un.org/en/2021/sc14445.doc.htm

Victor, C. R., Burholt, V., & Martin, W. (2012, 2012/03/01). Loneliness and ethnic minority elders in Great Britain: An exploratory study. Journal of Cross-Cultural Gerontology, 27(1), 65–78. doi:https://doi.org/10.1007/s10823-012-9161-6.

Willoughby, M., Kipsaina, C., Ferrah, N., Blau, S., Bugeja, L., Ranson, D., & Ibrahim, J. E. (2017). Mortality in nursing homes following emergency evacuation: A systematic review. *Journal of the American Medical Directors Association, 18*(8), 664–670. https://doi.org/10.1016/j.jamda.2017.02.005

World Health Organization (2014). *Gender, climate change and health.* World Health Organization chrome-extension: //efaidnbmnnnibpcajpcglclefindmkaj/https://iris.who.int/bitstream/10665/144781/1/9789241508186_eng.pdf

Yin, L., Zachary, M., Zheng, Y., & Zhang, X. (2020). The impacts of climate change on the traditional agriculture of ethnic minority in China. *Journal of Environmental Science and Engineering A, 43*. https://doi.org/10.17265/2162-5298/2020.02.001

Zeigler, A. (2019). How to stop climate change and never be lonely again. *Communities, 183*, 59–63.

Zuelsdorff, M., & Limaye, V. S. (2024). A framework for assessing the effects of climate change on dementia risk and burden. *The Gerontologist, 64*(3), gnad082. https://doi.org/10.1093/geront/gnad082

Liat Ayalon, PhD, is a Professor in the School of Social Work, at Bar Ilan University, Israel. Prof. Ayalon is currently funded by the Israel Science Foundation to study intergenerational relations in the context of climate change (ISF 217–20). She consults both national and international organizations concerning the development and evaluation of programs and services for older adults. In recognition of her work, Prof. Ayalon was selected by the UN Decade of Healthy Ageing as one of 50 world leaders working to transform the world to be a better place in which to grow older.

Open Access This chapter is licensed under the terms of the Creative Commons Attribution 4.0 International License (http://creativecommons.org/licenses/by/4.0/), which permits use, sharing, adaptation, distribution and reproduction in any medium or format, as long as you give appropriate credit to the original author(s) and the source, provide a link to the Creative Commons license and indicate if changes were made.

The images or other third party material in this chapter are included in the chapter's Creative Commons license, unless indicated otherwise in a credit line to the material. If material is not included in the chapter's Creative Commons license and your intended use is not permitted by statutory regulation or exceeds the permitted use, you will need to obtain permission directly from the copyright holder.

Chapter 10
The Influence of Societal Crises on Social Integration and Loneliness

Lisa J. Klasen, Mareike Bünning, Nadiya Kelle, Clemens Tesch-Römer, and Oliver Huxhold

10.1 Introduction

Societal crises significantly impact social integration and loneliness. However, there is currently no model that outlines the multiple pathways through which these crises influence social integration, while accounting for life circumstances such as differences between social groups based on age, gender, and socioeconomic status. Developing such a model is crucial, especially since European societies have faced an increasing number of societal crises in recent decades, profoundly affecting people's lives (Handler, 2024a). For instance, the Great Recession in 2007 and the subsequent European debt crisis were accompanied by job losses and income reduction, threatening prosperity and growth in many countries (Busch et al., 2013; Verick & Islam, 2010). The European migration crisis in 2015 caused far-reaching debates on refugees and societal values (Handler, 2024b; Sola, 2018). The COVID-19 pandemic threatened the health of many people and drastic countermeasures severely restricted social interactions (Kersten & Rixen, 2022). The war in Ukraine has had and continues to have a massive and fundamental impact on the Ukrainian people by killing thousands and destroying the basis of life of large parts of the population (Liadze et al., 2023; United Nations, 2022b). At the same time, the war affects Europe as a whole as it threatens peace in the region, increases living costs, and drives inflation (United Nations, 2022a). Lastly, as an omnipresent example, climate change progressively affects life in the European region through

L. J. Klasen (✉)
German Centre of Gerontology, Berlin, Germany

Department of Psychology, Humboldt-Universität zu Berlin, Berlin, Germany
e-mail: lisa.klasen@dza.de

M. Bünning · N. Kelle · C. Tesch-Römer · O. Huxhold
German Centre of Gerontology, Berlin, Germany

© The Author(s) 2025
M. Aartsen et al. (eds.), *Macro Social Influences on Loneliness in Later Life*, International Perspectives on Aging 47,
https://doi.org/10.1007/978-3-031-94565-6_10

weather extremes and threatens the livelihood of large parts of the population (IPCC, 2023). In retrospect and overall, these societal crises have most likely had a greater impact on social integration and the development of loneliness than has been recognized so far.

Financial aspects of societal crises were often among the first impacts that became salient in the public awareness and were therefore one of the focal topics of discussion (Damstra & Vliegenthart, 2018; Greussing & Boomgaarden, 2017). Disturbances in other areas of life tended to develop more gradually and often faded into the background of the political and scientific debate on new events or societal crises (United Nations, 2011). Yet, analyses of past societal crises reveal that the impacts on other life domains are also widespread and profound. This became particularly evident in light of the COVID-19 pandemic, as government-imposed countermeasures such as contact restrictions and physical distancing measures intended to contain the virus, did not only had consequences for finances but also brought people's social integration to public awareness.

Recognising that societal crises impact social relationships is crucial, as people fundamentally need to be socially integrated (Baumeister & Leary, 1995). Social integration involves maintaining strong ties with close confidants, engaging with a broader network of friends and acquaintances, and participating in social activities or voluntary work. When individuals perceive their social integration as insufficient, loneliness occurs, contributing to mental and physical dysfunctions over time (Cacioppo et al., 2015). Negative consequences of societal crises on social relationships can thus lead to further harmful developments in other life areas.

Despite the relevance of this topic, to date no framework has been developed that captures the breadth and development of effects of a given societal crisis on social integration and its impacts on loneliness. Only singular studies have investigated the links between different societal crises and various aspects of social integration. These studies have shown that societal crises such as the Great Recession from 2007 (Iglič et al., 2021), the European debt crisis (Parmar et al., 2016), and most prominently, the COVID-19 pandemic (Entringer & Kröger, 2020; Huxhold & Tesch-Römer, 2021; Van Tilburg et al., 2021), have had detrimental effects on important aspects of people's social integration and the development of loneliness. However, without a comprehensive theoretical framework it is difficult to classify and integrate different empirical findings. Moreover, such a theoretical framework may also help to manage future societal crises, for example, by providing a theoretical foundation for interventions to avoid and reduce loneliness (Pitas & Ehmer, 2020).

Therefore, our aim here is to fill this research gap by introducing a theoretical framework—the DIRe-Crises-Model. For this purpose, the Differential Investment of Resources Model (DIRe-Model) by Huxhold and colleagues (2022), is placed in the context of societal crises and further developed to capture the effects of societal crises on social integration and their implications for loneliness. To illustrate the general applicability of the model, the adapted framework is discussed in the context of different societal crises in Europe.

10.2 Defining Societal Crises

Based on our review of the literature, we define societal crises as long-term and far-reaching disruptions to fundamental structures or values of a given society (e.g., Boin et al., 2018; Rosenthal et al., 1989; Schubert & Klein, 2020). Societal crises differ in many ways; such as their causes, development over time, severity of impact on people's life, or in terms of the applied countermeasures. However, our review of crisis definitions has revealed that, at their core, all societal crises are characterized by the following five criteria: First, societal crises are triggered by the (potential) loss of elementary resources, such as health or money (e.g., Schubert & Klein, 2020). Second, since a loss of an elementary resource has a broad impact on many life domains, these situations have the potential to escalate and impact various areas of society. Third, such situations develop into a long-term disturbance when the negative consequences of these losses can no longer be mitigated with the usual means and additional countermeasures become necessary (Schubert & Klein, 2020). However, in contrast to a catastrophe, an escalating event can be prevented by effective decisions and measures (Boin et al., 2018). Thus, a crisis does not necessarily have to end in a catastrophe. Fourth, these situations cause *threat* (i.e., subjectively perceived danger), *uncertainty* (i.e., lack of necessary information) and *urgency* (i.e., need to act quickly) (Boin et al., 2018; Schäfers, 2018; Shaluf et al., 2003). Fifth, a situation can only evolve into a societal crisis when the *majority* of people and the public discourse *perceive* this situation as critical and subsequently declare it a crisis (Boin et al., 2018; Rosenthal & Kouzmin, 1997). This defining feature explains why some difficult situations are categorized as societal crises while similar others are not (Boin et al., 2018). Ultimately, for a difficult situation to be recognised as a crisis, all five criteria must be met.

10.3 DIRe-Crises-Model

To delineate the impacts of societal crises on social integration, we build on the Differential Investment of Resources Model (DIRe-Model, for more information see Huxhold et al., 2022a). The DIRe-Model views the development of social relationships as an interplay of individual behaviour and contextual conditions at the macro- and meso-level of a given society. The macro-level context includes societal institutions (e.g., welfare state type), cultural norms of societies (e.g., level of ageism or filial piety) and also—as we will outline—societal crises that affect these societies (e.g., Great Recession from 2007, COVID-19 pandemic, climate change).

Regarding the meso-level, a precise definition remains a challenge in aging research, as no universally agreed-upon framework exists. However, the common denominator across different definitions is that the meso-level connects individuals with the broader society (e.g., Bronfenbrenner, 1977; Bronfenbrenner & Morris, 2008; Silverstein & Giarrusso, 2011; Staggenborg, 2002). In our approach, we define meso-level factors more narrowly as intermediary contextual conditions that moderate the impact of macro-level societal structures on individual outcomes. These factors include dimensions of social inequality—such as age, gender, and socioeconomic status — that not only influence individual characteristics (e.g., health, financial resources) but also constrain individual agency through, for example, different social norms and unequal opportunity structures. Thus, we consider them contextual rather than purely individual factors, aligning with the biographical-institutional-societal model (Silverstein & Giarrusso, 2011) and the sociology-of-age framework (Barrett, 2022).

The distinction between the macro-level of the societal crises and the meso-level of the life circumstances is necessary to understand the moderating influence of social inequality. In other words, it is important to note that while societal crises may impact the social integration of all people, their effects are not uniform (Heisig, 2021; Ohlbrecht & Jellen, 2021; Wachtler & Hoebel, 2020). Negative effects of societal crises and unintended consequences of countermeasures are often disproportionately harmful for socially disadvantaged individuals in comparison to people with better coping resources (Kiess et al., 2023). For instance, crises may amplify pre-existing inequalities, reinforcing disadvantages for those with fewer economic or health-related capacities.

Although other meso-level factors and thus life circumstances stem from an individual's immediate environment—such as neighbourhood cohesion, urbanity, and local opportunity structures for leisure activities (see also Chap. 4 of this book; Van Regenmortel et al., 2025)—this chapter focuses specifically on social inequality as a meso-level factor. By narrowing our focus, we aim to emphasize how structural disparities shape individuals' experiences of societal crises while leaving aspects of the physical and social environment for future research.

Building on the DIRe-Model, the DIRe-Crises-Model defines social ties as "all persons for whom the ego has: (a) subjective awareness; (b) a mental representation of how they relate; and (c) a belief in their mutual influence on each other" (Huxhold et al., 2022a, p. 59). Social ties differ in terms of perceived closeness and kinship. In the DIRe-Crises-Model, we assume in line with previous research that one's social ties can be structured in three concentric circles surrounding the individual that differ in their perceived closeness (Antonucci et al., 2014; Cacioppo et al., 2015; Huxhold et al., 2020; Reynolds et al., 2020). Specifically, the perceived closeness of ties decreases across these circles from the inside to the outside (Antonucci et al., 2014). Thus, the inner circle includes one's closest ties (i.e., strong ties), like close family and close friends, who are the primary providers of emotional and instrumental support (Fuller et al., 2020; Huxhold et al., 2020). The perceived absence of intimate connections can lead to emotional loneliness (Cacioppo et al., 2015). The middle circle represents an individual's wider network, consisting of ties whom one sees regularly and shares interests and experiences with, such as friends or extended family (Dunbar, 2014; Fuller et al., 2020). These ties can provide stimulation and fun in the form of social activities (Huxhold & Fiori, 2024). The perceived absence of these connections can lead to social loneliness (Cacioppo et al., 2015). The outer circle includes all weak ties, which are less emotionally close, but still have an impact on one's general well-being, such as neighbors or work colleagues (Fingerman, 2009; Granovetter, 1973). Activities with members from this circle regularly incorporate participation in the community, for example, in voluntary groups (Reynolds et al., 2020). The outer circle mainly provides novelty, information, and access to other social networks (Fingerman, 2009; Granovetter, 1973). The perceived absence of a wider network can lead to collective loneliness (Cacioppo et al., 2015). From a theoretical perspective, it is suggested that to increase one's sense of belonging, avoid the different dimensions of loneliness, and gain access to different social functions, people generally establish a wide array of ties spanning all three circles (Cacioppo et al., 2015; Fingerman, 2009; Huxhold et al., 2022a).

As in the DIRe-Model, we assume that people have to invest time and energy in their social ties to maintain a certain level of social integration, as shown in the Individual Network Feedback Loop of the DIRe-Crises-Model (see Fig. 10.1). Time is understood as the free time available for social interactions while energy is the perceived potential (behaviourally, emotionally and cognitively) to engage in a social interaction (e.g., measured with the level of fatigue or vitality) (Hall & Merolla, 2020). To maintain close ties, people have to invest on *average* more time, but less energy due to a higher level of familiarity. In contrast, weaker ties need less time but more energy to maintain. These investments of time and energy are determined by capacities (influencing the available amount of investable time and energy), motivations (determining the direction and size of investments) and skills (specifying the effectiveness of investment). For example, an illness can reduce the individual's capacity (i.e., the available time and energy an individual can be invested in social relationships), while high social skills—such as high levels of empathy—can improve the effectiveness of these investments. In return for the invested time and energy, an individual derives a number of social functions from their social network—such as social support, stimulation, and the feeling of

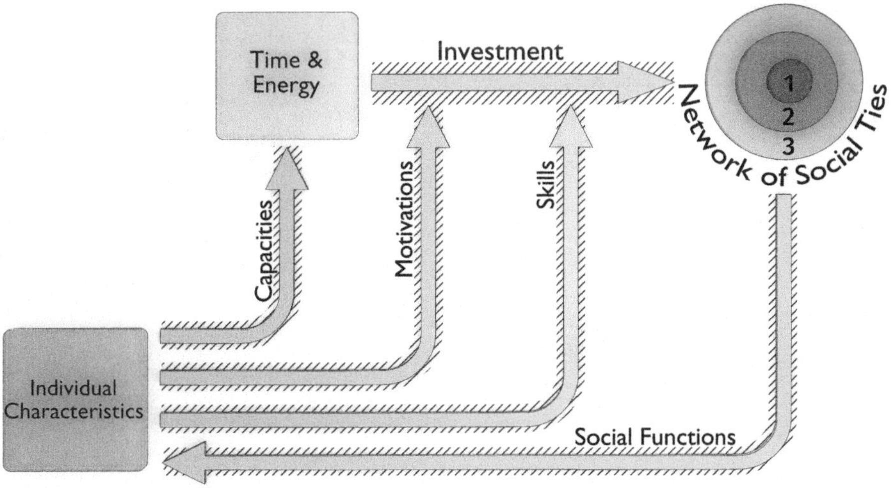

Fig. 10.1 Individual Network Feedback Loop in the DIRe-Crises-Model (Credit: Edzard Füllbrunn, Keypose Animation)

belonging. High-quality social networks can prevent loneliness and thereby help to maintain physical and mental health. Conversely, individuals who have a limited social network lack support and stimulation and may feel lonely. Moreover, low-quality social ties may even induce strain or may become overly controlling. Ultimately, support and stimulation, as well as strain and control stemming from social relationships influence the initial resources of time and energy that individuals can invest in their relationships, which creates a reinforcing feedback loop.

In the full DIRe-Crises-Model (see Fig. 10.2), societal crises are placed in the macro-level context and influence the social investment process via four different pathways by impacting:

(A) individual characteristics that are essential for resource investment,
(B) the available time and energy that can be invested in relationships,
(C) the social opportunity structure to interact with (potential) social contacts and
(D) the functions of social relationships.

While societal crises may differ in numerous ways, these pathways are effective in all societal crises, although to varying degrees.

In this process, the meso-level context, represented by the individual's life circumstances, as shaped by different dimensions of social inequality (e.g., socioeconomic status, age, or gender), moderates the effects of a societal crisis and can thus weaken or strengthen these effects for an individual. This moderating effect of the

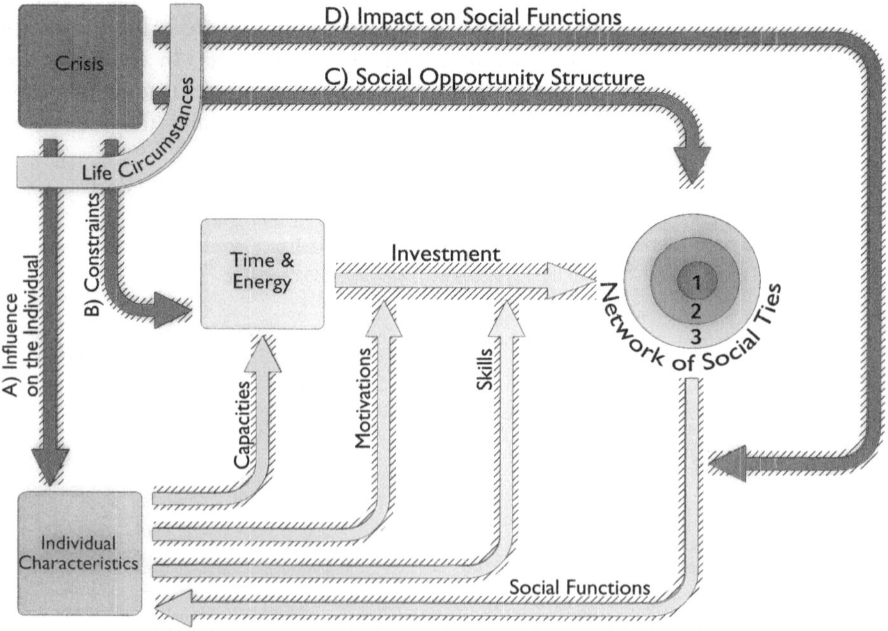

Fig. 10.2 DIRe-Crises-Model (Credit: Edzard Füllbrunn, Keypose Animation)

individual's life circumstances explains why societal crises often exacerbate pre-existing social inequalities (e.g., Bodea et al., 2021; Stok et al., 2021).

10.3.1 Path A: Impact on the Investment Process via Individual Characteristics

Individual characteristics such as capacities, motivations, and skills are crucial for social integration, as they determine the available time, energy, and how these resources are spent on social interactions. Societal crises are likely to impact these characteristics in affected populations, thereby indirectly influencing the social integration process.

Capacities—Capacities are individual characteristics that influence the available amount of investable time and energy (e.g., physical and psychological health) (Huxhold et al., 2022a). Societal crises are likely to impact the capacities because societal crises are threatening situations (Boin et al., 2018; Shaluf et al., 2003), which can cause anxiety and require coping. These conditions can place stress on both mind and body, potentially reducing an individual's capacity and therefore the time and energy available for social interactions.

This effect became apparent during the European debt crisis and the COVID-19 pandemic. In both societal crises a great number of workers experienced financial uncertainties, as unpredictable job losses and wage cuts became omnipresent (Bundeszentrale für politische Bildung (bpb), 2021; Busch et al., 2013). Such circumstances create existential fears and emotional stress (Blustein & Guarino, 2020). In the long term, such conditions can contribute to reduced relationship investments, as coping with the situation consumes too much energy. This assumption is supported by a study showing that social network sizes decreased during the financial crises in Europe, when individuals experienced economic strain (Iglič et al., 2021). The family stress model for romantic relationships (Conger et al., 2010) describes a comparable process in which economic hardship and feelings of economic pressure increase emotional distress. This, in turn, may lead to conflicts, withdrawal and distancing within romantic relationships, which can be interpreted as poor relationship investment. Ultimately, such behaviours negatively affect relationship quality and stability. Since societal crises, as described above, have the potential to cause financial uncertainties for many people, it is likely that similar negative processes affect a broad spectrum of different ties. Furthermore, climate change may impact individual characteristics as well, as it is accompanied by more frequent and severe heat waves. Over the past few decades, numerous scientific studies have shown that high temperatures put a strain on the body and mind, making it more difficult to perform tasks (Kjellstrom et al., 2016; Yeganeh et al., 2018). In terms of social interactions, it is conceivable that everyday life during heat waves may require more time and energy, leaving less for social interactions. This assumption is supported by a German study, which found that social interactions among older adults declined as temperatures increased (Lindemann et al., 2018).

Motivation—Motivations are individual characteristics like personality traits or perceptions of aging which determine in which social ties and to what extent time and energy are invested (Huxhold et al., 2022a). As described above, societal crises are likely to reduce time and energy available for social interactions. Therefore, people have to be more selective in terms of which relationships they invest in. We assume that in times of societal crises, people turn to their strong ties, as these ties especially provide emotional and instrumental support, which might be highly valued at the beginning of a societal crisis when uncertainty and threat are high. As a result, the inner circle consisting of strong ties is strengthened, while the outer circles of weaker ties shrink due to reduced investment of time and energy. So far, this 'turtling-up' mechanism has primarily been observed in lower-level crises, such as those affecting individual organizations, rather than in large-scale societal crises. For example, in organizational contexts facing extreme price changes, employees were more likely to increase their contacts within the company while reducing their contacts outside the organization. (Romero et al., 2016).

However, initial studies have also shown evidence for turtling-up during societal crises. For instance, it has been shown that in Slovenia during the financial crisis, networks of weak ties decreased while family networks were strengthened (Iglič, 2014). The authors explained this development with reduced trust in other people during times of economic uncertainty, leading to increased investments in trustworthy and reliable strong ties. Somewhat relatedly, another study found that during the financial crisis civic engagement, which is very often accompanied by interactions with weak ties, also declined (Cameron, 2021). This finding may hint at reduced investment of time and energy in the third circle of the social network. In addition, during the COVID-19 pandemic, several studies showed that the network of weak ties decreased significantly, while the closest ties, in particularly family connections, were strengthened (Kovacs et al., 2021; Steijvers et al., 2022; Völker, 2023). One might argue that in the case of the pandemic, this development was mainly due to countermeasures which severely restricted the contact with other people. While Völker (2023) argues that there were still opportunities to interact with people beyond the own household and family, such as the neighbourhood, her findings indicate that during the pandemic the neighbourhood did not become more important for social interactions whereas strong ties did.

Skills—Skills are characteristics that influence the effectiveness of the investment process. For example, high levels of social skills may enable an individual to interact and communicate more effectively. Societal crises can affect socially relevant skills in different ways. On the one hand, they can provide opportunities for the development of new skills or the improvement of existing ones in order to adapt to the crisis situation. On the other hand, societal crises can impair skills as the individual is confronted with increased demands.

For example, during the COVID-19 pandemic technical devices such as smartphones, enabled contact with one's ties even when strict contact restrictions were in place. In this context, it is possible that people became more engaged with their smartphones and related applications to interact more effectively with their ties (e.g., sending pictures, making video calls). This may have led to an improvement in technical skills especially within older age groups, which would have taken more time without the societal crisis. This assumption is supported by a qualitative study of German middle-class families, which found that the digital communication increased in all generations to stay in contact with one's social ties during the pandemic (Schad & Hense, 2023). Another qualitative study from Portugal showed, that older people used their smartphones more often, mainly to socialize with their ties during the contact restrictions (Murciano-Hueso et al., 2022). Some participants even reported that the pandemic was an opportunity to start using smartphones at all. However, the results remain ambiguous, as quantitative studies show only a small overall increase in internet access and usage and present mixed findings regarding its use for social interactions among older age groups during the COVID-19 pandemic (Bünning et al., 2023; Kortmann et al., 2021; Kung & Steptoe, 2023). In the long term, these technical skills can continue to be beneficial for one's social integration, as these enable an additional kind of communication and help people stay in contact with geographically distant friends (Antonucci et al., 2019).

However, societal crises may also hamper social skills through, for example, anxieties or demanding circumstances. For example, the heat hypothesis states that hot temperatures are associated with increases in antisocial behaviors such as assault or violence (Anderson, 2001). This also includes the assumption that heat negatively biases the interpretation of ambiguous social interactions as being more aggressive. According to Anderson, one explanation could be increased discomfort during heat periods, which might color social interaction more negatively. While laboratory-based studies report rather mixed results, population-based studies provide strong evidence for the heat-hypothesis (Anderson, 2001; Hsiang et al., 2013; Lynott et al., 2023). This development is particularly relevant in the context of climate change and the associated increase in the frequency of heat waves. In fact, predictions show that violence may increase in the face of climate change in many countries worldwide (Anderson, 2001; Mares & Moffett, 2015). However, even on a smaller scale, an aggressive bias in social interactions could have a huge impact on social integration by severely reducing the effectiveness of the investment of time and energy in social relationships.

10.3.2 Path B: Impact on the Available Time and Energy

Societal crises tend to reduce available time and energy for social interactions either due to their direct negative impacts or due to the government's countermeasures, which may increase demands on individuals. This reduction is significantly influenced by an increase in care work, which is generally provided for close family members (e.g., children, parents, in-laws) (Ehrlich & Kelle, 2019). During societal crises, the heightened need for care work may lead to more time being spent with these close ties, while interactions with weaker ties are limited, thus restricting interactions with the broader social world.

Government countermeasures significantly increased the amount of care work during the COVID-19 pandemic. For example, the German government implemented countermeasures like homeschooling and closing kindergartens, requiring many people to care for and support their children alongside their usual work (Bujard et al., 2020; Grote et al., 2021). Additionally, the closure of day care facilities for older people and the loss of professional carers intensified the burden of caring for relatives at home (Brandt et al., 2021; Ehrlich et al., 2022). This may have significantly reduced the time and energy available for social interactions beyond immediate family.

Crises themselves also increase demands on people. Climate change, for instance, brings extreme weather events like heatwaves and floods, which may require significant time and energy for protective measures and repairs, detracting from social interactions. These events also heighten the need for care work; during heatwaves, it is advised to check on vulnerable family members, such as older adults and young children, who are at higher risk of heat-related health issues and may need additional assistance (Arsad et al., 2022; UNICEF, 2023; WHO, 2018).

Overall, societal crises and the measures taken to address them can lead to an increase in care work, reducing the time and energy available for social interactions, especially with weaker social ties.

10.3.3 Path C: Impact on the Social Opportunity Structure

The social opportunity structure, meaning all ties with which an individual could (potentially) interact, and invest time and energy, is entirely determined by the context (Huxhold et al., 2022a). Therefore, disturbances, such as societal crises, can massively impact the opportunity structure. In particular, negative consequences of societal crises and their countermeasures have the potential to minimize opportunities and increase the costs to socially interact with others. Even though it is often assumed that societal crises may spark solidarity, motivating people to seek solutions through volunteering and mutual assistance—such as the widespread support for those fleeing the war in Ukraine (Höltmann et al., 2022) and the activation of informal support networks during the early stages of the COVID-19 pandemic (Bertogg & Koos, 2021)—negative effects on the social opportunity structure seem to outweigh positive ones. Empirical evidence from several studies suggests that the proportion of engagement decreases in times of societal crises or at best remain stable (Cameron, 2021; Ramaekers et al., 2022; Simonson & Kelle, 2023). For example, despite governmental calls for solidarity, neighbourhood-based mutual aid did not increase significantly during the COVID-19 pandemic (Ramaekers et al., 2023). Hence, the negative effects on the social opportunity structure suggest that societal crises pose a major obstacle to social interactions. We propose, that this especially affects the maintenance of weak ties, which one meets in larger settings (e.g., clubs, sports activities) or by chance outside one's home (e.g., on the street, at work), as these public places are particularly impacted by societal crises. This reduced availability of weaker ties would further increase the effect of turtling-up within the social network during societal crises.

These processes have been observed in different societal crises. Most prominently, during the COVID-19 pandemic, the social opportunity structure was massively impacted, as countermeasures severely restricted most social interactions. Due to the implementation of homeschooling and home office, contact restrictions, and closures of a wide range of public and cultural facilities, people had barely any possibilities to interact in person with others besides their household members (Grote et al., 2021). These circumstances made contact with non-household ties and especially weak ties more difficult. Climate change, accompanied by more frequent extreme weather events such as heat waves, droughts, or floods due to heavy rainstorms (IPCC, 2023), increasingly unfolds its negative consequences on social opportunity structures. For instance, during long-lasting heat waves, outside activities are hardly possible in some regions of Europe, restricting the timing and places for interactions with others. In the long-term, droughts and water shortages are increasingly threatening green spaces, such as forests or parks (Esperon-Rodriguez et al., 2022). This development might be especially relevant for urban areas where green spaces not only function as a space for social interactions but are also crucial for temperature regulation and well-being (Reyes-Riveros et al., 2021). In the future, these effects of climate change on the social opportunity structure will further increase as extreme weather events become more frequent and even more pronounced (IPCC, 2023). As described above, these circumstances will likely affect weak ties the most, as people, for example, stay at home during heat waves and avoid outdoor places. Thus, decreasing the possibility of meeting those ties by chance or in their normal setting.

10.3.4 Path D: Impact on the Functions of Social Relationships

The influence of specific social ties on the individual can change over historical time for example due to historical changes in gender roles and family structure (Bühler & Nikitin, 2020; Hughes & Waite, 2007). For example, one study found that the relationship between loneliness and partnership status was less pronounced in later-born cohorts than in earlier-born cohorts (Böger & Huxhold, 2020). However, not only can changes over long periods of time reshape the importance of social ties; sudden disruptions such as societal crises can have an impact as well. We assume that societal crises can change the significance of specific ties within one's social network, as certain individuals may become more important when others are absent (Pinquart, 2003). In the context of societal crises, it might be expected that strong ties would compensate for the absence of weak ties, i.e., people might engage in more social activities with their family instead of with their absent friends. In addition, societal crises may also alter the importance of ties by changing the relevance of certain network functions. For example, it is conceivable that companionship and emotional support, which are typically provided by strong ties, become more necessary in uncertain and threatening times. At the same time, typical weak tie functions, like exploration and stimulation, might decrease in importance, making these ties less relevant, and strong ties more relevant for well-being and for avoiding loneliness. Only a few studies investigated these changes in the context of societal crises. One study from Singapore found that the relationship between social support from close ties and well-being temporarily increased during the COVID-19 pandemic (Lee et al., 2023). Another study examined the changing impact of grandchild care on well-being and loneliness during the COVID-19 pandemic (Bünning & Huxhold, 2024). While grandparents who provided grandchild care reported lower levels of loneliness even prior to the crisis, this association was particularly pronounced for grandfathers during the pandemic, and grandchild care was only positively related to grandmothers' life satisfaction during the pandemic. These results provide evidence for the increased importance of strong ties during societal crises. However, currently there are not enough empirical studies investigating the reweighting of social functions under different contextual conditions to allow for the precise derivation of broader hypotheses regarding *Path D*.

10.3.5 The Moderating Influence of Life Circumstances

Societal crises do not affect every person to the same extent (Heisig, 2021; Ohlbrecht & Jellen, 2021; Wachtler & Hoebel, 2020). In general, the burdens of societal crises, as well as the resources that help to minimize negative effects on social integration or to take advantage of new developmental opportunities, are unevenly distributed across societies and vary with individual life circumstances such as socioeconomic status (SES) or other social group memberships. Note that we define those group memberships as part of the social-structural context as those characteristics significantly shape the life circumstances beyond the individual's sphere of influence (Huxhold et al., 2022a). For example, life circumstances are structured by age, as major life transitions are closely bound to chronological age (e.g., parenthood, retirement) (Heckhausen & Buchmann, 2019). Generally speaking, life circumstances can weaken or strengthen the effects of a given societal crisis on social integration. Recognizing this fact is particularly important for the identification of risk groups.

It should be noted that the relevance and the impact direction of life circumstances may differ between different societal crises, i.e., in one societal crisis a certain life circumstance may have an especially strong impact, while in another societal crisis this particular context is less important. It is therefore essential to reassess the relevance of life circumstances when looking at the impact of different societal crises.

However, SES may be an exception to this rule, as this characteristic always seems to be relevant, meaning every societal crisis has a particularly strong impact on people with a lower SES. This may be explained by unequal access to resources to cope with societal crises and their related hazards. For example, compared to people with a high SES, people with a lower SES have fewer financial resources to cope with temporary income reductions during societal crises (Romeu Gordo et al., 2023). In addition, they often face higher job insecurity (Landsbergis et al., 2014), which may further increase during economic downturns. Furthermore, people with a lower SES often live in smaller homes, making overcrowding a relevant issue (EUROSTAT, 2024; Wachtler & Hoebel, 2020), especially when spaces outside the home are inaccessible, as experienced, for example, during the COVID-19 pandemic (e.g. homeschooling) or weather extremes (e.g. heat waves) due to climate change. These circumstances may exacerbate the effects of societal crises on time and energy for social interaction or the social opportunity structure (*Path A and C*). Research suggests that individuals with lower SES experience a greater reduction in social network size and an increase in loneliness during societal crises compared to those with higher SES, as exemplified by studies on the COVID-19 crisis (Steijvers et al., 2022; Völker, 2023, but note diverging/opposing findings by Bertogg & Koos, 2022). This is particularly crucial, since network diversity and size generally differ between groups of different SES even without a societal crises (Ajrouch et al., 2005; Antonucci, 2001; Van Groenou & Van Tilburg, 2003). Developments during societal crises may therefore further intensify socio-economic differences in social networks.

Besides SES, other differences in life circumstances such as gender or age also shape the effects of societal crises on social integration. In terms of gender, although much has been accomplished in recent decades in terms of gender equality in Europe, there are still significant differences between men and women in various areas of life. Among other things, this is reflected in sectoral and occupational segregation in the labour market (e.g., women are more likely to work in the health and social sector, while men are more likely to work in construction or manufacturing) (Matysiak & Cukrowska-Torzewska, 2021). Furthermore, women are still the main provider of care- and housework, while men on average spend more time in paid work (Pailhé et al., 2021; Panova et al., 2017). Such societal differences between women and men can significantly alter the impact of societal crises on social integration. For example, during the COVID-19 pandemic, mothers in particular faced an increase in parenting stress and psychological distress (Li et al., 2022). In addition, it was often assumed that systemically relevant professions, such as medicine and education, experienced a particularly sharp increase in stress and workload during the pandemic—professions in which predominantly women work. However, the results regarding this assumption are quite mixed (e.g., Hipp & Bünning, 2020; Magnavita et al., 2021), potentially reflecting variations in the quality of the samples. Overall, these circumstances probably led to a greater reduction in time and energy for social interactions for women (*Path A and B*). This assumption is consistent with findings that women reported losing more friends during the pandemic than men (Bertogg & Koos, 2022). However, the impact of gender can also vary across different societal crises. For example, at the beginning of the financial crisis in 2008, men were more likely to lose their jobs, as male-dominated sectors were especially affected by the crises (Bettio et al., 2013). However, during the COVID-19 pandemic women were not only more likely to be working in occupations that probably faced a sharp increase in stress, but also in sectors that faced greater job insecurity such as the hospitality and catering industry, making women also more vulnerable to job losses during the pandemic (Barbieri et al., 2021). Since the occupational context is important for socializing in middle-adulthood, the opportunity structure for social interactions was more reduced for men during the financial crisis and more diminished for women during the Covid-19 pandemic (*Path C*). Moreover, as job insecurity and loss are often accompanied by higher levels of fear (*Path A*), it is likely that coping with these conditions took up more time and required more emotional support which might lead to a turtling-up of the network for the respective gender.

Looking at age, diverse processes emerge as the impact of age on social integration varies across societal crises as well as across paths. Older age can act as a protective factor during societal crises. For example, older people possess more and better problem-solving strategies to cope with critical life events, such as societal crises, due to their greater life experience (Blanchard-Fields, 2007; Lind et al., 2021). In addition, older people are less dependent on the labour market, as the majority are already retired (Crößmann et al., 2018). Consequently, fears of job losses due to crises, such as those experienced during the financial crises or the COVID-19 pandemic, do not affect older people as much as younger people. These circumstances may result in older people having a smaller decline in their capacities for social interactions (*Path A*). Furthermore, as individuals age, their network size decreases and becomes more focused on strong ties (Carstensen et al., 1999; Wrzus et al., 2013). These findings indicate that compared to younger people, older people have diverse advantages to protect themselves against the risk of loneliness due to societal crises. In addition, it is possible that crisis-related turtling-up of networks do not affect the influence of networks on older adults' well-being as much, as they already have fewer weak ties in their network (*Path D*). However, older age may also act as a risk factor. If older adults become lonely, they are more likely to remain so (Huxhold & Henning, 2023). Old age is often associated with a decline in health (Cezard et al., 2021; Spuling et al., 2019), making older people more vulnerable in physically demanding situations, such as heat waves due to climate change. These circumstances not only decrease their capacities and possibly also their motivation for social interactions (*Path A*), but also their social opportunity structure, as their personal mobility radius decreases sharply (*Path C*). During economic downturns with high inflation old age is a risk factor for (enduring) loneliness because it is difficult for retirees to adjust their own income situation (Deeken & Freudenberg, 2023). This might also increase their risk of financial difficulties and their anxieties (*Path A*) and therefore their risk of becoming lonely. Overall, the experiences of past societal crises highlight the complex influence of age on social integration during societal crises and make it necessary to assess the impact of age in each specific societal crisis separately.

In addition to SES, age and gender, other group memberships may also moderate the impact of crises on social integration. For instance, several crises, such as climate change or wars (e.g., in Ukraine or the Middle East), drive migration. As a result of migration from crisis regions, European societies are becoming more diverse. These new population groups often face multiple challenges, such as limited access to resources, coping with the crisis in their country of origin, experiencing hostility or discrimination, and developing new network ties while integrating into a new society (Hajak et al., 2021; Hannafi & Marouani, 2022).

10.4 Discussion

Europe has been hit by various societal crises over the past decades, which have had a great impact on people's social integration. However, despite increased research that underlines the impact of societal crises on people's social integration, so far no model has been introduced which explains the impact pathways of societal crises on social integration and loneliness. The DIRe-Crises-Model fills this gap. The model introduces multiple pathways linking macro-level disruptions to social processes and the development of loneliness while also integrating life circumstances at the meso level as moderators of these pathways. This approach highlights the diverse effects of societal crises on social integration and enables a more precise identification of underlying issues. Therefore, the model enables future research to classify and synthesize empirical findings on societal crises, social integration and loneliness. Additionally, the model can offer a theoretical basis for developing targeted interventions to avoid or reduce loneliness and thus ensure better support for vulnerable groups.

One major conclusion of the model is that societal crises can lead to "turtling-up" of social networks, with people turning to their strong ties for emotional and instrumental support (Taylor, 2011), while often diminishing their weak ties. Such a focus on strong ties can have a downside, as information accessed through weak ties (Granovetter, 1973) can become particularly valuable in times of uncertainty (Pitas & Ehmer, 2020). Additionally, the sense of social belonging can be reinforced through weak ties, especially during times of crisis (Kelle et al., 2025).

Moreover, during societal crises, when stress and anxiety are high, networks also risk decreasing in quality. As suggested by the family stress model (Conger et al., 2010), increased emotional distress reduces capacities and skills for investing in relationships. While weak ties may be lost, strong ties are maintained but risk becoming dysfunctional. Since it's harder to break negative strong ties than weak ones, these harmful relationships may persist in the network. Over time, these dynamics may lead to a smaller, lower-quality network. In the long term, the disruptions due to crises and the accompanying turtling-up of the social network will most likely decrease the individual's well-being and especially increase the risk of loneliness.

Research shows that loneliness may lead to feelings of social exclusion, as social relationships shape one's sense of belonging within society (Huxhold et al., 2022b). Therefore, if these circumstances persist and the reduced network structures become entrenched, it is possible that societal crises may also lead to an increase in feelings of social exclusion as people lose contact with the wider society. This may reduce the overall cohesion of society, while at the same time reducing important social functions that are most needed in times of societal crisis, such as volunteering. It can therefore be argued that the impact of societal crises on social integration has the potential to negatively affect not only individuals but indirectly also society as a whole. The consequences of crises for social integration may exacerbate the direct negative effects of crises on society.

But social networks can recover from crisis-related disruptions when crises situations ease or when people are able to adapt to the crisis. The DIRe-Crises-Model is a helpful framework in this regard, as the incorporated feedback loops allow for the assessment of not only immediate impacts but also long-term impacts on social integration. We assume that when conditions of high anxiety and stress decrease or people adapt, they have greater capacities, higher motivation, and more opportunities to invest time and energy in social interactions—especially in their wider network. However, it should be acknowledged that forming new relationships or deepening existing ones is time and energy consuming (Hall & Davis, 2017; Hall et al., 2023). This may be particularly problematic for people who have become lonely over the course of a societal crisis, since they face higher psychological and structural obstacles to reconnect with others (Hawkley & Cacioppo, 2010; Huxhold & Henning, 2023). In addition, life circumstances may shape the recovery process, as certain social groups, such as individuals with low socioeconomic status, often face greater disruption from societal crises and possess fewer resources, leading to a slower recovery. Currently, we do not know much about long-term recoveries of social integration after a societal crisis. Regarding the COVID-19 pandemic, only a few studies have investigated these developments with mixed results (Rebechi et al., 2024; van Tilburg, 2024). However, these assumptions regarding the recovery of social networks may need to be reconsidered, as the current interplay of multiple crises and ongoing structural challenges continues to give rise to new and increasing stressors for individuals. As a result, a subsiding of the crisis situation seems unlikely, and adapting to prevailing circumstances becomes more difficult. Our considerations regarding social cohesion, individual recovery, and the interplay of multiple crises highlight the importance of observing the long-term effects of crises. In a rapidly changing world, only long-term studies can capture the full scope of consequences, beyond those that are immediately apparent.

Acknowledgement We thank Nadja Keller for supporting us with literature research, technical editing, and proof reading of the final manuscript and Willi Bredereck for supporting us with literature research.

Competing Interests The authors have no conflicts of interest to declare that are relevant to the content of this chapter.

References

Ajrouch, K. J., Blandon, A. Y., & Antonucci, T. C. (2005). Social networks among men and women: The effects of age and socioeconomic status. *The Journals of Gerontology Series B: Psychological Sciences and Social Sciences, 60*(6), 311–317. https://doi.org/10.1093/geronb/60.6.S311

Anderson, C. A. (2001). Heat and violence. *Current Directions in Psychological Science, 10*(1), 33–38. https://doi.org/10.1111/1467-8721.00109

Antonucci, T. C. (2001). Social relations: An examination of social networks, social support and sense of control. In J. E. Birren & K. W. Schaie (Eds.), *Handbook of the psychology of ageing* (5th ed., pp. 427–453). Academic.

Antonucci, T. C., Ajrouch, K. J., & Birditt, K. S. (2014). The convoy model: Explaining social relations from a multidisciplinary perspective. *The Gerontologist, 54*(1), 82–92. https://doi.org/10.1093/geront/gnt118

Antonucci, T. C., Ajrouch, K. J., Webster, N. J., & Zahodne, L. B. (2019). Social relations across the life span: Scientific advances, emerging issues, and future challenges. *Annual Review of Developmental Psychology, 1*(1), 313–336. https://doi.org/10.1146/annurev-devpsych-121318-085212

Arsad, F. S., Hod, R., Ahmad, N., Ismail, R., Mohamed, N., Baharom, M., Osman, Y., Radi, M. F. M., & Tangang, F. (2022). The impact of heatwaves on mortality and morbidity and the associated vulnerability factors: A systematic review. *International Journal of Environmental Research and Public Health, 19*(23), 16356. https://doi.org/10.3390/ijerph192316356

Barbieri, D., Cazorla, A. G., Thil, L., Mollard, B., Ochmann, J., Peciukonis, V., Reingardė, J., & Salanauskaitė, L. (2021). *Gender equality index 2021: Health.* https://doi.org/10.2839/834132

Barrett, A. E. (2022). Centering age inequality: Developing a sociology-of-age framework. *Annual Review of Sociology, 48*(1), 213–232. https://doi.org/10.1146/annurev-soc-083121-043741

Baumeister, R. F., & Leary, M. R. (1995). The need to belong: Desire for interpersonal attachments as a fundamental human motivation. *Psychological Bulletin, 117*(3), 497–529. https://doi.org/10.1037/0033-2909.117.3.497

Bertogg, A., & Koos, S. (2021). Socio-economic position and local solidarity in times of crisis: The COVID-19 pandemic and the emergence of informal helping arrangements in Germany. *Research in Social Stratification and Mobility, 74*, 100612. https://doi.org/10.1016/j.rssm.2021.100612

Bertogg, A., & Koos, S. (2022). The making and breaking of social ties during the pandemic. Socio-economic position, demographic characteristics, and changes in social networks. *Frontiers in Sociology, 7*, 837968. https://doi.org/10.3389/fsoc.2022.837968

Bettio, F., Corsi, M., D'Ippoliti, C., Lyberaki, A., Lodovici, M. S., & Verashchagina, A. (2013). *The impact of the economic crisis on the situation of women and men and on gender equality policies: Synthesis report.* https://doi.org/10.2838/53123

Blanchard-Fields, F. (2007). Everyday problem solving and emotion: An adult developmental perspective. *Current Directions in Psychological Science, 16*(1), 26–31. https://doi.org/10.1111/j.1467-8721.2007.00469.x

Blustein, D. L., & Guarino, P. A. (2020). Work and unemployment in the time of COVID-19: The existential experience of loss and fear. *Journal of Humanistic Psychology, 60*(5), 702–709. https://doi.org/10.1177/0022167820934229

Bodea, C., Houle, C., & Kim, H. (2021). Do financial crises increase income inequality? *World Development, 147*, 105635. https://doi.org/10.1016/j.worlddev.2021.105635

Böger, A., & Huxhold, O. (2020). The changing relationship between partnership status and loneliness: Effects related to aging and historical time. *The Journals of Gerontology: Series B, 75*(7), 1423–1432. https://doi.org/10.1093/geronb/gby153

Boin, A., Hart, P., & t., & Kuipers, S. (2018). The crisis approach. In H. Rodríguez, W. Donner, & J. E. Trainor (Eds.), *Handbook of disaster research* (pp. 23–38). Springer. https://doi.org/10.1007/978-3-319-63254-4_2

Brandt, M., Garten, C., Grates, M., Kaschowitz, J., Quashie, N., & Schmitz, A. (2021). Veränderungen von Wohlbefinden und privater Unterstützung für Ältere: Ein Blick auf die Auswirkungen der COVID-19-Pandemie im Frühsommer 2020. *Zeitschrift für Gerontologie und Geriatrie, 54*(3), 240–246. https://doi.org/10.1007/s00391-021-01870-2

Bronfenbrenner, U. (1977). Toward an experimental ecology of human development. *American Psychologist, 32*(7), 513–531. https://doi.org/10.1037/0003-066x.32.7.513

Bronfenbrenner, U., & Morris, P. A. (2008). The bioecological model of human development. In W. Damon & R. M. Lerner (Eds.), *Handbook of child psychology* (pp. 793–828). Wiley Online Library.

Bühler, J. L., & Nikitin, J. (2020). Sociohistorical context and adult social development: New directions for 21st century research. *American Psychologist, 75*(4), 457–469.

Bujard, M., Laß, I., Diabaté, S., Sulak, H., & Schneider, N. F. (2020). *Eltern während der Corona-Krise: Zur Improvisation gezwungen*. Bundesinstitut für Bevölkerungsforschung (BiB). https://doi.org/10.12765/bro-2020-01

Bundeszentrale für politische Bildung (bpb). (2021). Auswirkungen der Coronapandemie: Auszug aus dem Datenreport 2021. In *Datenreport 2021: Ein Sozialbericht für die Bundesrepublik Deutschland* (pp. 463–503).

Bünning, M., & Huxhold, O. (2024). Grandchild care and grandparents' well-being in context: The impact of the Covid-19 pandemic. *Innovation in Aging, 8*(12). https://doi.org/10.1093/geroni/igae101.

Bünning, M., Schlomann, A., Memmer, N., Tesch-Römer, C., & Wahl, H.-W. (2023). Digital gender gap in the second half of life is declining: Changes in gendered internet use between 2014 and 2021 in Germany. *The Journals of Gerontology: Series B, 78*(8), 1386–1395. https://doi.org/10.1093/geronb/gbad079

Busch, K., Hermann, C., Hinrichs, K., & Schulten, T. (2013). *Euro crisis, austerity policy and the European social model: How crisis policies in southern Europe threaten the EU's social dimension* (International Policy Analysis, Issue. F. E. Foundation).

Cacioppo, S., Grippo, A. J., London, S., Goossens, L., & Cacioppo, J. T. (2015). Loneliness: Clinical import and interventions. *Perspectives on Psychological Science, 10*(2), 238–249. https://doi.org/10.1177/1745691615570616

Cameron, S. (2021). Civic engagement in times of economic crisis: A cross-national comparative study of voluntary association membership. *European Political Science Review, 13*(3), 265–283. https://doi.org/10.1017/S1755773921000060

Carstensen, L. L., Isaacowitz, D. M., & Charles, S. T. (1999). Taking time seriously: A theory of socioemotional selectivity. *American Psychologist, 54*(3), 165–181. https://doi.org/10.1037/0003-066x.54.3.165

Cezard, G., McHale, C. T., Sullivan, F., Bowles, J. K. F., & Keenan, K. (2021). Studying trajectories of multimorbidity: A systematic scoping review of longitudinal approaches and evidence. *BMJ Open, 11*, e048485. https://doi.org/10.1136/bmjopen-2020-048485

Conger, R. D., Conger, K. J., & Martin, M. J. (2010). Socioeconomic status, family processes, and individual development. *Journal of Marriage and Family, 72*(3), 685–704. https://doi.org/10.1111/j.1741-3737.2010.00725.x

Crößmann, A., Mischke, J., & Hoffmann, J. (2018). Arbeitsmarkt auf einen Blick: Deutschland und Europa. *Statistisches Bundesamt (Destatis)*.

Damstra, A., & Vliegenthart, R. (2018). (Un) covering the economic crisis? Over-time and inter-media differences in salience and framing. *Journalism Studies, 19*(7), 983–1003. https://doi.org/10.1080/1461670X.2016.1246377

Deeken, T., & Freudenberg, C. (2023). Inflation trifft Rente: Welche Maßnahmen haben unsere Nachbarländer im Vergleich zu Deutschland ergriffen? *Deutsche Rentenversicherung, 2023*(2), 133–151.

Dunbar, R. I. M. (2014). The social brain: Psychological underpinnings and implications for the structure of organizations. *Current Directions in Psychological Science, 23*(2), 109–114. https://doi.org/10.1177/0963721413517118

Ehrlich, U., & Kelle, N. (2019). Pflegende Angehörige in Deutschland: Wer pflegt, wo, für wen und wie? *Zeitschrift für Sozialreform, 65*(2), 175–203. https://doi.org/10.1515/zsr-2019-0007

Ehrlich, U., Kelle, N., Klaus, D., & Möhring, K. (2022). How did the COVID-19 pandemic impact family caregivers well-being? A longitudinal study of older adults in Germany. *Ageing and Society*, 1–18. https://doi.org/10.1017/S0144686X22000873

Entringer, T. M., & Kröger, H. (2020). Einsam, aber resilient: Die Menschen haben den Lockdown besser verkraftet als vermutet. *DIW aktuell, 46*, 1–6. https://hdl.handle.net/10419/222876

Esperon-Rodriguez, M., Tjoelker, M. G., Lenoir, J., Baumgartner, J. B., Beaumont, L. J., Nipperess, D. A., Power, S. A., Richard, B., Rymer, P. D., & Gallagher, R. V. (2022). Climate change increases global risk to urban forests. *Nature Climate Change, 12*, 950–955. https://doi.org/10.1038/s41558-022-01465-8

EUROSTAT. (2024). *Overcrowding rate by age, sex and poverty status – total population – EU-SILC survey*. Retrieved 14.08.2024 from https://data.europa.eu/data/datasets/wf1zsq4hldrrfc6z5zxa?locale=en

Fingerman, K. L. (2009). Consequential strangers and peripheral ties: The importance of unimportant relationships. *Journal of Family Theory & Review, 1*(2), 69–86. https://doi.org/10.1111/j.1756-2589.2009.00010.x

Fuller, H. R., Ajrouch, K. J., & Antonucci, T. C. (2020). The convoy model and later-life family relationships. *Journal of Family Theory & Review, 12*(2), 126–146. https://doi.org/10.1111/jftr.12376

Granovetter, M. S. (1973). The strength of weak ties. *American Journal of Sociology, 78*(6), 1360–1380. https://doi.org/10.1086/225469

Greussing, E., & Boomgaarden, H. G. (2017). Shifting the refugee narrative? An automated frame analysis of Europe's 2015 refugee crisis. *Journal of Ethnic and Migration Studies, 43*(11), 1749–1774. https://doi.org/10.1080/1369183X.2017.1282813

Grote, U., Arvand, M., Brinkwirth, S., Brunke, M., Buchholz, U., Eckmanns, T., von Kleist, M., Niebank, M., Ruehe, B., Schulze, K., Stoliaroff-Pépin, A., Thanheiser, M., Schaade, L., Said, D., & Haas, W. (2021). Maßnahmen zur Bewältigung der COVID-19-Pandemie in Deutschland: Nichtpharmakologische und pharmakologische Ansätze. *Bundesgesundheitsblatt – Gesundheitsforschung – Gesundheitsschutz, 64*(4), 435–445. https://doi.org/10.1007/s00103-021-03306-z

Hajak, V. L., Sardana, S., Verdeli, H., & Grimm, S. (2021). A systematic review of factors affecting mental health and well-being of asylum seekers and refugees in Germany. *Frontiers in Psychiatry, 12*, 643704. https://doi.org/10.3389/fpsyt.2021.643704

Hall, J. A., & Davis, D. C. (2017). Proposing the communicate bond belong theory: Evolutionary intersections with episodic interpersonal communication. *Communication Theory, 27*(1), 21–47. https://doi.org/10.1111/comt.12106

Hall, J. A., & Merolla, A. J. (2020). Connecting everyday talk and time alone to global well-being. *Human Communication Research, 46*(1), 86–111. https://doi.org/10.1093/hcr/hqz014

Hall, J. A., Dominguez, J., Merolla, A. J., & Otmar, C. D. (2023). Social bandwidth: When and why are social interactions energy intensive? *Journal of Social and Personal Relationships, 40*(8), 2614–2636. https://doi.org/10.1177/02654075231154937

Handler, H. (2024a). Krisen formen Europa. In *Krisengeprüftes Europa: Die EU auf dem Weg zu einer neuen Identität* (2nd ed., pp. 1–9). Springer Fachmedien Wiesbaden. https://doi.org/10.1007/978-3-658-42924-9

Handler, H. (2024b). Migrationspolitik der EU zwischen Abwehr und Integration. In *Krisengeprüftes Europa: Die EU auf dem Weg zu einer neuen Identität* (2nd ed., pp. 75–109). Springer Fachmedien Wiesbaden. https://doi.org/10.1007/978-3-658-42924-9

Hannafi, C., & Marouani, M. A. (2022). Social integration of Syrian refugees and their intention to stay in Germany. *Journal of Population Economics, 36*(2), 581–607. https://doi.org/10.1007/s00148-022-00913-1

Hawkley, L. C., & Cacioppo, J. T. (2010). Loneliness matters: A theoretical and empirical review of consequences and mechanisms. *Annals of Behavioral Medicine, 40*(2), 218–227. https://doi.org/10.1007/s12160-010-9210-8

Heckhausen, J., & Buchmann, M. (2019). A multi-disciplinary model of life-course canalization and agency. *Advances in Life Course Research, 41*, 100246. https://doi.org/10.1016/j.alcr.2018.09.002

Heisig, J. P. (2021). Soziale Ungleichheit und gesundheitliches Risiko in der Pandemie. In *Corona. Pandemie und Krise* (pp. 332–344). Bundeszentrale für politische Bildung (bpb). https://hdl.handle.net/10419/234052

Hipp, L., & Bünning, M. (2020). Parenthood as a driver of increased gender inequality during COVID-19? Exploratory evidence from Germany. *European Societies, 23*(1), 658–673. https://doi.org/10.1080/14616696.2020.1833229

Höltmann, G., Hutter, S., & Rößler-Prokhorenko, C. (2022). *Solidarität und Protest in der Zeitenwende: Reaktionen der Zivilgesellschaft auf den Ukraine-Krieg*. WZB Discussion Paper No. ZZ 2022–601. https://hdl.handle.net/10419/265547.

Hsiang, S. M., Burke, M., & Miguel, E. (2013). Quantifying the influence of climate on human conflict. *Science, 341*, 1235367. https://doi.org/10.1126/science.1235367

Hughes, M. E., & Waite, L. J. (2007). The aging of the second demographic transition. In K. W. Schaie & P. Uhlenberg (Eds.), *Social structures: The impact of demographic changes on the well-being of older persons* (pp. 179–211). Springer.

Huxhold, O., & Fiori, K. L. (2024). Understanding loneliness in late life. *Current Opinion in Psychology, 57*, 101801. https://doi.org/10.1016/j.copsyc.2024.101801

Huxhold, O., & Henning, G. (2023). The risks of experiencing severe loneliness across middle and late adulthood. *The Journals of Gerontology: Series B, 78*(10), 1668–1675. https://doi.org/10.1093/geronb/gbad099

Huxhold, O., & Tesch-Römer, C. (2021). *Einsamkeit steigt in der Corona-Pandemie bei Menschen im mittleren und hohen Erwachsenenalter gleichermaßen deutlich* (DZA Aktuell, Issue 04/2021).

Huxhold, O., Fiori, K. L., Webster, N. J., & Antonucci, T. C. (2020). The strength of weaker ties: An underexplored resource for maintaining emotional well-being in later life. *The Journals of Gerontology Series B: Psychological Sciences and Social Sciences, 75*(7), 1433–1442. https://doi.org/10.1093/geronb/gbaa019

Huxhold, O., Fiori, K. L., & Windsor, T. D. (2022a). Rethinking social relationships in adulthood: The differential investment of resources model. *Personality and Social Psychology Review, 26*(1), 57–82. https://doi.org/10.1177/10888683211067035

Huxhold, O., Suanet, B., & Wetzel, M. (2022b). Perceived social exclusion and loneliness: Two distinct but related phenomena. *Sociological Science, 9*, 430–453. https://doi.org/10.15195/v9.a17

Iglič, H. (2014). The crumbling or strengthening of social capital? The economic crisis' impact on social networks and interpersonal trust in Slovenia. *Journal Družboslovne Razprave, 77*, 7–26.

Iglič, H., Rözer, J., & Volker, B. G. M. (2021). Economic crisis and social capital in European societies: The role of politics in understanding short-term changes in social capital. *European Societies, 23*(2), 195–231. https://doi.org/10.1080/14616696.2020.1765406

IPCC. (2023). *Climate change 2023: Synthesis report: A report of the intergovernmental panel on climate change*. https://www.ipcc.ch/report/ar6/syr/

Kelle, N., Bünning, M., & Simonson, J. (2025). COVID-19 pandemic, volunteering, and well-being: Volunteering's role in mitigating depressive symptoms, loneliness, and perceived social exclusion during the pandemic. *Social Indicators Research* (Online first).

Kersten, J., & Rixen, S. (2022). Leben in der Krise. In *Der Verfassungsstaat in der Corona-Krise* (3rd ed., pp. 25–64). C.H.BECK.

Kiess, J., Preunkert, J., Seeliger, M., & Steg, J. (2023). Krisen erkennen, Krisen analysieren: Die Soziologie in Zeiten multipler Krisenkonstellationen. In J. Kiess, J. Preunkert, M. Seeliger, & J. Steg (Eds.), *Krisen und Soziologie* (pp. 7–19). Beltz Juventa.

Kjellstrom, T., Briggs, D., Freyberg, C., Lemke, B., Otto, M., & Hyatt, O. (2016). Heat, human performance, and occupational health: A key issue for the assessment of global climate change impacts. *Annual Review of Public Health, 37*(1), 97–112. https://doi.org/10.1146/annurev-publhealth-032315-021740

Kortmann, L., Hagen, C., Endter, C., Riesch, J., & Tesch-Römer, C. (2021). *Internetnutzung von Menschen in der zweiten Lebenshälfte während der Corona-Pandemie: Soziale Ungleichheiten bleiben bestehen* (DZA Aktuell, Issue 05/2021).

Kovacs, B., Caplan, N., Grob, S., & King, M. (2021). Social networks and loneliness during the COVID-19 pandemic. *Socius, 7*, 1–16. https://doi.org/10.1177/2378023120985254

Kung, C. S., & Steptoe, A. (2023). Changes in Internet use patterns among older adults in England from before to after the outbreak of the COVID-19 pandemic. *Scientific Reports, 13*, 3932. https://doi.org/10.1038/s41598-023-30882-8

Landsbergis, P. A., Grzywacz, J. G., & LaMontagne, A. D. (2014). Work organization, job insecurity, and occupational health disparities. *American Journal of Industrial Medicine, 57*(5), 495–515. https://doi.org/10.1002/ajim.22126

Lee, S. S., Shim, Y., Choi, J., & Choi, I. (2023). Paradoxical impacts of social relationship on well-being during the covid-19 pandemic. *Journal of Happiness Studies, 24*, 745–767. https://doi.org/10.1007/s10902-022-00614-2

Li, J., Bünning, M., Kaiser, T., & Hipp, L. (2022). Who suffered most? Parental stress and mental health during the initial phase of the COVID-19 pandemic in Germany. *JFR – Journal of Family Research, 34*(1), 281–309. https://doi.org/10.20377/jfr-704

Liadze, I., Macchiarelli, C., Mortimer-Lee, P., & Sanchez Juanino, P. (2023). Economic costs of the Russia-Ukraine war. *The World Economy, 46*(4), 874–886. https://doi.org/10.1111/twec.13336

Lind, M., Bluck, S., & McAdams, D. P. (2021). More vulnerable? The life story approach highlights older people's potential for strength during the pandemic. *The Journals of Gerontology: Series B, 76*(2), e45–e48. https://doi.org/10.1093/geronb/gbaa105

Lindemann, U., Skelton, D. A., Oksa, J., Beyer, N., Rapp, K., Becker, C., & Klenk, J. (2018). Social participation and heat-related behavior in older adults during heat waves and on other days. *Zeitschrift für Gerontologie und Geriatrie, 51*(5), 543–549. https://doi.org/10.1007/s00391-017-1338-8

Lynott, D., Corker, K., Connell, L., & O'Brien, K. (2023). The effects of temperature on prosocial and antisocial behaviour: A review and meta-analysis. *British Journal of Social Psychology, 62*, 1177–1214. https://doi.org/10.1111/bjso.12626

Magnavita, N., Soave, P. M., & Antonelli, M. (2021). Prolonged stress causes depression in frontline workers facing the COVID-19 pandemic—a repeated cross-sectional study in a COVID-19 Hub-hospital in central Italy. *International Journal of Environmental Research and Public Health, 18*(14), 7316.

Mares, D. M., & Moffett, K. W. (2015). Climate change and interpersonal violence: A "global" estimate and regional inequities. *Climatic Change, 135*(2), 297–310. https://doi.org/10.1007/s10584-015-1566-0

Matysiak, A., & Cukrowska-Torzewska, E. (2021). Gender and labour market outcomes. In N. F. Schneider & M. Kreyenfeld (Eds.), *Research handbook on the sociology of the family*. Edward Elgar Publishing. https://doi.org/10.4337/9781788975544.00032

Murciano-Hueso, A., Martín-García, A.-V., & Cardoso, A. P. (2022). Technology and quality of life of older people in times of COVID: A qualitative study on their changed digital profile. *International Journal of Environmental Research and Public Health, 19*, 10459. https://doi.org/10.3390/ijerph191610459

Ohlbrecht, H., & Jellen, J. (2021). Unequal tensions: The effects of the coronavirus pandemic in light of subjective health and social inequality dimensions in Germany. *European Societies, 23*(1), 905–922. https://doi.org/10.1080/14616696.2020.1852440

Pailhé, A., Solaz, A., & Stanfors, M. (2021). The great convergence: Gender and unpaid work in Europe and the United States. *Population and Development Review, 47*(1), 181–217. https://doi.org/10.1111/padr.12385

Panova, R., Sulak, H., Bujard, M., & Wolf, L. (2017). Die Rushhour des Lebens im Familienzyklus: Zeitverwendung von Männern und Frauen. In S. Bundesamt (Ed.), *Wie die Zeit vergeht. Analysen zur Zeitverwendung in Deutschland* (pp. 45–63). Statistisches Bundesamt.

Parmar, D., Stavropoulou, C., & Ioannidis, J. P. (2016). Health outcomes during the 2008 financial crisis in Europe: Systematic literature review. *BMJ, 354*, i4588. https://doi.org/10.1136/bmj.i4588

Pinquart, M. (2003). Loneliness in married, widowed, divorced, and never-married older adults. *Journal of Social and Personal Relationships, 20*(1), 31–53.

Pitas, N., & Ehmer, C. (2020). Social capital in the response to COVID-19. *American Journal of Health Promotion, 34*(8), 942–944. https://doi.org/10.1177/0890117120924531

Ramaekers, M. J. M., Verbakel, E., & Kraaykamp, G. (2022). Informal volunteering and socialization effects: Examining modelling and encouragement by parents and partner. *VOLUNTAS: International Journal of Voluntary and Nonprofit Organizations, 33*, 347–361. https://doi.org/10.1007/s11266-021-00315-z

Ramaekers, M. J., Verbakel, E., & Kraaykamp, G. (2023). Decline in informal helping during the first COVID-19 lockdown: A longitudinal analysis of Dutch data. *European Societies, 26*(3), 690–717. https://doi.org/10.1080/14616696.2023.2200503

Rebechi, A., Lepintuer, A., Clark, A. E., Rohde, N., Vögele, C., & D'ambrosio, C. (2024). Loneliness during the COVID-19 pandemic: Evidence from five European countries. *Economics & Human Biology, 55*, 101427. https://doi.org/10.1016/j.ehb.2024.101427

Reyes-Riveros, R., Altamirano, A., De La Barrera, F., Rozas-Vásquez, D., Vieli, L., & Meli, P. (2021). Linking public urban green spaces and human well-being: A systematic review. *Urban Forestry & Urban Greening, 61*, 127105. https://doi.org/10.1016/j.ufug.2021.127105

Reynolds, R. M., Meng, J., & Dorrance Hall, E. (2020). Multilayered social dynamics and depression among older adults: A 10-year cross-lagged analysis. *Psychology and Aging, 35*(7), 948–962. https://doi.org/10.1037/pag0000569

Romero, D. M., Uzzi, B., & Kleinberg, J. (2016). *Social networks under stress*. Proceedings of the 25th International Conference on World Wide Web, Montreal, Canada.

Romeu Gordo, L., Simonson, J., & Lozano Alcántara, A. (2023). Financial consequences of COVID-19 in Germany: Living standards of older people during the first year of the pandemic. *Journal of Aging & Social Policy*, 1–18. https://doi.org/10.1080/08959420.2023.22575

Rosenthal, U., & Kouzmin, A. (1997). Crises and crisis management: Toward comprehensive government decision making. *Journal of Public Administration Research and Theory, 7*(2), 277–304. https://doi.org/10.1093/oxfordjournals.jpart.a024349

Rosenthal, U., Charles, M. T., & Hart, P.T. (Eds.). (1989). *Coping with crisis: The management of disasters, riots and terrorism*. Charles C. Thomas Publisher.

Schad, M., & Hense, A. (2023). Covid-19's effects on strong and weak ties in middle-class families: Insights from intergenerational qualitative longitudinal data. *Soziale Welt, 74*(1), 40–63. https://doi.org/10.5771/0038-6073-2023-1-40

Schäfers, B. (2018). Krise. In J. Kopp & A. Steinbach (Eds.), *Grundbegriffe der Soziologie* (pp. 245–247). Springer VS. https://doi.org/10.1007/978-3-658-20978-0_49

Schubert, K., & Klein, M. (2020). Krise. In *Das Politiklexikon* (7th ed.). Bundeszentrale für politische Bildung. https://www.bpb.de/kurz-knapp/lexika/politiklexikon/17759/krise/

Shaluf, I. M., Ahmadun, F. I. R., & Mat Said, A. (2003). A review of disaster and crisis. *Disaster Prevention and Management, 12*(1), 24–32. https://doi.org/10.1108/09653560310463829

Silverstein, M., & Giarrusso, R. (2011). Aging individuals, families, and societies: Micro–meso–macro linkages in the life course. In R. Settersten & J. Angel (Eds.), *Handbook of sociology of aging* (pp. 35–49). Springer. https://doi.org/10.1007/978-1-4419-7374-0_3

Simonson, J., & Kelle, N. (2023). Volunteering in organisations by people in the second half of life during the Covid-19 pandemic. In J. Simonson, J. Wünsche, & C. Tesch-Römer (Eds.), *Ageing in times of the COVID-19 pandemic* (pp. 201–214). Springer VS. https://doi.org/10.1007/978-3-658-40487-1_11

Sola, A. (2018). The 2015 refugee crisis in Germany: Concerns about immigration and populism. *SOEPpaper, 966*, 1–34. https://doi.org/10.2139/ssrn.3169243

Spuling, S. M., Cengia, A., & Wettstein, M. (2019). Funktionale und subjektive Gesundheit bei Frauen und Männern im Verlauf der zweiten Lebenshälfte. In C. Vogel, M. Wettstein, & C. Tesch-Römer (Eds.), *Frauen und Männer in der zweiten Lebenshälfte: Älterwerden im sozialen Wandel* (pp. 35–52). Springer Fachmedien Wiesbaden. https://doi.org/10.1007/978-3-658-25079-9_3

Staggenborg, S. (2002). The "meso" in social movement research. In D. S. Meyer, N. Whittier, & B. Robnett (Eds.), *Social movements: Identity, culture, and the state* (pp. 124–139). Oxford University Press. https://doi.org/10.1093/oso/9780195143553.003.0009

Steijvers, L. C., Brinkhues, S., van Tilburg, T., Hoebe, C. J., Stijnen, M. M., Vries, N. D., Crutzen, R., & Dukers-Muijrers, N. H. (2022). Changes in structure and function of social networks of independently living middle-aged and older adults in diverse sociodemographic subgroups

during the COVID-19 pandemic: A longitudinal study. *BMC Public Health, 22*, 2253. https://doi.org/10.1186/s12889-022-14500-2
Stok, F. M., Bal, M., Yerkes, M. A., & De Wit, J. B. (2021). Social inequality and solidarity in times of COVID-19. *International Journal of Environmental Research and Public Health, 18*(12), 6339. https://doi.org/10.3390/ijerph18126339
Taylor, S. E. (2011). Social support: A review. *The Oxford Handbook of Health Psychology, 1*, 189–214.
van Tilburg, T. G. (2024). Residual loneliness in the Netherlands after the COVID-19 pandemic: An application of the single interrupted time series design with pre-, peri- and post-pandemic observations. *Public Health, 237*, 238–244. https://doi.org/10.1016/j.puhe.2024.10.023
UNICEF. (2023). *Protecting children from heat stress: A technical note*. https://www.unicef.org/media/139926/file/Protecting-children-from-heat-stress-A-technical-note-2023.pdf
United Nations. (2011). *The global social crisis: Report on the world social situation 2011*. U. N. Publications.
United Nations. (2022a). *Global impact of the war in Ukraine: Billions of people face the greatest cost-of-living crisis in a generation*. U. N. Publications.
United Nations. (2022b). *Six month of war in Ukraine*. United Nations Publications. Retrieved 03.05.2024 from https://unric.org/en/six-months-of-war-in-ukraine/
Van Groenou, M. I. B., & Van Tilburg, T. (2003). Network size and support in old age: Differentials by socio-economic status in childhood and adulthood. *Ageing and Society, 23*(5), 625–645. https://doi.org/10.1017/S0144686X0300134X
Van Regenmortel, S., Tiilikainen, E., Ristolainen, H., Burholt, V., & Dahlberg, L. (2025). Social exclusion perspective on loneliness in later life. In M. Aartsen, I. Precupetu, & B. Suanet (Eds.), *Macro social influences on loneliness in later life: Towards a better understanding of the loneliness paradox in later life*. Springer.
Van Tilburg, T. G., Steinmetz, S., Stolte, E., van der Roest, H., & de Vries, D. H. (2021). Loneliness and mental health during the COVID-19 pandemic: A study among Dutch older adults. *The Journals of Gerontology: Series B, 76*(7), e249–e255. https://doi.org/10.1093/geronb/gbaa111
Verick, S., & Islam, I. (2010). *The great recession of 2008–2009: Causes, consequences and policy responses*. IZA Discussion Paper No. 4934.
Völker, B. (2023). Networks in lockdown: The consequences of COVID-19 for social relationships and feelings of loneliness. *Social Networks, 72*, 1–12. https://doi.org/10.1016/j.socnet.2022.08.001
Wachtler, B., & Hoebel, J. (2020). Soziale Ungleichheit und COVID-19: Sozialepidemiologische Perspektiven auf die Pandemie. *Gesundheitswesen, 82*, 670–675. https://doi.org/10.1055/a-1226-6708
WHO. (2018). *Heat and health*. Retrieved 07.09.2023, from https://www.who.int/news-room/fact-sheets/detail/climate-change-heat-and-health
Wrzus, C., Hänel, M., Wagner, J., & Neyer, F. J. (2013). Social network changes and life events across the life span: A meta-analysis. *Psychological Bulletin, 139*(1), 53–80. https://doi.org/10.1037/a0028601
Yeganeh, A. J., Reichard, G., McCoy, A. P., Bulbul, T., & Jazizadeh, F. (2018). Correlation of ambient air temperature and cognitive performance: A systematic review and meta-analysis. *Building and Environment, 143*, 701–716. https://doi.org/10.1016/j.buildenv.2018.07.002

Lisa Joanne Klasen is a psychologist, a PhD student at Humboldt University Berlin and works at the German Centre of Gerontology (DZA) in the CoESI project "Social Integration of Older People During the COVID-19 Pandemic", funded by the German Ministry of Education and Research. Her research focuses on social integration, with particular interest in macro-level influences on loneliness and individual-level factors affecting social well-being.

Mareike Bünning is a sociologist and senior scientist at the German Centre of Gerontology (DZA). She works on the German Ageing Survey (DEAS) and is a principal investigator on several projects, including the project CoESI "Social Integration of Older People During the COVID-19 Pandemic," funded by the German Ministry of Education and Research. Her research focuses on families, social integration, social support and social inequality. She is also interested in survey methodology. Her work has been published in *Journals of Gerontology: Series B*, *Innovation in Aging*, *European Sociological Review*, and *Journal of Marriage and Family*.

Nadiya Kelle is a sociologist and senior scientist at the German Centre of Gerontology (DZA). She is a principal investigator on several projects at DZA, focusing on social inequalities over the life course, loneliness, and social integration, including the project CoESI "Social Integration of Older People During the COVID-19 Pandemic," funded by the German Ministry of Education and Research. Her research interests include gender inequalities, social participation, as well as the relationships between employment, caregiving, and volunteering. Her work has been published in *Social Indicators Research*, *Voluntas*, and *Ageing & Society*.

Clemens Tesch-Römer, Director Retired of the German Centre of Gerontology (1998 to 2023), has been Adjunct Professor of Psychology at the Freie Universität Berlin (since 2023 Lecturer in psychology). PI of European and German surveys and networks, e.g. German Ageing Survey (2001–2023), German Survey on Volunteering (2012–2021), and COST Action IS 1402 on Ageism (2014–2018). Member of the German Federal Government's Third to Ninth Expert Commissions on Older Persons. Served as president of the German Society for Gerontology and Geriatrics (2008–2010) and IAGG-ER (2015–2019). Research interests: social inequality, quality of life, social integration, and societal participation in the second half of life.

Oliver Huxhold is a psychologist and senior scientist, currently serving as the head of research on social relationships and health at the German Centre of Gerontology. He is a principal investigator on several projects, including the CoESI project "Social Integration of Older People During the COVID-19 Pandemic," funded by the German Ministry of Education and Research. His research interests focus on lifespan psychology, with a particular emphasis on social relationships and social integration (including loneliness) in older adults. He also investigates issues related to social inequality and social exclusion. His work has been published in *Journals of Gerontology: Series B*, *Psychology and Aging*, and *Personality and Social Psychology Review*, among others.

Open Access This chapter is licensed under the terms of the Creative Commons Attribution 4.0 International License (http://creativecommons.org/licenses/by/4.0/), which permits use, sharing, adaptation, distribution and reproduction in any medium or format, as long as you give appropriate credit to the original author(s) and the source, provide a link to the Creative Commons license and indicate if changes were made.

The images or other third party material in this chapter are included in the chapter's Creative Commons license, unless indicated otherwise in a credit line to the material. If material is not included in the chapter's Creative Commons license and your intended use is not permitted by statutory regulation or exceeds the permitted use, you will need to obtain permission directly from the copyright holder.

Part V
Future Directions

Chapter 11
Macro-Level Influences on Loneliness in Later Life: An fsQCA Analysis

Iuliana Precupetu, Cosmina Pop, and Marja Aartsen

11.1 On the Problem of Analyzing Macro-Level Influences

In 1990, Jylhä and Jokela discovered significant variations in loneliness prevalence among European countries, a phenomenon that could not be solely explained by individual variables related to life situations. Countries with the highest levels of loneliness were those where living alone was least common, and community ties were strongest (Jylhä & Jokela, 1990). This puzzling pattern, later referred to as the "cultural paradox of loneliness" (Heu et al., 2021, p. 60), has been reported in several subsequent European studies (Sundström et al., 2009; Dykstra, 2009; De Jong Gierveld & Tesch-Römer, 2012; Hansen & Slagsvold, 2016; Swader, 2019), and is often explained in terms of differences in individual versus collectivistic values (see van Tilburg, 2025 for more details). However, studies incorporating data from other continents, such as Asia and America, find that individualistic countries exhibit higher rates of loneliness compared to collectivistic countries (Taniguchi & Kaufman, 2021; Barreto et al., 2021). This inconsistency may be attributed to overlapping other macro-factors also prevalent in countries where living alone is more common, such as demographic characteristics and health (Fokkema et al., 2012), or social wealth and type of welfare regime (Hansen & Slagsvold, 2016). Hence, results from cross-national studies on loneliness prevalence may be misleading if

I. Precupetu (✉)
Research Institute for Quality of Life, Romanian Academy, Bucharest, Romania

Research Institute of the University of Bucharest, Bucharest, Romania
e-mail: iuliana@iccv.ro

C. Pop
Research Institute for Quality of Life, Romanian Academy, Bucharest, Romania

M. Aartsen
Norwegian Social Research (NOVA), Oslo Metropolitan University, Oslo, Norway

© The Author(s) 2025

M. Aartsen et al. (eds.), *Macro Social Influences on Loneliness in Later Life*, International Perspectives on Aging 47,
https://doi.org/10.1007/978-3-031-94565-6_11

competing macro-level explanations are not considered (see also Suanet & Pavlidis, 2025).

There may be multiple pathways from macro-level factors to individual level loneliness, and interactions between macro-level characteristics may exert different impacts on loneliness (de Jong Gierveld & Tesch-Römer, 2012; Tufă, 2025; Suanet & Aartsen, 2025). However, this is seldom empirically investigated. Moreover, risk factors or conditions for low loneliness and high loneliness may not be symmetrical, that is, factors associated with high loneliness may not be the same as for low loneliness. Hence, understanding country differences in loneliness is complex and requires an analytical technique that can deal with these causal complexities. To tackle this complexity, Qualitative Comparative Analysis (QCA; Ragin, 1987; Schneider & Wagemann, 2012; Rihoux & Ragin, 2009) seems a promising approach. In a nutshell, QCA is a family of research methods that facilitates the examination of complex causal relationships. It combines quantitative and qualitative analysis through developing set-theoretic relations that are dependent on both theory and empirical knowledge (Ragin, 2008). QCA examines how conditions (called risk-factors in inferential statistics) or different combinations of conditions (called configurations or pathways) lead to a certain outcome–in our case, low loneliness. The outcome of the analysis is a list of conditions or combination of conditions that are necessary and/or sufficient for low loneliness to occur, or not occur (Ragin, 2008) (see Methods for a more detailed explanation).

While the number of studies applying QCA is increasing, it has seldom been used in loneliness research, except for two notable examples. The first is a study by Yang (2018), who employed this method to identify the necessary and sufficient causal individual conditions associated with loneliness among adults residing in the UK. The researcher examined the configurations of five micro-level conditions frequently found to be associated with loneliness: being female, old age, not living with a spouse or partner, poor health, and not being frequently social with others. While advanced age alone is not a necessary condition, it becomes necessary when combined with any of the other conditions. Gender, on the other hand, was found to be neither necessary nor sufficient for loneliness. In the second study, researchers investigated six macro-social conditions: five infrastructures (commercial, public, internet, accessibility of social groups, relational pluralism) and strong personal connections, which is an aggregated condition (Swader & Moraru, 2023). Out of these six conditions, only high internet access and active participation in associations emerged as necessary conditions for low loneliness.

This chapter provides another application of QCA to shed more light on the macro-social influences on loneliness in later life. Our leading research question is: What are the necessary and sufficient macro-conditions that are fundamental to understanding country-level differences in loneliness in European countries? Given the focus of the book, we select cases within Europe and concentrate on older adults. For the selection of conditions, we rely on previous empirical and theoretical studies on macro-social influences on loneliness. We include macro-social factors, in line with the scope of the book. We do not aim for the largest possible selection of conditions, as a large number of conditions can make the results incomprehensible and difficult to understand. Often, five or six different conditions are investigated with QCA. Other legitimate reasons for limiting the number of conditions include the lack of data, factors that do not vary across the cases, the absence of theoretical support for the condition (Mello, 2021), and the case-to-factor ratio. Including too many conditions and too few cases can lead to the problem of overdetermination (Marx & Dusa, 2011). Before moving to the analyses, we present prevailing evidence for macro-level factors and previous theoretical models for the understanding of macro-level influences on loneliness in later life.

11.2 Macro-Social Factors and Previous Theoretical Models on Loneliness

Earlier explanations for the country variations in loneliness prevalence often relied on post-hoc interpretations, such as variations in demographic characteristics and poor health (Fokkema et al., 2012), and differences in social wealth and type of welfare regime (Hansen & Slagsvold, 2016). These post-hoc explanations were followed by more theory-based explanations, such as in the study on interpersonal and generalized trust (Rapolienė & Aartsen, 2021). An interesting theoretical approach to further understanding country-level variations in loneliness is to consider the interaction between micro and macro social factors and their impact on loneliness (De Jong Gierveld & Tesch-Römer, 2012). Studies on the impact of these interactions on loneliness are still rare, but there are some notable exceptions. A study among older adults living in European countries and China (Wu et al., 2022) investigates how income inequality and welfare generosity moderate the association between socio-economic status and loneliness. The authors conclude that the association between socio-economic status and loneliness is stronger in countries with high income inequality but weaker in more welfare-generous societies. Another study investigates the moderating impact of collectivism on the associations between living situation and loneliness in countries from all continents of the world. It was found that the well-known negative association between marriage and loneliness is attenuated for those living in more collectivistic countries (Taniguchi & Kaufman, 2021).

11.3 Analytical Framework: Selection of Macro-Level Conditions

The empirical and theoretical studies presented above guide us in the selection of conditions that we apply in our study. Based on the scientific principle of parsimony and the interpretability of the findings, we limit the total number of conditions to five: digitalization, poverty, trust, individualism, and community safety. We formulate the following research question: What are the possible combinations of structural conditions leading to low loneliness in Europe?

11.3.1 Digitalization

A recent scoping review showed that the use of Information and Communication Technologies (ICT) among older people is associated with lower loneliness through both the enhancement of existing social connections and the establishment of new relationships, while also facilitating intergenerational connections (Petersen et al., 2023). Internet use can enable access to resources like information, health and social services, social events, shopping, online support groups, thus providing improved opportunities for quality of life and well-being. The effects of ICT technologies on the well-being of older adults include better self-efficacy, self-esteem, autonomy, and independence (Petersen et al., 2023). Even though technology can also have negative consequences for loneliness, especially in the case of older people who might not have the skills to use it effectively, or when exposing them to negative experiences (for a detailed discussion, see Seifert, 2025), it can be a positive factor to the extent that it does not replace face-to-face interactions. At the macro level, digitalization has the capacity to reshape public services and policy frameworks to better meet the needs of aging populations. Societies that prioritize digital infrastructure and accessibility not only empower older individuals but also create more inclusive environments that have the potential to foster social interactions and support overall well-being. Here, we argue that **digitalization**, as a process of adoption of digital technologies in everyday life, is associated with low loneliness in older people, either individually or in conjunction with other relevant macro conditions.

11.3.2 Poverty

Societal wealth and welfare can influence loneliness levels by providing better living conditions, social services, and opportunities for social engagement (Hansen & Slagsvold, 2016; De Jong Gierveld & Tesch-Römer, 2012; Tufă, 2025). The different levels of loneliness in European societies, especially those between Eastern and Western countries, can be explained, according to De Jong Gierveld and Tesch-Römer (2012), by the different levels in average incomes and wealth. In the case of Eastern European societies, there is a direct pathway between the socio-economic country level of inequalities and people's well-being (including loneliness) through the individual level of material resources, as well as an indirect pathway connecting the macro context in terms of poverty and social exclusion, which diminishes trust and increases negative outcomes. Based on the model proposed by De Jong Gierveld and Tesch-Römer (2012) we include **low poverty** as a key condition for low levels of loneliness in European countries.

11.3.3 Trust

A key feature of social capital, namely trust, was found to be linked to loneliness at individual level (Nyqvist et al., 2016; van Tilburg et al., 2020; Luhmann & Hawkley, 2016). At country level, in Eastern European countries, a low level of trust in other people and in the system was linked to individuals' loneliness through social disengagement (Rapolienė & Aartsen, 2021). The study, which was based on data from the European Social Survey, illuminates that loneliness is partly constructed by the social–cultural and historical–political characteristics of the countries in which people live. Living under totalitarian regimes has undermined the trust people have in other people and the government, a feeling that remained even after the fall of the communist regime. This lower trust leads to social disengagement, which in turn creates feelings of loneliness. In fact, trust illustrates a reciprocal relationship between society and individuals, as societal systems can contribute to loneliness by affecting trust and social engagement, while individuals, through their participation and engagement, actively shape society in return (Suanet & Pavlidis, 2025). Institutional trust, capturing the relation between individual and the macro level of society through political institutions, plays a crucial role in influencing civic engagement, social cohesion, and the stability of social interactions (Justino & Samarin, 2025). Aggregate levels of institutional trust were shown to be generally higher in Nordic and Western countries and lower in Eastern and Southern countries (Boda et al., 2018). High institutional trust fosters the development of the networks and frameworks that facilitate collaboration and collective action within communities, enabling thus cooperation and strengthening societal bonds. We use **trust in parliament** as a condition for low loneliness.

11.3.4 Individualism

A comprehensive explanation of how individualism as a societal value can influence loneliness is provided in Chap. 3 (van Tilburg, 2025). In short, individualism refers to a value system where autonomy and self-reliance are higher valued than being member of a group, and expectations from others with respect to personal contact or support are generally low. In countries where individualism is the norm, ties between individuals are rather loose and people are focused on themselves and their immediate family (Hofstede et al., 2010). People in individualistic countries who also have individualistic values are less likely to become lonely if they have little social contact. However, since people develop their own values in their formative years and remain the same throughout their life (Inglehart, 2009) they may also develop loneliness in later life if they live in individualistic countries. Nevertheless, we see that individualistic countries have lower levels of loneliness in general (Swader, 2019). We include **individualism** in our analysis as a key condition for low loneliness.

11.3.5 Community Safety

Opportunities for social interaction and low loneliness arise in the communities where people live. Community integration is a significant predictor of social loneliness (Dahlberg & McKee, 2013), while urbanization and socio-economic circumstances at neighborhood level were found to be associated with loneliness (Scharf & De Jong Gierveld, 2008). According to Scharf and De Jong Gierveld (2008), objective characteristics of neighborhoods as well as perceived characteristics (e.g., satisfaction, feelings of safety during the daytime and at night) are key to investigating loneliness. Although community safety is usually considered a meso-level factor, here we examine the role of community characteristics in terms of their broader societal role. We are interested in the implications that a certain type of social structure has in shaping individual outcomes like loneliness. In fact, community characteristics are the result of policies at national level (e.g. housing, urban planning) focused or not on minimizing social and area-based inequalities, thereby mirroring macro level efforts. Based on these arguments, we include **community safety** in our analysis as a condition of low loneliness.

11.4 Methods

11.4.1 QCA and fsQCA

QCA can analyze complex causal situations with the following three features: *equifinality*, signifying that different pathways can lead to the same outcome; *asymmetry*, meaning that the explanation for the presence of loneliness does not also account for the absence of the phenomenon; and *conjunctural causation*, denoting that outcomes are often the result of combinations of conditions, not isolated factors (Ragin, 2008). QCA relies on set-theoretic relationships and Boolean logic and operations (AND, OR, NOT) to analyze causal relationships and configurations in qualitative data. The outcome of a QCA is a list of necessary (that is that the condition is always present when the outcome occurs) and sufficient (that is if the condition occurs, the outcome occurs) conditions that are logically conducive to a given outcome (Schneider & Wagemann, 2012).

As a set-theoretic analysis, QCA begins by defining cases as members in sets. A set is a group of elements that share certain characteristics (Mello, 2021), such as countries with high economic affluence or high individualism. The degree of membership in sets of each case (country) is determined either in so-called *crisp sets* by assigning a value 1 to indicate presence or 0 to indicate absence of each condition, or in *fuzzy sets* that reflect varying degrees of membership in a set, with numerical values ranging between 0 and 1. The process of assigning values to the fuzzy sets is called calibration. If fuzzy sets are used, the method is called fuzzy-set QCA or fsQCA. Cases can concomitantly belong to different sets in various degrees such as high economic affluence AND high individualism, creating configurations of conditions that are causally linked to the outcome of low loneliness. Schneider and Wagemann (2012) argue that fsQCA should be used whenever possible.

All possible core configurations of causal conditions linked to the outcome are included in the "truth table," enabling the logical analysis of the various combinations of conditions contributing to low loneliness. Configurations describe the shared attributes of a group of cases/countries resulting in a process of classification (Yang, 2018). As an approach and as a set of techniques, QCA is case-oriented to the extent that it is based on case knowledge and allows for the identification of cross-case patterns (Ragin, 2000; Rihoux & Lobe, 2015). QCA is the appropriate method for macro level analysis when dealing with a small or medium N (usually 20 to 50 cases) where traditional statistical methods might not be appropriate due to limited sample size (Ragin, 2008; Mello, 2021).

However, fsQCA has not been without critiques, mainly related to its capability to capture complex causality, and to analytical robustness of QCA results, especially regarding its sensitivity to changes in the number of cases, the arbitrary calibration of conditions, and the potential measurement errors (Lucas & Szatrowski, 2014; Arel-Bundock, 2019). Several authors have addressed these highlighted issues and proposed various ways to overcome them (Gerrits & Pagliarin, 2020; Thiem, 2019; Mello, 2021), and currently the method is growing in relevance, changing from a niche to a mainstream method especially in sociology, political science, and business studies (Rihoux et al., 2013). Usually analyses employ thorough robustness checks (e.g., Swader & Moraru, 2023; Paykani et al., 2018), the recommendation being that all types of robustness tests should be applied (test-sets) (Oana & Schneider, 2024). Most importantly, the transparency of the approach allowing replication of results, including calibration thresholds and analytical procedure, is key to all QCA (Mello, 2021). In our analysis, we use fsQCA version 4.1 software.[1]

[1] https://sites.socsci.uci.edu/~cragin/fsQCA/software.shtml

11.4.2 Data

Our analysis includes 27 cases, covering all European countries for which data were available for all selected indicators. We use statistical data, mainly derived from Eurostat 2020–2023 (see Annex for the list of indicators and raw data), as well as survey data. Survey data come from the European Quality of Life Survey (EQLS) (2016). The EQLS is a repeated cross-sectional survey carried out in European countries every years among people aged 18 or older who reside in private households in the country at the time of data collection. As a highly reliable set of data extensively used in research, EQLS 2016 was the best choice of available data for our study as the dataset is the most recent one to use a stratified sampling design by geo-administrative region (NUTS) and level of urbanization (Eurostat's DEGURBA to select respondents), giving all members of the survey population a chance of being included in the sample (Eurofound, 2018).

11.4.3 Outcomes

Our outcome is *low loneliness,* which was derived from the direct measure of loneliness as the percentage of 50+ people who indicated that they have been feeling lonely over the last two weeks. Answer categories range from (1) All of the time to (6) At no time. Loneliness was assumed to be present if people said they were at least more than half of the time lonely. A country-level aggregate based on weighted data is calculated. Our data show that the lowest prevalence of loneliness among people aged 50 and over is in Denmark (3.6%), Sweden (5.3%) and the Netherlands (5.6%). The highest levels are in Romania (22.4%) and Greece (25.2%), where almost a quarter of the older population feel lonely. In general, Eastern European countries tend to have the highest prevalence of loneliness except for Slovenia (8.8%) and Slovakia (9.6%). Among Western countries, Ireland (7.7%), UK (8.3%) and Germany (9.9%) register lower degrees of loneliness (Fig. 11.1).

11.4.4 Conditions

Our conditions capture unique societal features that are linked to our outcome, loneliness. We expect meaningful configurations of our five conditions to be associated with low loneliness in European countries. For **digitalization,** we use the Eurostat indicator *Individuals with basic or above basic overall digital skills.* The indicator is based on data from the EU survey on the use of ICT in households and by individuals (Eurostat, 2023a; all EU countries). This indicator measures the share of people aged 16 to 74 who have at least basic digital skills. It is a composite indicator based on selected activities performed by individuals on the internet in specific

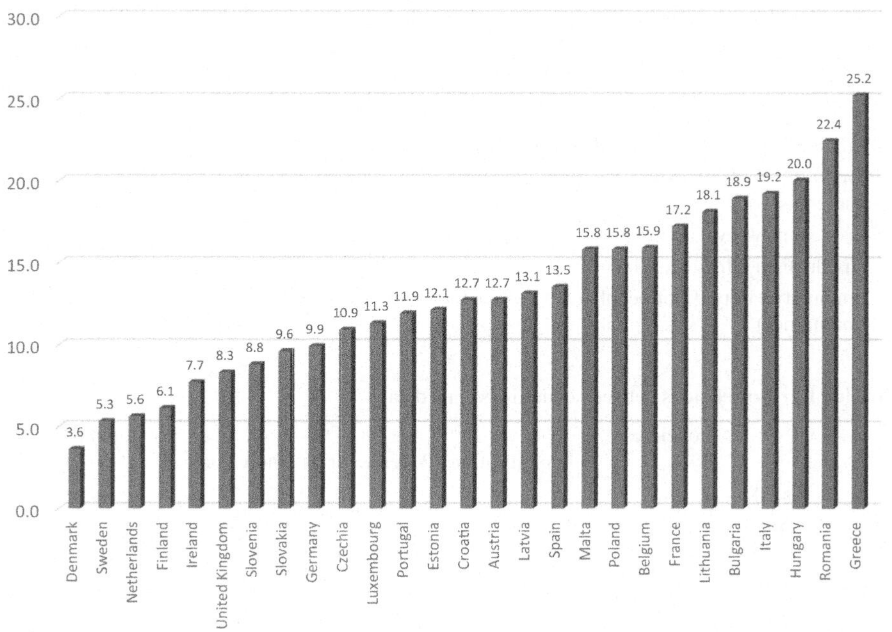

Fig. 11.1 Loneliness in 50+ older adults (2016) (%). Source: EQLS 2016. Note: Share of 50+ people who answered they felt lonely all of the time, most of the time or more than half of the time. Weighted data

areas. For the UK, we use Essential Digital Skills Report 2021.[2] Hence, we define the set **High digitalization**. For **Poverty** we use the *At risk of poverty rate* with the cut-off point of 60% of median equivalised income after social transfers. The indicator is based on the European Union Statistics on Income and Living Conditions (EU-SILC). The values for this indicator are from 2022 for all European Union countries and from 2018 for the UK (Eurostat, 2023b). The set **Low poverty** is defined. For **Trust,** we use the indicator *trust in the parliament* from EQLS 2016 measured on a scale from 1 to 10. A country-level average based on weighted data is calculated, we define the set **High trust**. For **Individualism,** we use Hofstede's Individualism index[3] 2015 measuring the integration of individuals into groups and ranging from 0 to 100. We define the set **High individualism**. Community safety is measured with an item from EQLS survey data showing the share of people who declared they feel safe in their communities (strongly agree+agree). We define the set **High community safety**. Table 11.1 provides descriptives for the outcome and all conditions, and Table 11.2 shows correlations between conditions.

[2] Essential Digital Skills Report 2021 Third Edition – Benchmarking the Essential Digital Skills of the UK https://www.lloydsbank.com/consumer-digital-index.html

[3] https://geerthofstede.com/research-and-vsm/dimension-data-matrixIndividualism

Table 11.1 Descriptives for the outcome and conditions

	Max	Median	Min
Loneliness (% of 50+ year old people feeling lonely more than half of the time)	25.2	12.7	3.6
Digitalization (% of people with at least basic digital skills)	81.0	56.4	27.8
Poverty (% of people below the 60% of median equivalized income after social transfers)	22.9	16.0	10.1
Trust (country-level average)	6.5	4.4	2.8
Individualism (Hofstede's index)	89.0	60.0	27.0
Community safety (% of people who declare they feel safe in their communities)	89.9	74.3	53.7

Table 11.2 Correlations between conditions (raw data)

	Loneliness 50+	Digitalisation	Poverty	Trust	Individualism	Community safety
Loneliness 50+	1					
Digitalization	−.71[a]	1				
Poverty	.45[b]	−.37	1			
Trust	−.63[a]	.60[a]	−.41[b]	1		
Individualism	−.32	.50[a]	−.23	.60[a]	1	
Community safety	−.54[a]	.50[a]	−.30	.48[b]	.08	1

Note: own calculations based on EQLS survey and Eurostat data

[a] Correlation is significant at the 0.01 level (2-tailed)

[b] Correlation is significant at the 0.05 level (2-tailed)

11.4.5 Calibration

Calibration is a purposeful and thoughtful tool, involving both quantitative and qualitative assessments in the attempt to transform interval-scale measures into fuzzy sets (Ragin, 2008). Both case knowledge and the empirical distribution of data are used to achieve meaningful calibration (Schneider & Wagemann, 2012). We use the direct method of calibration (Ragin, 2008) by first setting three anchors at 1 (full membership in the set), 0.5 (cross-over point; maximum ambiguity) and 0 (full non-membership). A logistic function is used in fsQCA4.1 software to fit the raw data in-between the three qualitative anchors so that the corresponding fuzzy scores are 0.95, 0.5, and 0.05. First, we employ a calibration based on theoretical knowledge of cases and the distribution of data (the threshold values for calibration are included in Table 11.3). Second, as a robustness test for our analysis, we employ an alternative theoretical calibration and vary calibration anchors for our conditions and outcome. Raw values of all indicators, together with calibration anchors are provided in the Annex.

Table 11.3 Thresholds values for calibration

Set conditions	1 - Fully in	0.5 - Cross-over point	0 - Fully out
Low levels of loneliness 50+	6.1	12.5	18.1
High digitalization	78.9	61.5	31.2
Low poverty	13.4	18.9	22.5
High trust	6.0	4.3	3.2
High individualism	74.0	59.5	35.0
High community safety	84.7	74.4	60.7

Table 11.4 Analysis of necessary conditions

	Consistency	Coverage
High digitalization	0.732	0.843
Low poverty	0.896	0.657
High trust	0.612	0.757
High individualism	0.720	0.654
High community safety	0.742	0.750

11.5 Results

11.5.1 Necessary Conditions for Low Loneliness

QCA's analytical protocol requires starting the analysis with the identification of necessary conditions tested individually. A condition is necessary if the outcome (for example, low loneliness) can only be present if the condition is also present (e.g., high digitalization); in other words, the outcome cannot occur without the condition being present. Necessity is determined by the consistency statistic and the coverage of a condition. Consistency refers to the degree to which the presence of the condition is associated with the outcome. The coverage of a condition measures how many instances of the outcome are accounted for by the condition. Necessity is proven when the fuzzy-set scores of a condition are consistently equal to or higher than the fuzzy-set scores of the outcome (Ragin, 2017).

The analysis of necessary conditions (Table 11.4) reveals that low poverty has the highest consistency (0.896) and substantial coverage (0.657), indicating that, despite being at the limit of the accepted consistency threshold (0.9 according to Ragin, 2006; Paykani et al., 2018), it is a necessary condition for low loneliness. High digitalization has high coverage (0.843), suggesting that a significant number of cases of low loneliness can be attributed to this condition. High community safety is associated with the outcome (consistency 0.742) and is relevant to the outcome across a sufficient number of cases (coverage 0.750). High trust and high individualism show moderate associations with the outcome (0.612 and 0.720 respectively), while high trust covers a significant portion of the cases (coverage 0.757) indicating that their role is significant in low loneliness. However, none of the conditions, except low poverty, can be considered, on their own, necessary conditions for low loneliness.

11.5.2 The Truth Table and the Sufficient Conditions for Low Loneliness

Sufficiency tests aim to assess whether, if the causal condition occurs, the outcome also occurs. When the fuzzy-set scores of a condition or configuration (a combination of conditions) are consistently less than or equal to their fuzzy-set membership scores on the outcome, it can be assessed that we have a sufficient condition (Ragin, 2017). All possible conditions and configurations of conditions linked to the outcome are included in the truth table. Each row in the truth table displays the logically possible combinations of conditions and the distribution of the empirical cases across the rows. A number of 2^k combinations, where k is the number of conditions included in the study, are possible. In our case, there are 5 conditions and hence 32 possible rows in the truth table.

The truth table tool in the fsQCA software that we used produces three solutions: complex, parsimonious, and intermediate (the first two are included in the Annex). The software allows for a minimization procedure that simplifies the number of configurations. We describe the intermediate solution (Table 11.5), which is easily interpretable, in line with recommendations by Dușa (2022). The intermediate solution identifies only the configurations of those conditions that are deemed relevant based on theoretical or empirical considerations (Ragin, 2008).

The solution has good overall consistency (0.838) and explains 74.2% of the cases of low loneliness across all countries. The analysis of sufficient conditions shows three possible pathways to low loneliness (Table 11.6). Low poverty is present in all solutions, reinforcing that it constitutes a necessary condition for low loneliness. For Nordic countries and Luxembourg, the pathways to a low degree of loneliness are alternative: either through the configuration of low poverty AND high digitalization AND high trust, or through the pathway of low poverty AND high digitalization AND high individualism. A third pathway, including low poverty AND no high individualism AND high community safety explains low loneliness in countries like Slovenia, Portugal, Croatia, and Malta. All countries with low loneliness have low poverty, except for Spain, which emerges as a contradictory case in this type of calibration.[4]

[4]Spain does not align with the three identified pathways, suggesting it can be explained by an alternative combination of factors. While community safety and digitalization are present and might be key to low loneliness, it is probably its unique context that explains why the country appears as an outlier. For example, the strong familial structures and values, the informal community networks and cultural emphasis on social interaction can justify better this particular case. The country is also classfied in the negated solution, suggesting that, while it meets criteria for the main solution it simultaneously exhibits characteristics that align with the conditions leading to the negated outcome, pointing thus to the complex nature of causality.

Table 11.5 Truth table for low loneliness. Distribution of cases across configurations of conditions

P	D	T	I	C	N	Out	Cases	Raw consist.	PRI consist.
1	1	1	0	0	1	1	AT	0.975	0.851
1	1	0	0	1	1	1	HR	0.975	0.849
0	1	0	0	1	1	1	ES	0.904	0.111
1	0	0	0	1	2	1	PT, SI	0.895	0.725
1	1	1	1	1	5	1	DK, ND, FI, SE, LU	0.874	0.807
1	0	1	0	1	1	1	MT	0.867	0.455
1	1	0	1	1	2	1	IE, FR	0.813	0.607
1	1	0	1	0	1	1	UK	0.803	0.611
1	0	0	0	0	3	0	CZ, GR, SK	0.762	0.463
1	0	1	1	0	3	0	BE, DE, HU	0.706	0.423
1	0	0	1	1	1	0	PL	0.700	0.235
0	0	0	1	0	4	0	EE, IT, LT, LV	0.550	0.007
0	0	0	0	0	2	0	BG, RO	0.454	0.024

Note: Raw consistency is a measure used to evaluate how consistently a specific condition or combination of conditions is associated with the outcome. PRI consistency is an alternative measure of consistency for fuzzy sets based on a quasi-proportional reduction in error calculation. The raw with low PRI consistency (0.111) was eliminated from the truth table and not included in the standard analysis

Conditions: P – Low poverty, D – High digitalization, T – High trust, I – High individualism, C – Community safety

Cases: AT – Austria, BE – Belgium, BG – Bulgaria, HR – Croatia, CZ – Czech Republic, DK – Denmark, EE – Estonia, FI – Finland, FR – France, DE – Germany, EL – Greece, HU – Hungary, IE – Ireland, IT – Italy, LV – Latvia, LT – Lithuania, LU – Luxembourg, MT – Malta, NL – Netherlands, PL – Poland, PT – Portugal, RO – Romania, SK – Slovakia, SI – Slovenia, ES – Spain, SE – Sweden, UK – United Kingdom

Table 11.6 Intermediate solution for low loneliness

Pathways/causal mechanisms	Countries	Consistency	Coverage	Unique coverage
Pathway 1 P*D*T	FI, NL, DK, SE, LU, AT	0.892	0.506	0.029
Pathway 2 P*D* I	NL, IE, DK, SE, FI, UK, LU, FR	0.846	0.549	0.082
Pathway 3 P* ~ I*C	SI, PT, HR, MT	0.848	0.373	0.134
Solution consistency	0.838			
Solution coverage	0.742			

Note: ~the lack of a condition, * AND

Conditions: P – Low poverty, D – High digitalization, T – High trust, I – High individualism, C – Community safety

Cases: AT – Austria, HR – Croatia, DK – Denmark, FI – Finland, FR – France, IE – Ireland, LU – Luxembourg, MT – Malta, NL – Netherlands, PT – Portugal, SI – Slovenia, SE – Sweden, UK – United Kingdom

The first pathway we label "Trusting societies" represents socially connected countries where economic security combines with digital inclusion and high institutional trust. The second is the pathway of "Individualistic societies" where individual autonomy is supported by economic wellbeing and digital connectivity, enabling various forms of social connection and ultimately low loneliness. These two configurations of conditions share the infrastructure of economic affluence and high digitalization as hard components but differ in the soft social constituents of trust and individualism. The third pathway labeled "Communal ties societies" represents countries where economic security combines with safe communities, creating protective social environments against loneliness. Pathway 3 stands out as the most distinct configuration, emphasizing community cohesion as a key driver in less individualistic societies.

11.5.3 Negated Outcome Analysis

The intermediate solution for negated low loneliness shows that poverty AND low trust AND low community safety explain higher levels of loneliness in Bulgaria, Romania, Latvia, Italy, Lithuania, and Estonia. The negated outcome analysis highlights the lack of both hard and soft components of low loneliness and the need for identifying the specific configurations for high loneliness in the case of these countries (Table 11.7).

Table 11.7 Intermediate solution for negated low loneliness

Pathways/causal mechanisms	Countries	Consistency	Coverage	Unique coverage
Pathway 1 ~P* ~ T* ~ C	BG, RO, LV, IT, LT, EE	0.893	0.444	0.236
Pathway 2 ~P * ~ D * ~ T* ~ I	ES	0.976	0.217	0.023
Pathway 3 P* ~ D* ~ T*I	PL	0.865	0.297	0.151
Solution consistency	0.866			
Solution coverage	0.638			

Note: ~the lack of a condition, * AND

Conditions: P – Low poverty, D – High digitalization, T – High trust, I – High individualism, C – Community safety

Cases: BG, RO, LV, IT, LT, EE, ES, PL

11.5.4 Robustness

Robustness checks include several types of possible tests: changes to calibration, to frequency cutoff for the truth table raws, to raw consistency, and changes to the set of cases or conditions under analysis (Oana & Schneider, 2024). We conducted a first robustness test by applying an alternative calibration to adjust the thresholds for fuzzy set membership (Ragin, 2008). We established alternative theoretical anchors where possible for the outcome and conditions (thresholds used and results are included in the Annex). Analysis of necessary conditions shows, similarly to the analysis based on the first version of theoretical calibration, good consistency and coverage. None of the conditions emerge as necessary on their own for the outcome of low loneliness. The intermediate solution, although slightly different from the one based on theoretical calibration, shows the importance of digitalization for low loneliness and classifies in the same configuration Denmark, Sweden, the Netherlands, Finland, and Luxembourg, while creating unique paths towards low loneliness.

The second robustness test changed the cutoff for raw consistency within the truth table from 0.803 to 0.867 (Annex). The intermediate solution created unique pathways and reinforced the robust core of our analysis of low loneliness, which is the configuration low poverty AND digitalization AND high trust present in Finland, the Netherlands, Denmark, Sweden, Luxembourg, and Austria. The pathway we named "Trusting societies" consistently achieves a low degree of loneliness in the respective countries.

11.6 Discussion

Wealth acts as a foundational macro-level condition for low levels of loneliness. Affluent countries in Europe provide better living conditions and welfare provisions that allow individuals to thrive while shielding them from negative circumstances and life events. Whereas this condition is valid for many social outcomes (e.g. life satisfaction, mental health) it is not trivial to regard it as the basic ground for low levels of loneliness, given the key role of wealth in creating the infrastructure needed for social engagement at both community and macro level. The different levels of loneliness in European countries can be explained by the different levels of economic resources. As described by de Jong Gierveld and Tesch-Römer (2012), wealthier nations tend to have structures in place that promote social integration of older people, thereby decreasing the likelihood of loneliness. Economic circumstances are connected to loneliness both directly and by influencing other conditions, such as trust, either encouraging social interaction or impeding relations. Societal contexts characterized by economic stability usually foster supportive environments, eventually encouraging social interactions.

Digitalization emerges as a key factor in low loneliness, pointing in line with other studies (Swader & Moraru, 2023), to the role of technological underpinnings in explaining low levels of loneliness in Nordic and Western European countries. Highly digitized societies provide the proper infrastructure in terms of various tools and platforms that enhance social interactions, access to services, and support systems. Digital tools have the potential to cultivate positive relationships among older adults (Chopik, 2016), allowing them to stay in touch with family and friends, helping them maintain and strengthen social connections that could otherwise weaken due to physical distance. Access to online communities that share experiences and interests as well as engagement in various activities (e.g., online classes) can also promote social interaction. Most importantly for older people, digitalization has made access to various support services easier, including health services (Zubatsky et al., 2020), mental health resources, community programs, and assistance for daily living.

Political trust is part of a main pathway to low loneliness, along with economic affluence and digitalization. Trust captures here a structural feature representing a key societal resource for solidarity, participation in society, and well-functioning democracies. While a previous study (Yang, 2018) found that the association between individual level political trust and loneliness is significant in societies like the Nordic countries, the United Kingdom, Germany, Austria and insignificant in Eastern European countries, we discovered that trust as macro-condition is an integral part of the different pathways leading to loneliness in all these countries.[5] While high trust is linked to low loneliness in Finland, Netherlands, Denmark, Sweden, Luxembourg, and Austria, low trust is related, in a different pathway, to loneliness in Bulgaria, Romania, Latvia, Italy, Lithuania, and Estonia. In line with what was suggested before (Langenkamp, 2022), political trust can significantly influence people's sense of belonging and social integration. When individuals feel disconnected from political institutions or perceive a lack of trust in their leaders, feelings of loneliness can intensify. Conversely, high levels of political trust might foster community engagement and social cohesion, potentially reducing loneliness.

High individualism, together with low poverty and high digitalization, renders a pathway towards reduced loneliness in the Netherlands, Ireland, Denmark, Sweden, Finland, the United Kingdom, Luxembourg, and France. Countries where individualist values like autonomy, self-orientation and achievement prevail were shown to have lower prevalence of loneliness (Stegen et al., 2024). Our results point to the role of social ties in loneliness. Social relations in individualist countries based on personal choice with a focus on family and other bonds that are rather diffuse coupled with low expectations towards those relations contribute to lower loneliness.

Low individualism is an integral part of another pathway towards reduced loneliness, together with low poverty and high community safety in case of Slovenia, Portugal, Croatia, and Malta. Positive community circumstances can foster more engagement in social activities, provide the arenas for building social connections and social support, offer access to resources such as community centers, parks, and social services, facilitate mobility, allowing older adults to access social opportunities and maintain relationships.

[5] Except for Germany

The three pathways we identified highlight various mechanisms towards low loneliness that are currently present in European countries. The "Trusting societies" path, based on the configuration of wealth, digital inclusion, and high trust in institutions, captures the role of the hard infrastructure of loneliness in combination with trust in political institutions, creating environments where individuals can easily connect and engage with others, thereby mitigating feelings of loneliness. This suggests that promoting digital literacy and trust in governance (through the proper functioning of these institutions) could be effective strategies for addressing loneliness. The alternative pathway, "Individualistic societies," based on the same infrastructure of the first path but including a soft cultural factor, emphasises a configuration where individualism is, in the right combination of factors that promote personal connections and communication, conducive to low loneliness. Finally, the third and unique pathway, "Communal ties societies," points to the importance of cohesive and safe community structures that foster social bonds and a sense of belonging in reducing loneliness. This underscores the need for policies that enhance community safety and encourage collective participation.

Our analysis has some limitations. Due to its focus on complex causal structures, fsQCA offers precise insights about which further steps could be undertaken in subsequent (comparative) case studies (Schneider & Wagemann, 2010, p. 17). Hence, the explorative character of QCA results requires they should be followed by additional analyses. The analysis was designed to explain low loneliness, while for countries with high loneliness, it is possible that factors other than those included here to be crucial. For example, the nature of analysis (negated outcome and conditions) does not allow us to take account of collectivism, which might rather be key in high loneliness in (some) Southern and Eastern European countries. Individualism and collectivism are not placed on the same continuum but stem from different societal circumstances, having distinct effects on loneliness (as also noted by van Tilburg, 2025). A future analysis that includes collectivism might shed better light on the conditions of loneliness in these countries.

The QCA-methodology applied in this chapter offers a unique understanding of macro-level influences on loneliness, and that some factors associated with low loneliness are country specific. To conclude, while there is no clear and unique recipe for low loneliness in European countries, possible pathways point to combinations of conditions that have proven successful in the countries with reduced loneliness among the older people. Economic, cultural and social factors at the macro level are closely linked together in influencing loneliness in later life in European countries.

Acknowledgements The authors would like to thank Adrian Dușa and the reviewers for their helpful and constructive comments and suggestions.

Competing Interests The authors have no conflicts of interest to declare that are relevant to the content of this chapter.

11.7 Annex

11.7.1 Raw Data and Calibration

Outcome Variable: Low Loneliness

Table 11.8 Loneliness for people 50+ years old (%) and two versions of calibrations

Country	Loneliness (%)	V1 theoretical	V2 alternative theoretical
DK	3.6		
SE	5.3		
NL	5.6		
FI	6.1	*Fully in*	
IE	7.7		
UK	8.3		*Fully in*
SI	8.8		
SK	9.6		
DE	9.9		
CZ	10.9		
LU	11.3		
PT	11.9		
EE	12.1		
		Cross over point 12.5	*Cross over point 12.5*
HR	12.7		
AT	12.7		
LV	13.1		
ES	13.5		
MT	15.8		
PL	15.8		
BE	15.9		
FR	17.2		*Fully out*
LT	18.1	*Fully out*	
BG	18.9		
IT	19.2		
HU	20.0		
RO	22.4		
GR	25.2		

Source: EQLS (2016)

Countries: AT—Austria, BE—Belgium, BG—Bulgaria, CZ—Czechia, DE—Germany, EE—Estonia, ES—Spain, FI—Finland, FR—France, GR—Greece, HR—Croatia, HU—Hungary, IE—Ireland, IT—Italy, LT—Lithuania, LU—Luxembourg, MT—Malta, NL—Netherlands, PL—Poland, PT—Portugal, RO—Romania, SE—Sweden, SI—Slovenia, SK—Slovakia, UK—United Kingdom

Digitalization

Table 11.9 Individuals with basic or above basic overall digital skills in 2021 (%) and two versions of calibration

Country	Individuals with basic or above basic overall digital skills (%)	V1 theoretical	V2 alternative theoretical
UK	81.0		
FI	79.2		
NL	78.9	*Fully in*	
IE	70.5		
DK	68.7		
SE	66.6		
ES	64.2		*Fully in*
LU	63.8		
HR	63.4		
AT	63.3		
FR	62.0		
		Cross over point 61.5	
MT	61.2		
CZ	59.7		
			Cross over point 56.5
EE	56.4		
PT	55.3		
SK	55.2		
BE	54.2		
GR	52.5		
LV	50.8		
SI	49.7		
HU	49.1		
DE	48.9		
LT	48.8		*Fully out*
IT	45.6		
PL	42.9		
BG	31.2	*Fully out*	
RO	27.8		

Source: Eurostat (2023a), Essential Digital Skills Report (2021) (UK)
Countries: AT—Austria, BE—Belgium, BG—Bulgaria, CZ—Czechia, DE—Germany, EE—Estonia, ES—Spain, FI—Finland, FR—France, GR—Greece, HR—Croatia, HU—Hungary, IE—Ireland, IT—Italy, LT—Lithuania, LU—Luxembourg, MT—Malta, NL—Netherlands, PL—Poland, PT—Portugal, RO—Romania, SE—Sweden, SI—Slovenia, SK—Slovakia, UK—United Kingdom

Poverty

Table 11.10 At risk of poverty rate in 2022 (cut-off point: 60% of median equivalised income after social transfers) (%) and two versions of calibration

Country	At risk of poverty rate	V1 theoretical	V2 alternative theoretical
CZ	10.2		
HU	12.1		
SI	12.1		
DK	12.4		
FI	12.7		
BE	13.2		
IE	13.4	*Fully in*	*Fully in*
PL	13.7		
SK	13.7		
NL	14.5		
DE	14.8		
AT	14.8		
FR	15.6		
SE	16		
			Cross over point 16.2
PT	16.4		
MT	16.7		
LU	17.3		
HR	18		
UK	18.6		
GR	18.8		
		Cross over point 18.9	
IT	20.1		*Fully out*
ES	20.4		
LT	20.9		
RO	21.2		
LV	22.5	*Fully out*	
EE	22.8		
BG	22.9		

Source: Eurostat (2023b)

Countries: AT—Austria, BE—Belgium, BG—Bulgaria, CZ—Czechia, DE—Germany, EE—Estonia, ES—Spain, FI—Finland, FR—France, GR—Greece, HR—Croatia, HU—Hungary, IE—Ireland, IT—Italy, LT—Lithuania, LU—Luxembourg, MT—Malta, NL—Netherlands, PL—Poland, PT—Portugal, RO—Romania, SE—Sweden, SI—Slovenia, SK—Slovakia, UK—United Kingdom

Trust in Parliament

Table 11.11 Trust in Parliament (mean) and two version of calibrations

Country	Trust in Parliament (mean)	V1 theoretical	V2 alternative theoretical
FI	6.5		
SE	6.4		
DK	6.2		
LU	6.0	*Fully in*	
NL	5.7		
AT	5.6		
DE	5.5		*Fully in*
MT	5.1		
HU	5.0		
BE	5.0		
EE	4.9		
UK	4.9		
IE	4.7		
FR	4.4		
		Cross over point 4.3	*Cross over point 4.3*
PT	4.2		
CZ	4.2		
PL	4.1		
SK	4.1		
LT	3.9		
ES	3.8		*Fully out*
LV	3.8		
RO	3.7		
IT	3.7		
SI	3.2	*Fully out*	
HR	3.2		
BG	3.2		
GR	2.8		

Source: EQLS (2016)

Countries: AT—Austria, BE—Belgium, BG—Bulgaria, CZ—Czechia, DE—Germany, EE—Estonia, ES—Spain, FI—Finland, FR—France, GR—Greece, HR—Croatia, HU—Hungary, IE—Ireland, IT—Italy, LT—Lithuania, LU—Luxembourg, MT—Malta, NL—Netherlands, PL—Poland, PT—Portugal, RO—Romania, SE—Sweden, SI—Slovenia, SK—Slovakia, UK—United Kingdom

Individualism

Table 11.12 Individualism (2015) and two versions of calibration

Country	Individualism	V1 theoretical	V2 alternative theoretical
UK	89		
HU	80		
NL	80		
IT	76		
BE	75		
DK	74	*Fully in*	
FR	71		*Fully in*
SE	71		
IE	70		
LV	70		
DE	67		
FI	63		
EE	60		
LT	60		
LU	60		
PL	60		
		Cross over point 59.5	*Cross over point 59.5*
MT	59		
CZ	58		
AT	55		
SK	52		
ES	51		*Fully out*
GR	35	*Fully out*	
HR	33		
BG	30		
RO	30		
PT	27		
SI	27		

Source: Hofstede (2015) https://osf.io/4gb8e

Countries: AT—Austria, BE—Belgium, BG—Bulgaria, CZ—Czechia, DE—Germany, EE—Estonia, ES—Spain, FI—Finland, FR—France, GR—Greece, HR—Croatia, HU—Hungary, IE—Ireland, IT—Italy, LT—Lithuania, LU—Luxembourg, MT—Malta, NL—Netherlands, PL—Poland, PT—Portugal, RO—Romania, SE—Sweden, SI—Slovenia, SK—Slovakia, UK—United Kingdom

Community Safety

Table 11.13 Perceptions of safety in the neighborhood (%) and two versions of calibratation

Country	Community safety (%)	V1 theoretical	V2 alternative theoretical
ES	89.9		
FI	87.6		
DK	85.2		
SE	84.7	*Fully in*	
SI	82.8		
PL	81.9		
NL	80.8		*Fully in*
PT	79.3		
MT	78.7		
LU	78.2		
FR	77.7		
IE	77.4		
HR	76.2		
		Cross over point 74.4	*Cross over point 74.4*
EE	74.3		
AT	74		
BE	72.4		
HU	71.5		
SK	70.8		
RO	70.4		
UK	70.3		
LV	66.5		*Fully out*
DE	66.2		
IT	60.7	*Fully out*	
GR	60		
LT	59.6		
BG	56.2		
CZ	53.7		

Source: EQLS (2016)

Countries: AT—Austria, BE—Belgium, BG—Bulgaria, CZ—Czechia, DE—Germany, EE—Estonia, ES—Spain, FI—Finland, FR—France, GR—Greece, HR—Croatia, HU—Hungary, IE—Ireland, IT—Italy, LT—Lithuania, LU—Luxembourg, MT—Malta, NL—Netherlands, PL—Poland, PT—Portugal, RO—Romania, SE—Sweden, SI—Slovenia, SK—Slovakia, UK—United Kingdom

11.7.2 Complex and Parsimonious Solutions (V1 Theoretical Calibration)

Table 11.14 Complex solution

Frequency cutoff: 1 Consistency cutoff: 0.803				
	Cases	Consistency	Coverage	Raw unique coverage
P* ~ D* ~ I*C	SI, PT, MT	0.860	0.330	0.069
P*D* ~ T*I	IE, UK, FR	0.800	0.301	0.039
P*D*I*C	NL, DK, IE, SE, FI, LU, FR	0.855	0.468	0.190
P*D*T* ~ I* ~ C	AT	0.975	0.199	0.007
P*D* ~ T*C	IE, HR, FR	0.852	0.314	0.008
Solution coverage: 0.692				
Solution consistency: 0.842				

Note: ~the lack of a condition, * AND
P—Low Poverty, D—High Digitalization, T– High Trust, I—High Individualism, C—High Community Safety
Cases: AT—Austria, HR—Croatia, CZ—Czechia, DK—Denmark, FI—Finland, FR—France, IE—Ireland, LU—Luxembourg, MT—Malta, NL—Netherlands, PL—Poland, PT—Portugal, SI—Slovenia, ES—Spain, SE—Sweden, UK—United Kingdom

Table 11.15 Parsimonious solution

Frequency cutoff: 1 Consistency cutoff: 0.803				
	Cases	Consistency	Coverage	Raw unique coverage
D	UK, NL, FI, IE, DK, SE, ES, HR, LU, AT, FR	0.842	0.732	0.403
~I*C	SI, PT, ES, HR, MT	0.806	0.414	0.085
Solution coverage: 0.817				
Solution consistency: 0.805				

Note: ~the lack of a condition, * AND
D—High Digitalization, I—High Individualism, C—High Community Safety
Cases: AT—Austria, DK—Denmark, ES—Spain, FI—Finland, FR—France, HR—Croatia, IE—Ireland, LU—Luxembourg, MT—Malta, NL—Netherlands, PT—Portugal, SE—Sweden, SI—Slovenia, UK—United Kingdom
D—High Digitalization, I—High Individualism, C—High Community Safety

11.7.3 Solution for Negated Outcome

Table 11.16 Intermediate solution

Frequency cutoff: 1 Consistency cutoff: 0.907				
	Countries	Consistency	Coverage	Raw unique coverage
~P* ~ T* ~ C	LV, RO, IT, LT, EE	0.893	0.444	0.236
~P*D* ~ T* ~ I	ES	0.976	0.217	0.023
P* ~ D* ~ T*I	PL	0.865	0.297	0.151
Solution coverage: 0.638				
Solution consistency: 0.866				

Note: ~the lack of a condition, * AND
P—Low Poverty, D—High Digitalization, T– High Trust, I—High Individualism, C—High Community Safety
Cases: E—Estonia, ES—Spain, IT—Italy, LV—Latvia, LT—Lithuania, PL—Poland, RO—Romania

11.7.4 Robustness Test 1: V2 Alternative Theoretical Calibration

Table 11.17 Analysis of Necessary Conditions for low loneliness

	Consistency	Coverage
High digitalization	0.749	0.766
Low poverty	0.743	0.702
High individualism	0.640	0.630
High trust	0.515	0.724
High community safety	0.698	0.734

Table 11.18 Intermediate solution for low loneliness

Frequency cutoff: 1 Consistency cutoff: 0.829				
	Countries	Consistency	Coverage	Raw unique coverage
P* ~ I	SI, SK, AT, CZ, PT, MT	0.815	0.367	0.247
D*I* ~ C	UK	0.898	0.203	0.080
D*I*	DK, SE, NL, FI, LU	0.910	0.367	0.226
Solution coverage: 0.713				
Solution consistency: 0.873				

Note: ~the lack of a condition, * AND
P—Low Poverty, D—High Digitalization, T– High Trust, I—High Individualism, C—High Community Safety
Cases: AT—Austria, CZ—Czechia, DK—Denmark, EE—Estonia, FI—Finland, LT—Lithuania LU—Luxembourg, MT—Malta, NL—Netherlands, PL—Poland, PT—Portugal, SI—Slovenia, SK—Slovakia, SE—Sweden, UK—United Kingdom

11.7.5 Robustness Test 2: Change in Consistency Threshold (V1 Theoretical Calibration)

Table 11.19 Intermediate solution. Chnage in consistency threshold from 0.803 to 0.867

Frequency cutoff: 1 Consistency cutoff: 0.867				
	Countries	Consistency	Raw coverage	Unique coverage
P *D*T	FI, Nl, DK, SE, LU, AT	0.892	0.505	0.287
P* ~ I*C	SI, PT, HR, MT	0.846	0.373	0.154
Solution coverage: 0.660				
Solution consistency: 0.860				

Note: ~the lack of a condition, * AND

P—Low Poverty, D—High Digitalization, T- High Trust, I—High Individualism, C—High Community Safety

Cases: AT—Austria, HR—Croatia, DK—Denmark, EE—Estonia, FI—Finland, LU—Luxembourg, MT—Malta, NL—Netherlands, PL—Poland, PT—Portugal, SI—Slovenia, SE—Sweden

References

Arel-Bundock, V. (2019). The double bind of qualitative comparative analysis. *Sociological Methods & Research, 51*(3), 963–982. https://doi.org/10.1177/0049124119882460

Barreto, M., Victor, C., Hammond, C., Eccles, A., Richins, M. T., & Qualter, P. (2021). Loneliness around the world: Age, gender, and cultural differences in loneliness. *Personality and Individual Differences, 169*, 110066. https://doi.org/10.1016/j.paid.2020.110066

Boda, Z., Medgyesi, M., Fondeville, N., & Özdemir, E. (2018). Societal change and trust in institutions. Publications Office of the European Union. Eurofound.

Chopik, W. J. (2016). The benefits of social technology use among older adults are mediated by reduced loneliness. *Cyberpsychology, Behavior and Social Network, 19*(9), 551–559. https://doi.org/10.1089/cyber.2016.0151

Dahlberg, L., & McKee, K. J. (2013). Correlates of social and emotional loneliness in older people: Evidence from an English community study. *Aging & Mental Health, 18*(4), 504–514. https://doi.org/10.1080/13607863.2013.856863

De Jong Gierveld, J., & Tesch-Römer, C. (2012). Loneliness in old age in eastern and Western European societies: Theoretical perspectives. *European Journal of Ageing, 9*(4), 285–295. https://doi.org/10.1007/s10433-012-0248-2

Dușa, A. (2022). Critical tension: Sufficiency and parsimony in QCA. Sociological Methods & Research, 51(2), 541–565. https://0511ixyoi-y-https-doi-org.z.e-nformation.ro/https://doi.org/10.1177/0049124119882456.

Dykstra, P. A. (2009). Older adult loneliness: Myths and realities.c), 91–100. https://doi.org/10.1007/s10433-009-0110-3

Essential Digital Skills Report. (2021). *Third Edition – Benchmarking the Essential Digital Skills of the UK*. https://www.lloydsbank.com/consumer-digital-index.html

Eurofound. (2018). *European quality of life survey 2016: Technical and field- work report*. https://www.eurofound.europa.eu/en/publications/eurofound-paper/2018/european-quality-life-survey-2016-technical-and-fieldwork-report

European Quality of Life Survey (EQLS) (2016) from/using European Quality of Life Survey Integrated Data File, 2003–2016. [Data set]. *3rd Edition*. UK Data Service. SN: 7348, https://doi.org/10.5255/UKDA-SN-7348-3

Eurostat. (2023a). *Individuals' level of digital skills by sex and age eq_dskl07* [Data set]. https://ec.europa.eu/eurostat/databrowser/product/page/EQ_DSKL07.

Eurostat. (2023b). *At-risk-of-poverty rate by poverty threshold, age and sex - EU-SILC and ECHP surveys Eurostat ilc_li02* [Data set]. https://ec.europa.eu/eurostat/databrowser/product/page/ILC_LI02.

Fokkema, T., De Jong Gierveld, J., & Dykstra, P. A. (2012). Cross-national differences in older adult loneliness. *The Journal of Psychology, 146*(1–2), 201–228. https://doi.org/10.1080/00223980.2011.631612

Gerrits, L., & Pagliarin, S. (2020). Social and causal complexity in qualitative comparative analysis (QCA): Strategies to account for emergence. *International Journal of Social Research Methodology, 24*(4), 501–514. https://doi.org/10.1080/13645579.2020.1799636

Hansen, T., & Slagsvold, B. (2016). Late-life loneliness in 11 European countries: Results from the generations and gender survey. *Social Indicators Research, 129*(1), 445–464. https://doi.org/10.1007/s11205-015-1111-6

Heu, L. C., van Zomeren, M., & Hansen, N. (2021). Does loneliness thrive in relational freedom or restriction? The culture-loneliness framework. *Review of General Psychology, 25*(1), 60–72. https://doi.org/10.1177/1089268020959033

Hofstede, G. (2015). *Dimension data matrix*. https://geerthofstede.com/research-and-vsm/dimension-data-matrix/

Hofstede, G., Hofstede, G. J., & Minkov, M. (2010). *Cultures and organizations: Software of the mind* (3rd ed.). McGraw Hill Professional.

Inglehart, R. (2009). Postmaterialist values and the shift from survival to self-expression values. In R. J. Dalton & H.-D. Klingemann (Eds.), *The Oxford handbook of political behavior*. Oxford Academic, Oxford University Press. https://doi.org/10.1093/oxfordhb/9780199270125.003.0012

Justino, P., & Samarin, M. (2025). Trust in a changing world: Social cohesion and the social contract in uncertain times [World Social Report 2025]. University of California at Berkeley.

Jylhä, M., & Jokela, J. (1990). Individual experiences as cultural—a cross-cultural study on loneliness among the elderly. *Ageing and Society, 10*(3), 295–315. https://doi.org/10.1017/S0144686X00008308

Langenkamp, A. (2022). The influence of loneliness on perceived connectedness and trust beliefs—Longitudinal evidence from The Netherlands. *Journal of Social and Personal Relationships, 40*(7), 2298–2322. https://doi.org/10.1177/02654075221144716

Lucas, S. R., & Szatrowski, A. (2014). Qualitative comparative analysis in critical perspective. *Sociological Methodology, 44*(1), 1–79. https://doi.org/10.1177/0081175014532763

Luhmann, M., & Hawkley, L. C. (2016). Age differences in loneliness from late adolescence to oldest old age. *Developmental Psychology, 52*(6), 943–959. https://doi.org/10.1037/dev0000117

Marx, A., & Dusa, A. (2011). Crisp-set qualitative comparative analysis (csQCA), contradictions and consistency benchmarks for model specification. *Methodological Innovations Online, 6*(2), 103–148. https://doi.org/10.4256/mio.2010.0037. Original work published 2011.

Mello, P. A. (2021). *Qualitative comparative analysis: An introduction to research design and application*. Georgetown University Press.

Nyqvist, F., Victor, C. R., Forsman, A. K., & Cattan, M. (2016). The association between social capital and loneliness in different age groups: A population-based study in Western Finland. *BMC Public Health, 16*(1), 542. https://doi.org/10.1186/s12889-016-3248-x

Oana, I.-E., & Schneider, C. Q. (2024). A robustness test protocol for applied QCA: Theory and R software application. *Sociological Methods & Research, 53*(1), 57–88. https://doi.org/10.1177/00491241211036158

Paykani, T., Rafiey, H., & Sajjadi, H. (2018). A fuzzy set qualitative comparative analysis of 131 countries: Which configuration of the structural conditions can explain health better? *International Journal for Equity in Health, 17*(1), 10. https://doi.org/10.1186/s12939-018-0724-1

Petersen, B., Khalili-Mahani, N., Murphy, C., Sawchuk, K., Phillips, N., Li, K. Z. H., & Hebblethwaite, S. (2023). The association between information and communication technologies, loneliness and social connectedness: A scoping review. *Frontiers in Psychology, 14*. https://doi.org/10.3389/fpsyg.2023.1063146

Ragin, C. C. (1987). The comparative method: Moving beyond qualitative and quantitative strategies. *University of California Press*. http://www.jstor.org. https://doi.org/10.1525/j.ctt1pnx57

Ragin, C. C. (2000). *Fuzzy-set social science*. University of Chicago Press.

Ragin, C. C. (2006). Set relations in social research: Evaluating their consistency and coverage. *Political Analysis, 14*(3), 291–310. https://doi.org/10.1093/pan/mpj019

Ragin, C. C. (2008). *Redesigning social inquiry: Fuzzy sets and beyond*. University of Chicago Press. https://doi.org/10.7208/chicago/9780226702797.001.0001

Ragin, C. C (2017). USER'S GUIDE TO Fuzzy-Set / Qualitative Comparative Analysis. Available at https://sites.socsci.uci.edu/~cragin/fsQCA/download/fsQCAManual.pdf.

Rapolienė, G., & Aartsen, M. (2021). Lonely societies: Low trust societies? Further explanations for national variations in loneliness among older Europeans. *European Journal of Ageing, 19*(3), 485–494. https://doi.org/10.1007/s10433-021-00649-z

Rihoux, B., Álamos-Concha, P., Bol, D., Marx, A., & Rezsöhazy, I. (2013). From Niche to mainstream method? A comprehensive mapping of QCA applications in journal articles from 1984 to 2011. *Political Research Quarterly, 66*(1), 175–184. http://www.jstor.org/stable/23563600

Rihoux, B., & Lobe, B. (2015). The case-orientedness of qualitative comparative analysis (QCA): Glass half-empty or half-full? DOI: https://doi.org/10.13140/RG.2.1.1919.1529.

Rihoux, B., & Ragin, C. C. (2009). *Configurational comparative methods: Qualitative comparative analysis (QCA) and related techniques* (Vol. 1–51). SAGE Publications, Inc. https://doi.org/10.4135/9781452226569

Scharf, T., & De Jong Gierveld, J. (2008). Loneliness in urban neighbourhoods: An Anglo-Dutch comparison. *European Journal of Ageing, 5*(2), 103–115. https://doi.org/10.1007/s10433-008-0080-x

Schneider, C. Q., & Wagemann, C. (2010). Standards of good practice in qualitative comparative analysis (QCA) and fuzzy-sets. *Comparative Sociology, 9*(3), 397–418. https://doi.org/10.1163/156913210X12493538729793

Schneider, C. Q., & Wagemann, C. (2012). Set-theoretic methods for the social sciences. *Cambridge University Press*. https://doi.org/10.1017/cbo9781139004244

Seifert, A. (2025). Information and communication technologies and the risk to loneliness. In M. Aartsen, I. Precupetu, & B. Suanet (Eds.), *Macro social influences on loneliness in later life. Towards of a better understanding of loneliness paradox in later life*. Springer.

Stegen, H., Duppen, D., Savieri, P., Stas, L., Pan, H., Aartsen, M., Callewaert, H., Dierckx, E., & De Donder, L. (2024). Loneliness prevalence of community-dwelling older adults and the impact of the mode of measurement, data collection, and country: A systematic review and meta-analysis. *International Psychogeriatrics, 36*(9), 747761. https://doi.org/10.1017/S1041610224000425.

Suanet, B., & Aartsen, M. (2025). Linking life course theory to multi-level explanations of loneliness: Towards a sociology of loneliness. In M. Aartsen, I. Precupetu, & B. Suanet (Eds.), *Macro social influences on loneliness in later life. Towards of a better understanding of loneliness paradox in later life*. Springer.

Suanet, B., & Pavlidis, G. (2025). And, you know: There's such a thing as society': Towards a clarification of the 'loneliness paradox' by a macrofication of loneliness studies. In M. Aartsen, I. Precupetu, & B. Suanet (Eds.), *Macro social influences on loneliness in later life. Towards of a better understanding of loneliness paradox in later life*. Springer.

Sundström, G., Fransson, E., Malmberg, B., & Davey, A. (2009). Loneliness among older Europeans. *European Journal of Ageing, 6*(4), 267–275. https://doi.org/10.1007/s10433-009-0134-8

Swader, C. S. (2019). Loneliness in Europe: Personal and societal individualism-collectivism and their connection to social isolation. *Social Forces, 97*(3), 1307–1336. https://doi.org/10.1093/sf/soy088

Swader, C. S., & Moraru, A. V. (2023). Social infrastructure and the alleviation of loneliness in Europe. *Kölner Zeitschrift für Soziologie, 75*(Suppl 1), 387–414. https://doi.org/10.1007/s11577-023-00883-6

Taniguchi, H., & Kaufman, G. (2021). Family, collectivism, and loneliness from a cross-country perspective. *Applied Research in Quality of Life, 17*, 1555–1581. https://doi.org/10.1007/s11482-021-09978-8

Thiem, A. (2019). Beyond the facts: Limited empirical diversity and causal inference in qualitative comparative analysis. *Sociological Methods & Research, 51*(2), 527–540. https://doi.org/10.1177/0049124119882463

Tufă, L. (2025). The social infrastructure of loneliness. A scoping review of societal influences and their implications. In M. Aartsen, I. Precupetu, & B. Suanet (Eds.), *Macro social influences on loneliness in later life. Towards of a better understanding of loneliness paradox in later life*. Springer.

Van Tilburg, T. G. (2025). Unravelling the socio-cultural influence on loneliness. In M. Aartsen, I. Precupetu, & B. Suanet (Eds.), *Macro social influences on loneliness in later life. Towards of a better understanding of loneliness paradox in later life*. Springer.

Van Tilburg, T. G., Steinmetz, S., Stolte, E., Van Der Roest, H., & De Vries, D. H. (2020). Loneliness and mental health during the COVID-19 pandemic: A study among Dutch older adults. *The Journals of Gerontology Series B, 76*(7), e249–e255. https://doi.org/10.1093/geronb/gbaa111

Wu, J., Zhang, J., & Fokkema, T. (2022). The micro-macro interplay of economic factors in late-life loneliness: Evidence from Europe and China. *Frontiers in Public Health, 10*. https://doi.org/10.3389/fpubh.2022.968411

Yang, K. (2018). Longitudinal loneliness and its risk factors among older people in England. *Canadian Journal on Aging/La Revue Canadienne Du Vieillissement, 37*(1), 12–21. https://doi.org/10.1017/s0714980817000526

Zubatsky, M., Berg-Weger, M., & Morley, J. (2020). Using telehealth groups to combat loneliness in older adults through COVID-19. *Journal of American Geriatrics Society, 68*(8), 1678–1679. https://doi.org/10.1111/jgs.16553

Iuliana Precupetu, PhD, is a senior researcher at the Research Institute for Quality of Life, Romanian Academy, and the Research Institute of the University of Bucharest. She is a sociologist specializing in quality of life, health inequalities and social exclusion in later life. Her current interests include the relationship between social exclusion in older age and mental health, as well as the application of life course methods to quality of life research. Most recently, she coordinated the AMASE research project: A multidimensional approach to social exclusion in later life – health consequences for ageing populations.

Cosmina Pop is a sociologist and researcher at the Research Institute for Quality of Life, Romanian Academy. She earned her PhD in sociology from the Doctoral School of the Faculty of Sociology and Social Work at the University of Bucharest in 2010, completing her thesis on "Subjective Quality of Life." Her research focuses on subjective indicators of quality of life, social and health inequalities, the quality of life of children, and the life course perspective. She has actively participated in numerous international conferences and summer schools, as well as contributed to various research projects at both national and international levels.

Marja Aartsen, PhD, is currently research professor and social gerontologist at NOVA – Norwegian Social Research at OsloMet. She is specialized in longitudinal research on social relations, social exclusion, loneliness, and cognitive functioning in the second half of life. She is interested in social issues related to aging in place and active or successful ageing. Recent research projects and collaborations include gendered pathways to exclusion from social relations (GENPATH), reducing old-age social exclusion (ROSENET) and a multidimensional approach to social exclusion and its health consequences (AMASE). She was editor of the European Journal of Ageing from 2017 until summer 2022.

Open Access This chapter is licensed under the terms of the Creative Commons Attribution 4.0 International License (http://creativecommons.org/licenses/by/4.0/), which permits use, sharing, adaptation, distribution and reproduction in any medium or format, as long as you give appropriate credit to the original author(s) and the source, provide a link to the Creative Commons license and indicate if changes were made.

The images or other third party material in this chapter are included in the chapter's Creative Commons license, unless indicated otherwise in a credit line to the material. If material is not included in the chapter's Creative Commons license and your intended use is not permitted by statutory regulation or exceeds the permitted use, you will need to obtain permission directly from the copyright holder.

Chapter 12
'And, you know: there's such a thing as society': Towards a Clarification of the 'loneliness paradox' by a Macrofication of Loneliness Studies

Bianca Suanet and George Pavlidis

12.1 Introduction

In recent years, loneliness has increasingly been recognized as a significant societal and health issue, evidenced amongst others by the World Health Organization's prioritization of loneliness as a global public health concern along with heightened public discourse and media coverage for the topic (Booth, 2023; CNN, 2023). Additionally, the study of loneliness has garnered much more attention in science recently, with the number of publications on the topic increasing strongly (Web of Science). Nevertheless, the strong focus on micro-level factors in research on loneliness (Suanet & Aartsen, 2025) has led to what can be termed a 'microfication' of this field of gerontology, namely the tendency to focus on immediate aspects of everyday life while overlooking broader social contexts that define daily experiences (Hagestad & Dannefer, 2001). The 'microfication' of loneliness research may be linked to the rise of neoliberalism (Sagan, 2017), which often denies the existence of society beyond individual interests (consider Thatcher's famous line: "And, you know, there's no such thing as society"). This micro-focus has not only narrowed the scope of loneliness studies but has also hindered our understanding of loneliness as a fundamentally social and societal issue (Suanet & Aartsen, 2025). This lack of research on macro-level indicators has limited the development of adequate policy responses, often reducing loneliness to an issue requiring individual solutions. A recent systematic literature review showed that, even though there is attention for loneliness in national policies these days, the policies differ and have to move beyond social contact, support, and social skills to become more effective

B. Suanet (✉)
Amstelveen, The Netherlands
e-mail: biancasuanet@gmail.com

G. Pavlidis
Institute for Social and Psychological Studies, Karlstad University, Karlstad, Sweden

© The Author(s) 2025

M. Aartsen et al. (eds.), *Macro Social Influences on Loneliness in Later Life*,
International Perspectives on Aging 47,
https://doi.org/10.1007/978-3-031-94565-6_12

(Goldman et al., 2024). As such, policymakers can use the term "loneliness" to obscure its fundamentally structural undercurrents, framing it as a personal rather than a political and public issue requiring collective action to change institutions, culture, and structures in society. We build on Perlman and Peplau's (1981) definition of loneliness as a subjective emotional experience that arises when there is a perceived discrepancy between desired and actual social relationships, separating it from the more objective condition of social isolation.

Here we argue that while we tend to understand loneliness as a concept that is traditionally attributed to the individual level, it is vital to consider the context in which loneliness is experienced. We do not propose to relinquish the individual perspective entirely, but rather to shift attention more towards the macro level. It is only through the broadening of the scientific exploration of loneliness that we can understand better this challenge and effectively address it. The need for a macro-perspective on loneliness is further highlighted by seemingly puzzling findings in recent research, also termed the 'loneliness paradox.' Studies over the past few years have shown that loneliness is experienced less intensely and by fewer people in more individualistic countries in Northern and Continental Europe than in more collectivist countries in Southern Europe (Swader, 2019; Van Tilburg, 2025). These findings contradict long-held beliefs that individualization uniformly dissolves people's experience of social integration—a view still dominant in public debate and scientific discourse (Suanet et al., 2024). Moreover, increased social connectivity through digital means has coincided with relatively high rates of loneliness in some groups, but their relation is still far from clear. The origins of loneliness in a changing society need to be investigated more in depth and not only focus on individual characteristics but also on meso-level and macro-level factors. This raises questions about what accounts for the observed country differences in loneliness?

In this chapter, we aim to delve deeper into macro-level influences on loneliness. We will expand on perspectives that view loneliness as stemming solely from individual resources or through the individualism/collectivism continuum. These viewpoints often overlook the intricate interplay of various facets within the process of individualization and other structural societal characteristics. Moreover, the current macro-level approach to studying loneliness that looks at only one societal factor at a time does not adequately explain the observed differences across countries. Our exploration promises to shed light on the 'loneliness paradox,' revealing opportunities and challenges for advancing research on macro-level factors influencing loneliness in diverse societal settings. By examining the loneliness paradox, macro-micro relationships, and the current state of research on macro-level factors influencing loneliness in Europe, we aim to identify the plausibility of suggested underlying reasons behind the observed European country variations. Furthermore, we reframe the discussion by highlighting limitations in existing research and proposing methodological and theoretical improvements to generate more reliable evidence on the loneliness paradox, offering insights and implications for future studies. Our approach combines theoretical insights and methodological considerations, laying the groundwork for a nuanced, context-driven understanding of loneliness and its variations across different countries.

12.2 'The Loneliness Paradox': What Is It (Not)?

The exact meaning of the 'loneliness paradox' is itself a subject of study, as scholars and policymakers use the term in various ways. Overall, the paradox refers to the research findings that we have not found people lonelier in environments where one would expect them to be lonelier, for example, in individualist societies (Heu et al., 2021). Generally, it refers to the notion that societal changes like individualization and digitalization have shaped how people experience relationships or the lack of them, what they value in different types of social networks (cultural change), and the opportunities for building meaningful social networks (opportunity structure). The key aspects of this paradox are the trends towards individualism and digitalization in Western cultures. It is often believed by policy makers, laypeople and scholars alike that an increased emphasis on personal achievement, self-reliance, and mobilization weakens communal bonds and reduces the opportunities to build social support systems. Indeed, such societal shifts could make it harder for individuals to form and maintain close relationships, potentially increasing feelings of loneliness (Killeen, 1998). Studies show that digitalization is welcomed as a means of social participation (e.g. Fischl et al., 2020). Technology thus has offered greater connectivity in modern times, but an overreliance on digital communication is sometimes thought to hinder genuine connections (see also Chap. 8 of this book; Seifert, 2025).

Despite these beliefs about a loneliness paradox, what does scientific evidence actually have to say? First, cross-national studies on loneliness in Europe do not show higher loneliness rates in more individualistic and digitalized countries as in Northern and Western European countries loneliness is lower than in Southern and Eastern European countries (Swader, 2019; Nyqvist et al., 2021) Differences in loneliness prevalence are attributed to various factors, such as differences in social welfare systems (Nyqvist et al., 2021), political and democratic systems (Rapolienė & Aartsen, 2022), and cultural norms around family and community support (Swader, 2019; Heu et al., 2021; Van Tilburg, 2025). Second, studies that have looked at European changes in loneliness over historical time have found that loneliness has shifted to lower levels rather than to higher levels in later-born cohorts of older adults (Aunsmo et al., 2023; Dahlberg et al., 2018; Suanet & Van Tilburg, 2019; Suanet et al., 2024). Also, digitalization has made us rely on digital means of communication more, and this has changed how we communicate and what we see as our convoy of relationships (Seifert, 2025). Overall, these findings challenge long-held views on how social change influences loneliness, particularly the notion that individualization and digitalization uniformly pose a threat to feelings of social integration in later life. They underscore the need to further investigate the origins of this so-called 'loneliness paradox', as macro-level societal conditions and changes, such individualization and digitalization, have not necessarily emerged as primary causes of loneliness of the country differences nor the changes over historical time. This emerging puzzle highlights the importance of gaining a deeper understanding of the complex relationship between macro-level factors and loneliness.

12.3 Exploring the Interplay Between Macro-Level Factors and Individuals' Loneliness: Insights from Coleman's Boat Model

To better be able to understand the loneliness paradox, we use Coleman's boat (1990) model, originating from his book on the *Foundations of Social Theory*. This is a well-known and useful conceptual framework in sociology that can help us to better understand this relation between macro-level factors and loneliness and can help us clarify the paradox (Coleman, 1990). In the model, it is understood that the flow of resources or influences between different levels of analysis tends to be both upstream (from micro to macro) and downstream (from macro to micro). Overall, the loneliness paradox primarily concerns downstream factors—specifically, how and when societal changes impact individuals' experiences of loneliness. Consequently, the first arrow in the model is central to understanding the loneliness paradox. However, it is also essential to recognize that individuals' behavior shapes macro-level social outcomes. Fully comprehending the loneliness paradox requires acknowledging the bidirectional influence of macro- and micro-level factors in shaping loneliness (Fig. 12.1).

At the macro level, it is presumed that 'social facts' such as societal culture, structures, and policies play a crucial role in shaping the conditions and outcomes of individuals (1990). Applied to the topic of loneliness, social welfare policies and healthcare provisions can either mitigate or exacerbate loneliness by ensuring adequate support systems and mental health services (de Jong Gierveld & Tesch-Römer, 2012). This is not to say that macro-level factors only impact people's experiences of loneliness in one direction top-down. People themselves also shape the macro-level factors that are important to loneliness. For example, individuals' evolving attitudes towards social interactions and community engagement can gradually shape cultural norms at the macro-level. When more people openly discuss their experiences of loneliness and advocate for supportive communities, cultural narratives around loneliness can become more inclusive and understanding (Barreto et al., 2024). By acknowledging the dynamic interplay between the macro-level societal factors and the individual experiences, Coleman's boat model is instrumental for loneliness studies on macro-level factors by highlighting the bidirectional

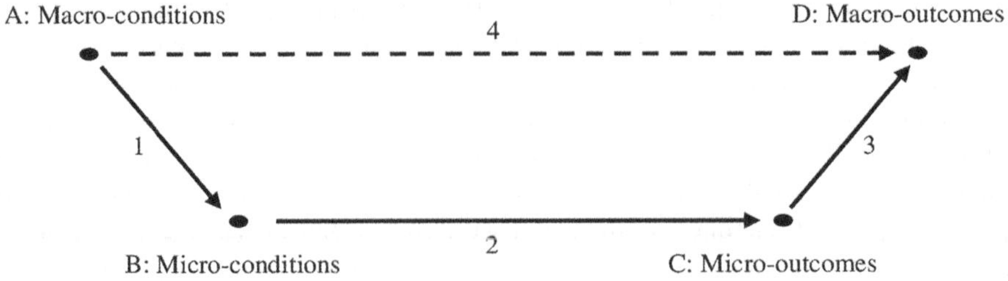

Fig. 12.1 Coleman's diagram

influence between 'social facts' and seemingly individual level outcomes such as loneliness, which are characteristic of all individual well-being outcomes. Taking away the veil of these always existing pathways can greatly help us to identify not only the origins of the paradox of loneliness better but also help us to find better and more effective ways to address it.

12.4 What Are the Relevant Theories and Findings that Help Us Clarify the Loneliness Paradox from a Macro Perspective?

Having described this bidirectional influence, what do we already know about the impact of macro-level factors in explaining the seemingly paradoxical finding that loneliness is particularly low in the more individualized Nordic and Continental European countries compared to Eastern and Southern Europe? Additionally, loneliness scores in the US and the UK, on average, tend to be higher than in Northern and Western Europe but lower than in Eastern and Southern Europe, even though they are just as individualized culturally (Hofstede Insights, 2024). Several key factors have been explored in research related to cultural, political, technological, and welfare state factors. Below, we briefly describe what has been found for each of these areas and how these findings help to understand the impact of macro influences in clarifying the loneliness paradox.

12.4.1 Cultural Explanations of Loneliness: Inglehart's Theory on Shifts in Cultural Values

In recent decades, Europe has experienced a profound shift in cultural values, which has significant implications for loneliness. Ronald Inglehart (2009) argued that as societies become more affluent and secure, their values shift from materialist concerns—focused on economic and physical security—to post-materialist values, which prioritize self-expression, quality of life, and individual autonomy. This cultural shift, driven by factors such as economic development, increased education, and a reduction in existential threats, enables people to focus more on higher-order needs. Countries that embrace post-materialist values tend to prioritize environmental protection, civil liberties, and gender equality, which influences social relations in ways that can contribute to loneliness. These values promote individualism and personal fulfillment over collective norms, meaning that people in post-materialist societies may have more freedom to define their relationships according to personal preferences. This greater relational freedom can lead to higher-quality relationships but also likely increases the vulnerability to social isolation (Heu et al., 2021). As such, the more adherence to post-materialist values and the more individualized a society is, the lower loneliness scores of people are likely to be.

Across Europe, cultural shifts have played out differently depending on historical, cultural, and socio-economic contexts (Inglehart, 2022). In Northern and Western Europe, especially in Protestant countries like Sweden and the Netherlands, there has been a pronounced embrace of self-expression and secular values. These values emphasize individual autonomy, expressiveness, and tolerance, reshaping social norms towards inclusivity and egalitarianism. Economic prosperity and progressive social policies further facilitated these values. Conversely, Southern European countries such as Italy and Spain, while experiencing economic development, maintained stronger traditional family and community ties alongside emerging postmodern values. They score slightly higher in survival and traditional values compared to Protestant Western and Northern Europe. In Eastern Europe, countries like Poland and Hungary have navigated rapid economic and political transformations post-socialism. They are neither very traditional nor very secular, but survival values remain important. In much of Southern Europe, self-expression is becoming more important than survival, but less so than in Northern and Continental Europe. On the world map, the US, UK, and much of the Anglo-Saxon world score higher on traditionalism than Europe but also score high on self-expression versus survival values. (Inglehart, 2022).

Given these variations, it is reasonable to conclude that countries in Northern and Western Europe, which place a greater emphasis on individualism and self-expression, would experience lower levels of loneliness, as the quality of relationships is generally higher. This has been supported by research to date focusing on country differences, as loneliness among older adults is lower in Northern and Western than Southern European countries (e.g. Swader, 2019). Overall, it therefore appears and is theoretically plausible that postmaterialist values generally align with lower loneliness scores by promoting supportive social structures, individual empowerment, increased relational freedom, and enhanced well-being. This makes postmodern values and individualization a compelling partial explanation for cross-country differences in loneliness, especially regarding relationship standards and the freedom to design social relationships as to the liking of the self (instead of that mandated by a higher authority). However, the exact mechanisms underlying the relationship between cultural context and loneliness remain unclear and require further investigation to identify specific pathways. For instance, is loneliness primarily reduced through differences in relationship standards, the quality of interpersonal ties, or a combination of both? Additionally, since postmaterialist values are closely linked to economic well-being, with more affluent countries tending to exhibit higher levels of economic prosperity, the actual underlying cause may lie more in economic factors than cultural values alone.

12.4.2 Governance and Structure and Functioning of Political Institutions as an Explanation for the Loneliness Paradox

More recently, this focus on culture as an explanation for country differences has been complemented by examining how political and democratic systems impact these differences and how loneliness affects the political system. Focusing on the link from macro to micro in Coleman's boat model, Rapolienė and Aartsen (2022) explored how the structure and functioning of political institutions influence individuals' loneliness in Europe. Their study delved into the idea that democratic governance, with its emphasis on individual rights, social equality, and civic participation, might mitigate loneliness through mechanisms such as trust and social engagement. They found that loneliness is partly shaped by the historical-political characteristics of the countries in which people live. The higher prevalence of loneliness in Eastern European post-totalitarian countries can be linked to a low level of trust in others and reduced social engagement. Here, the political history of these countries had an impact on people's societal trust over time. The authors concluded that the suppression from decades earlier is still visible in loneliness data years after these countries were no longer under Soviet control.

Focusing on the link from micro to macro, Langenkamp (2023) and Langenkamp and Bienstman (2022) pointed out that loneliness and a lack of social belonging are linked to increased voting for right-wing populist parties and lower voter turnout, impacting the political system. Here, we see the bidirectional impact of macro and micro as explained in Coleman's bathtub model. Over time, increased polarization in voting and lower voter turnout can diminish social cohesion, exacerbate group conflicts, especially between right-wing populist voters and migrants, and erode trust in the political system. Loneliness, akin to other adverse psychosocial outcomes, poses a risk to societal stability and democratic governance when individuals feel disconnected and disengaged, leading them to abstain from voting and civic participation. This underscores how societal systems contribute to loneliness by influencing trust and social engagement and how these individuals shape the society through their participation, engagement and trust, creating a reciprocal relationship where individuals both shape and are shaped by social change.

12.4.3 Technological Explanations: Is Digitalization in Society a Driver of the Loneliness Paradox?

It is often argued that digitalization also adversely impacts loneliness, even though people are more connected than ever before. Online interactions are often seen as lacking the depth and quality of face-to-face interactions. While social media allows for the maintenance of numerous connections, it might not typically foster the deep, meaningful relationships crucial for emotional well-being (Kraut et al., 2022).

Research indeed indicates anxious people use social media to compensate for a lack of face-to-face interactions, and that this association between anxiety, social media use and loneliness is not positive for the well-being of people (O'Day and Heimberg, 2021). However, its overall effects when moderately used are not so bad or even good, but at the same time, it seems that the impact of social media on loneliness is not that large and much more research is needed to actually prove a clear and strong association (Wiwatkunupakarn et al., 2021). As such, stereotypical statements that social media usage significantly heightens or lowers loneliness are just not very convincing, given the nuanced evidence that has been found regarding digitalization and its impact on people's loneliness. Overall, the impact of ICT on loneliness is complex, but it is unlikely to provide a strong explanation for the observed country differences, as the influence of social media on loneliness is not as significant in scientific findings as is often suggested in public debates.

12.5 Is It Truly a 'Loneliness Paradox', or Simply More Wealth and Better Life Conditions which Are more Equally Distributed?

What if the 'loneliness paradox' is not actually a paradox that can be explained mostly by culture, but is instead mostly a reflection of differences in the distribution of life chances in society, and the culture that develops dynamically in response? What if the structural constraints and opportunities that a society provide inevitably also become part of the personal experience in social relationships (Hansen & Slagsvold, 2016)? Considering this, it seems that having sufficient wealth and resources distributed among a substantial number of people within a politically legitimate system enables individuals to exercise more autonomy and choose their paths in life. This may contribute to lower loneliness rates in Northern and Western Europe compared to Eastern and Southern Europe. Cultural individualism might, in the end, be a sign of societal and collective privilege in the amount and distribution of resources, where the support of people around for survival is less needed and therefore less desired. Individualization does not necessarily lead people to devalue their ties but to invest in them more as they become important vehicles for identity and self-development and contribute to quality of life (Allan, 2008). Furthermore, social ties and belonging to others provides a natural need for people (Cacioppo & Cacioppo, 2018). As such, loneliness in individuals and societies is, just like other social capital outcomes, highly impacted by resources and how these are distributed across the population.

There is at least some clear evidence to support the claim that loneliness is quite like other social capital outcomes, in that it is highly impacted on by resources and how these are distributed. First, a study by Nyqvist et al. (2021) examined country differences in loneliness through the lens of different welfare state regimes. They argued and found that the more universal the social rights in a welfare state, the less loneliness people experience. Additionally, according to the study, those with fewer resources experience less loneliness in Nordic welfare states than people with fewer resources living in Southern and Eastern European countries, as these states tend to be more enabling. Second, even though this is not on older adults, a recent study of mid-life adults found that over historical time there have been reductions in the loneliness among European mid-life adults but not in the US, where the system is less redistributive and the policies for care and work are not as generous (Infurna et al., 2024). It needs to be investigated more in depth whether these findings also pertain to older adults. A recent study by Tapia-Muñoz et al. (2022) also found that higher income inequality within countries is associated with higher loneliness scores. Countries with more equal income distribution, often through redistributive policies, tend to report lower levels of loneliness. This is likely because less inequality not only ensures more equitable access to resources, fostering greater social participation, but also reduces feelings of social distance by making individuals feel more connected in terms of lifestyle, resources, and perceived worth. Fourth, it should be noted that theories on individualization and postmodern values all point to the importance of economic development as needed for changes in cultural values (Inglehart, 2022), which can impact loneliness by putting more emphasis on well-being and individual preferences in life over survival values.

12.6 Towards a Holistic View on Context: Constellations of Macro-Level Factors that Impact on Loneliness, and Multi-Level Intersectionality

Reviewing the perspectives just discussed, the question on what drives the loneliness paradox in Europe remains, for now. But it is becoming clear that macro-level impacts are important to unveil to fully understand it. As Inglehart's theory (2009) suggests, with economic change driving cultural change, these macro-level factors are not isolated or separate elements within society; instead, they are interconnected and collectively shape individuals' experiences of their social relationships. These macro-factors in culture, welfare states, political systems and technological innovation are fundamentally interconnected. Even though this is not acknowledged as much in current research, looking at constellations of macro factors that result in lower or higher loneliness might be much more fruitful than considering only separate aspects of a society for explaining country differences in loneliness.

One reason to focus more on constellations of factors is recent research on country differences in how societal change impacts loneliness, particularly by examining late-life developments over time. Most studies showed a decrease in loneliness among later-born cohorts across most Western and Northern European context among older adults, and a recent study showed that in the United States, loneliness scores are not lowering for mid-life older adults, but are increasing, whereas in Europe loneliness scores tend to decrease across birth cohort in Northern and

Continental European countries (Infurna et al., 2024). Both the US and Northern and Continental Europe have societies with an individualized culture, so that can hardly be the explanation of the differences in development of loneliness between the countries. However, in the United States, there is relatively little welfare support, whereas the European countries with the lowest levels of loneliness typically have strong welfare systems. So, having sufficient support as well as opportunities for social participation for those at the lower end of the socio-economic status spectrum might very well be the reason for lower loneliness rates overall and the positive development over historical time in European countries. Also, the more elaborate policies for care and work likely play a role in having enough time to nurture social ties across the life course. A plausible hypothesis could be that an individualized culture is good provided that actual tangible solidarity is located somewhere at the community or societal level. In other words, low expectations combined with good living conditions for many. The heightened risk of loneliness in an individualized society is obviously definitely present when resources are low for people and not distributed more equally to ensure enough for most to be able to be connected to society and participate. So, one could perhaps expect that loneliness incubating societies are those that are individualistic but do not have their solidarity located at the meso or macro level, or are collectivistic with limited resources.

Loneliness is a subjective experience that warrants deeper exploration of the relationship standards individuals hold. Cross-national studies have indicated that people tend to feel less lonely when their social networks align with cultural expectations. For instance, co-residence with children significantly reduces loneliness among older adults in Tuscany, but this effect is not observed in the Netherlands or Canada (Van Tilburg et al., 2004). De Jong Gierveld and Tesch-Römer (2012) further highlight that societal factors, including culture and economy, influence both loneliness and the standards for social relationships. While these standards are likely culture-dependent, they may also be shaped by the social networks individuals inhabit. Cacioppo et al.'s (2009) research suggests that individuals on the periphery of social networks often experience greater loneliness, yet the specific ways in which standards for relationships within a given context and network dynamics interact remain unclear. It could be that people in different parts of the network have different standards or these standards could be shared across networks. Gaining insights into how standards come about and how these are impacted by differences in micro, meso and macro-factors is an underexplored part of loneliness research.

The discussion of the "loneliness epidemic" or a paradox of loneliness takes away from the fact that there is a large heterogeneity within the respective populations as well and that loneliness tends to hit hard those with disadvantaged characteristics at micro, meso and macro factors in intersection. Risk factors for loneliness and perceived social exclusion, for example, have been found to be largely one and the same, even though the respective strengths of the effects differ between perceived social exclusion and loneliness (Huxhold et al., 2022). Social exclusion as a concept tends to point more to not feeling included in society. Therefore, combined with the observation above it might be better to conclude that loneliness has many characteristics of other more structural forms of social exclusion: loneliness disproportionality affects those with other disadvantageous characteristics, namely people living in poverty or with a lower socioeconomic status and people belonging to racial and ethnic minorities in their countries, and women. These are groups that tend to face a lot of discrimination in society and therefore might benefit less from an overall advantageous society. From this, we feel that more emphasis needs to be drawn to the very structural origins of loneliness among disadvantaged groups and individuals within even richer and more politically stable societies with a strong welfare state. As such, a focus on macro level is not complete without investigating how its effects differ across subgroups in the population.

Finally, a holistic view on loneliness demands more interdisciplinary integration. Most of the studies on loneliness come from the psychological field. However, other disciplines that can help us explain the loneliness paradox. For example, sociology can help unravel the role of social institutions and inequality in loneliness. Economics can help explain as well as look at the cost-benefit analysis of existing and proposed interventions. As such, we need to move towards an integration of different models of explaining loneliness, such as the social cognitive approach, evolutionary approach and welfare states theories, to better understand how and why loneliness arises as the result of intersections at the macro, meso and micro level. We will also better be able to gain a comprehensive picture of the mechanisms resulting in loneliness and shed more light on the actual reasons for a loneliness paradox in the sense that more individualized countries tend to be less lonely and whether this is not actually due to other non-observed factors or, as said before, a specific constellation of macro-factors. Third, we will be better able to understand how the psychological and social interact as loneliness is in its core a psycho-social issue. This demands both the focus on experiences of individuals as well as the cultural and structural underpinnings that results in them being more or less at risk of loneliness.

12.7 Methodological Considerations in Understanding the Impact of Macro-Level Factors on Loneliness Better to Help Solve the Paradox of Loneliness

In understanding the impact of societal context on loneliness better, it is important to shed further light on the policy implications of macro-level factors on loneliness, looking at how societal structures and policies impact on loneliness. First, next to diving more into European differences in loneliness and its origins, we need to use variation across the world to understand the impact of macro factors on loneliness and to see whether this paradox also arises similarly if one takes a global view. Deeper examination is warranted to ascertain the global applicability of findings in Europe and to understand why loneliness tends to be lower in 'individualized' countries in Europe (Infurna et al., 2024; Suanet & Aartsen, 2025). Economic, social, and cultural factors likely interact in complex, interconnected ways, and it is probable that the lower levels of loneliness in these countries result from a specific combination of factors at the macro, meso and micro level, including a welfare state that makes it easier for people to hold individualistic views and a path dependence in culture. Individualization as a process can be seen as a Western invention first and foremost, as also evidenced by findings of Inglehart (2009) on postmaterialist values. This correlation between wealth, individualism, and lower loneliness rates in affluent European countries merits further investigation on a global scale to really determine the impact of (constellations) of macro-level influences for loneliness. The field can move forward by including more directly (constellations of) macro-level indicators as predictors of differences in loneliness worldwide. What can be a solution is to create clusters of countries based on macro factors or other more innovative methods to separate necessary and sufficient macro factors to give rise to loneliness (Precupetu et al., 2025).

Second, it should be considered that definitions and measurement scales of loneliness are mostly of a western origin, and Western European and US origin predominantly. The most often deployed loneliness scales such as the UCLA and the De Jong-Gierveld scale are coming from the United States and Europe and are often used in other European as well as non-Western contexts. While some studies show no differential item functioning across European countries (Van Tilburg et al., 2004), this doesn't necessarily mean the experience of loneliness is identical across contexts and that the factors impacting on loneliness are similar. The construct validity of loneliness measures should be examined in various cultural contexts to ensure that differences in loneliness prevalence reflect true macro-level distinctions rather than cultural biases in measurement tools. This is not to say that the use of single direct questions is the way to go, because stigma is a huge problem, which likely tends to become larger if the country has a more collectivistic culture. The advantage is that it does use the word 'lonely,' so people understand it by their own definition, but then we need to know what that is. In short, to more fully understand loneliness in its context, it is important to bring in these more diverse perspectives from different cultures, see if there are common or distinct traits of loneliness in different macro-contexts.

The third major issue in loneliness research concerns sampling biases and their impact on estimating loneliness prevalence, which makes adequate conclusions about the loneliness paradox less secure. Studies based on panel data or large-scale surveys often struggle to reach socially isolated or lonely older adults, who may avoid participation. Scholars have raised concerns about the visibility of such groups in surveys, given their tendency to suffer in silence or avoid admitting feelings of loneliness. This sampling bias likely leads to an underestimation of loneliness in these populations. The prevalence of loneliness has often been estimated in relevant studies based on panel data or large-scale surveys, where participation is voluntary and probabilistic. These studies usually argue for the representativeness of their samples based on social indicators (e.g., gender, age, income, education), hence on indicators other than those of social isolation or loneliness (Surkalim et al., 2022). Yet, several scholars have expressed their reservations about the capacity of surveys to reach socially isolated or lonely older persons, even if these surveys are of large scale or population-based (Newall and Menec, 2019; Pavlidis et al., 2022). The invisibility of such individuals in research further complicates the estimation of loneliness prevalence.

Hansen and Slagsvold (2016) used the Generations and Gender Survey (GGS), which is a cross-national longitudinal study, to compare loneliness among older individuals across several European countries. The GGS survey aimed for representativeness by specifying random sampling of the non-institutionalized population aged 18–79, but Fokkema et al. (2016) noted that while response rates are comparable to those of other surveys and data are generally representative in terms of age, gender, region, and household size, there are issues with representativeness regarding marital status and educational attainment. Similarly, the Survey of Health, Ageing and Retirement in Europe (SHARE) has been used to compare loneliness prevalence among older persons in different countries. However, Börsch-Supan et al. (2013) acknowledged that despite a high overall response rate, there is significant unit nonresponse and panel attrition, which may introduce sample selection bias and limit the generalizability of results. The issue of underrepresentation of socially excluded older persons is not addressed or statistically corrected in SHARE data, as also highlighted by Surkalim et al. (2022).

Given these limitations, it is questionable whether differences in loneliness prevalence across European countries truly reflect national or cultural variations. Factors such as i) the varying capacities of national research teams to reach socially isolated and lonely individuals, and ii) cultural differences in the willingness of socially isolated older participants to engage in surveys could contribute to statistical artifacts. The 'loneliness paradox' observed in Europe, where the northern countries report lower loneliness despite having smaller social networks compared to the southern countries, might be a result of reluctance to participate in surveys or to admit loneliness, rather than genuine differences in loneliness levels (Ågren & Pavlidis, 2023).

In short, from a methodological perspective, we need to improve the research. Methodologically to be able to really say that we have a loneliness paradox. It demands a global approach for both scale and sufficient cultural, institutional and economic diversity at the macro level, but also attention to sampling bias and heterogeneity in loneliness measures.

12.8 The Need for Societal and Community Intervention Action on Loneliness

To address loneliness more effectively, it's crucial to shift our focus from individual experiences (the "I-frame") to the broader structural factors (the "S-frame") that contribute to this pervasive issue. Recent insights in policy research emphasize the importance of examining how our policies and approaches to societal issues are still focusing heavily on the individual level rather than on the societal level (Chater &

Loewenstein, 2023). When loneliness is framed solely as an individual problem, policymakers may overlook critical systemic issues such as socioeconomic disparities, inadequate community infrastructure, and insufficient mental health services. This narrow framing leads to incomplete solutions—like awareness campaigns or social initiatives—that may offer temporary relief but fail to tackle the root causes of isolation. In other words, by simplifying the complexities of loneliness, we risk perpetuating a cycle of neglect regarding the broader societal conditions that foster it. To combat this, interventions should focus on prevention and early intervention rather than the curation of already lonely individuals. This is even more so as the impact of loneliness interventions tends to be modest. Key societal institutions—such as schools, workplaces, and community organizations—can play vital roles in integrating individuals into social networks and in society by giving them social integration, a purpose, meaningful roles, etc., which are all known to be active elements in loneliness interventions (Bouwman & Van Tilburg, 2020). Educational systems can be designed to facilitate cooperation and build connections, while raising awareness about social health. By prioritizing systemic approaches that promote connection and address underlying disparities, we can create more meaningful and lasting solutions to loneliness, ultimately fostering a more cohesive society.

12.9 Conclusion and Discussion: What a Macrofication of Loneliness Studies Can Teach Us

With this chapter, we aim to provide a critical reflection on loneliness research to date and offer some new perspectives to move the field forward. We emphasize the significance of macro-social conditions and crises in understanding late-life loneliness, rather than focusing solely on often-invoked individual characteristics known to produce loneliness. In doing so, we aim to contribute to what we call a de-microfication and (re-)macrofication by highlighting the macro context as a core aspect of the production of loneliness. The micro level should not be neglected, but the focus needs to be balanced with a focus on relevant factors at meso and macro-levels. To do so, we first delve into the interconnected nature of social categories, such as gender, social class, birth cohort, and immigrant status, and contexts, recognizing the potential interdependent systems of disadvantage across micro, meso, and macro levels that individuals experience. Within this framework, a macro, meso, and micro intersectionality of loneliness emerges, suggesting that individuals' intersections of positioning within their networks, communities, and societies determine their likelihood of experiencing loneliness, rather than their individual traits alone. For instance, individuals from ethnic minority backgrounds or those with a low socio-economic status may reside in more disadvantaged neighbourhoods, and be less well embedded within institutions and social networks, the impact of which can vary depending on the prevailing welfare state and social policies in that context. By looking at loneliness as produced through the micro, meso, and macro context, we can unveil how context plays a role in loneliness, which has not been as central to the views of researchers, policymakers, and the public as might be desirable if we want to understand and address the issue.

While micro-level factors influencing loneliness, such as widowhood and transitions like moving, have been extensively studied, they are sometimes partly or even completely beyond individuals' control. Addressing loneliness effectively necessitates broader societal and communal interventions that also prevent loneliness from occurring in the first place, tailored to individuals' specific definitions and experiences of the problem, rather than relying on standardized individual programs targeting already lonely individuals only. An intersectional approach that considers characteristics at all levels is essential for comprehending why individuals experience loneliness in specific meso and macro contexts. Neglecting to account for standards for social relationships and their expected provision can lead to ambiguity in interpreting research findings, especially when differences stem from cultural ideals and stat provisions. Also, the failure to incorporate the experiences of lonely people make it difficult to let the voices of marginalized groups be heard and to make interventions more effective or accessible for these groups (Barreto et al., 2024). Effective intervention involves challenging stereotypes, stigma, and discrimination that contribute to social exclusion and loneliness among marginalized populations. In the end, this will necessitate advocating for structural changes at the institutional, community, and policy levels to address the root causes of loneliness and promote social inclusion and belonging for all individuals, including policies that address economic inequality, improve access to social services and support networks, and challenge discriminatory practices and attitudes.

Competing Interests The authors have no conflicts of interest to declare that are relevant to the content of this chapter.

References

Ågren, A., & Pavlidis, G. (2023). Sense-making of loneliness and exclusion from social relations among older adults in Sweden. *The Gerontologist, 63*(7), 1140–1148. https://doi.org/10.1093/geront/gnad005

Allan, G. (2008). Flexibility, friendship, and family. *Personal Relationships, 15*(1), 1–16. https://doi.org/10.1111/j.1475-6811.2007.00181.x

Aunsmo, R. H., Langballe, E. M., Hansen, T., Selbæk, G., & Strand, B. H. (2023). Time trends in loneliness from 1984 to 2019 among 27,032 older adults in Norway: A HUNT study. *Preventive Medicine, 175*, 107659. https://doi.org/10.1016/j.ypmed.2023.107659

Barreto, M., Doyle, D. M., & Qualter, P. (2024). Changing the narrative: Loneliness as a social justice issue. *Perspectives on Psychological Science*. https://doi.org/10.1111/pops.12965

Booth, R. (2023, November 16). WHO declares loneliness a 'global public health concern'. The Guardian. https://www.theguardian.com/global-development/2023/nov/16/who-declares-loneliness-a-global-public-health-concern. Accessed August 15, 2024.

Börsch-Supan, A., et al. (2013). Data resource profile: The survey of health, ageing and retirement in Europe (SHARE). *International Journal of Epidemiology, 42*(4), 992–1001. https://doi.org/10.1093/ije/dyt088

Bouwman, T. E., & Van Tilburg, T. G. (2020). Towards a more focused approach to loneliness: Seven active elements in loneliness interventions [Article in Dutch]. *Tijdschrift voor Gerontologie en Geriatrie, 51*(1). https://doi.org/10.1016/j.ypmed.2023.107659

Cacioppo, J. T., & Cacioppo, S. (2018). The need for interaction: An evolutionary perspective. *Perspectives on Psychological Science, 13*(1), 1–22. https://doi.org/10.1177/1745691617711453

Cacioppo, J. T., Fowler, J. H., & Christakis, N. A. (2009). Alone in the crowd: The structure and spread of loneliness in a large social network. *Journal of Personality and Social Psychology, 97*(6), 977–991. https://doi.org/10.1037/a0016076

Chater, N., & Loewenstein, G. (2023). The i-frame and the s-frame: How focusing on individual-level solutions has led behavioral public policy astray. *Behavioral and Brain Sciences, 46*, e147. https://doi.org/10.1017/S0140525X22002023

CNN. (2023). WHO makes loneliness a global health priority with new Commission on Social Connection. Retrieved from: https://edition.cnn.com/2023/11/15/health/who-loneliness-social-connection/index.html (July 5 2024).

Coleman, J. S. (1990). *Foundations of social theory*. Harvard University Press.

Dahlberg, L., Agahi, N., & Lennartsson, C. (2018). Lonelier than ever? Loneliness of older people over two decades. *Archives of Gerontology and Geriatrics, 75*, 96–103. https://doi.org/10.1016/j.archger.2017.11.004

de Jong Gierveld, J., & Tesch-Römer, C. (2012). Loneliness in old age in eastern and Western European societies: Theoretical perspectives. *European Journal of Ageing, 9*(4), 285–295. https://doi.org/10.1007/s10433-012-0248-2

Fischl, C., Lindelöf, N., Lindgren, H., & Nilsson, I. (2020). Older adults' perceptions of contexts surrounding their social participation in a digitalized society—an exploration in rural communities in northern Sweden. *European Journal of Ageing, 17*(3), 281–290. https://doi.org/10.1007/s10433-020-00558-7

Fokkema, T., et al. (2016). Generations and gender programme wave 1 data collection: An overview and assessment of sampling and fieldwork methods. *Demographic Research, 34*, 499–524. https://www.jstor.org/stable/26332044.

Goldman, N., Khanna, D., El Asmar, M. L., Qualter, P., & El-Osta, A. (2024). Addressing loneliness and social isolation in 52 countries: A scoping review of national policies. *BMC Public Health, 24*(1), 1207. https://doi.org/10.1186/s12889-024-18370-8

Hagestad, G. O., & Dannefer, D. (2001). Concepts and theories of aging: Beyond microfication in social science approaches. In R. Binstock & L. George (Eds.), *Handbook of aging and the social sciences* (2nd ed.). Academic.

Hansen, T., & Slagsvold, B. (2016). Late-life loneliness in 11 European countries: Results from the generations and gender survey. *Social Indicators Research, 129*(1), 445–464. https://doi.org/10.1007/s11205-015-1111-6

Heu, L. C., van Zomeren, M., & Hansen, N. (2021). Does loneliness thrive in relational freedom or restriction? The culture-loneliness framework. *Review of General Psychology, 25*(1), 60–72. https://doi.org/10.1177/1089268020959033

Hofstede Insights. (2024). *Country Scores.* Available online at: https://www.hofstede-insights.com/product/compare-countries/. July 8, 2024.

Huxhold, O., Suanet, B., & Wetzel, M. (2022). Perceived social exclusion and loneliness: Two distinct but related phenomena. *Sociological Science, 9*(17), 430–453. https://doi.org/10.15195/v9.a19

Infurna, F. J., Dey, N. E. Y., Gonzalez Avilés, T., Grimm, K. J., Lachman, M. E., & Gerstorf, D. (2024). Loneliness in midlife: Historical increases and elevated levels in the United States compared with Europe. *American Psychologist*. https://doi.org/10.1037/amp0001322

Inglehart, R. (2009). Postmaterialist values and the shift from survival to self-expression values. In R. J. Dalton & H.-D. Klingemann (Eds.), *The Oxford handbook of political behavior* (online ed.). Oxford Academic. https://doi.org/10.1093/oxfordhb/9780199270125.003.0012

Inglehart, R. (2022). *Cultural evolution: People's motivations are changing, and reshaping the world.* Cambridge University Press.

Killeen, C. (1998). Loneliness: An epidemic in modern society? *Journal of Advanced Nursing, 28*(4), 762–770. https://doi.org/10.1046/j.1365-2648.1998.00703.x

Kraut, R. E., Patterson, M., Lundmark, V., Kiesler, S., Mukopadhyay, T., & Scherlis, D. (2022). Internet paradox: A social technology that reduces social involvement and psychological well-being? *American Psychologist, 53*(9), 1017–1031. https://doi.org/10.1037/0003-066X.53.9.1017

Langenkamp, A. (2023). The influence of loneliness on perceived connectedness and trust beliefs—longitudinal evidence from The Netherlands. *Journal of Social and Personal Relationships, 40*(7), 2298–2322. https://doi.org/10.1177/02654075221144716

Langenkamp, A., & Bienstman, S. (2022). Populism and layers of social belonging: Support of populist parties in Europe. *Political Psychology, 43*(5), 931–949. https://doi.org/10.1111/pops.12835

Newall, N. E. G., & Menec, V. H. (2019). Loneliness and social isolation of older adults: Why it is important to examine these social aspects together. *Journal of Social and Personal Relationships, 36*(3), 925–939. https://doi.org/10.1177/0265407517749045

Nyqvist, F., Nygård, M., & Scharf, T. (2021). Social capital and loneliness in welfare state regimes before and after the global financial crisis: Results based on the European social survey. In A. Almakaeva, A. Moreno, & R. Wilkes (Eds.), *Social capital and subjective well-being. Societies and political orders in transition* (Societies and political orders in transition) (pp. 237–259). Springer. https://doi.org/10.1007/978-3-030-75813-4_12

O'Day, E. B., & Heimberg, R. G. (2021). Social media use, social anxiety, and loneliness: A systematic review. *Computers in Human Behavior Reports, 3*, 100070. https://doi.org/10.1016/j.chbr.2021.100070

Pavlidis, G., Motel-Klingebiel, A., & Aartsen, M. (2022). Exclusion from social relations in later life: On the gendered associations of social networks with mental wellbeing. *Aging & Mental Health, 27*(7), 1313–1321. https://doi.org/10.1080/13607863.2022.2116397

Perlman, D., & Peplau, L. A. (1981). Toward a social psychology of loneliness. In R. Gilmour & S. Duck (Eds.), *Personal relationships: 3. Relationships in disorder* (pp. 31–56). Academic Press.

Precupetu, I., Pop, C., & Aartsen, M. (2025). Macro-level influences on loneliness in later life: An fsQCA analysis. In M. Aartsen, I. Precupetu, & B. Suanet (Eds.), *Macro social influences on loneliness in later life: Towards a better understanding of the loneliness paradox in later life*. Springer.

Rapolienė, G., & Aartsen, M. (2022). Lonely societies: Low trust societies? Further explanations for national variations in loneliness among older Europeans. *European Journal of Ageing, 19*(3), 485–494. https://doi.org/10.1007/s10433-021-00649-z

Sagan, O. (2017). Narratives of loneliness and mental ill health in a time of neoliberalism. In O. Sagan & E. Miller (Eds.), *Narratives of loneliness: Multidisciplinary perspectives from the 21st century* (pp. 88–100). Routledge. https://doi.org/10.4324/9781315645582

Seifert, A. (2025). Information and communication technologies and the risk to loneliness. In M. Aartsen, I. Precupetu, & B. Suanet (Eds.), *Macro social influences on loneliness in later life* (Towards of a better understanding of loneliness paradox in later life). Springer.

Suanet, B., & Aartsen, M. (2025). Linking life course theory to multi-level explanations of loneliness: Towards a sociology of loneliness. In M. Aartsen, I. Precupetu, & B. Suanet (Eds.), *Macro social influences on loneliness in later life* (Towards of a better understanding of loneliness paradox in later life). Springer.

Suanet, B., Drewelies, J., Duezel, S., Eibich, P., Demuth, I., Steinhagen-Thiessen, E., Wagner, G. G., Lindenberger, U., Ram, N., Ghisletta, P., & Gerstorf, D. (2024). Historical change in trajectories of loneliness in old age: Older adults today are less lonely, but do not differ in their age trajectories. *Psychology and Aging, 39*(4), 350–363. https://doi.org/10.1037/pag0000803

Suanet, B., & Van Tilburg, T. G. (2019). Loneliness declines across birth cohorts: The impact of mastery and self-efficacy. *Psychology and Aging, 34*(8), 1134–1143. https://doi.org/10.1037/pag0000357

Surkalim, D. L., Luo, M., Eres, R., Gebel, K., van Buskirk, J., Bauman, A., & Ding, D. (2022). The prevalence of loneliness across 113 countries: Systematic review and meta-analysis. *BMJ, 376*, e067068. https://doi.org/10.1136/bmj-2021-067068

Swader, C. S. (2019). Loneliness in Europe: Personal and societal individualism-collectivism and their connection to social isolation. *Social Forces, 97*(3), 1307–1336. https://doi.org/10.1093/sf/soy088

Tapia-Muñoz, T., Staudinger, U. M., Allel, K., Steptoe, A., Miranda-Castillo, C., Medina, J. T., & Calvo, E. (2022). Income inequality and its relationship with loneliness prevalence: A cross-sectional study among older adults in the US and 16 European countries. *PLoS One, 17*(12), e0274518. https://doi.org/10.1371/journal.pone.0274518

van Tilburg, T. G. (2025). Unravelling the socio-cultural influence on loneliness. In M. Aartsen, I. Precupetu, & B. Suanet (Eds.), *Macro social influences on loneliness in later life: Towards a better understanding of the loneliness paradox in later life*. Springer.

Van Tilburg, T. G., Havens, B., & de Jong Gierveld, J. (2004). Loneliness among older adults in The Netherlands, Italy, and Canada: A multifaceted comparison. *Canadian Journal on Aging / La Revue Canadienne du Vieillissement, 23*(2), 169–180. https://doi.org/10.1353/cja.2004.0026

Wiwatkunupakarn, N., Pateekhum, C., Aramrat, C., Jirapornchaoren, W., Pinyopornpanish, K., & Angkurawaranon, C. (2021). Social networking site usage: A systematic review of its relationship with social isolation, loneliness, and depression among older adults. *Aging & Mental Health, 26*(7), 1318–1326. https://doi.org/10.1080/13607863.2021.1966745

Bianca Suanet, PhD, is a sociologist, specializing in loneliness, social relations, and care use among older adults, especially in relation to the impact of societal and policy changes. She was formerly Professor of Ageing and Social Change at the Linköping University in Sweden and Associate Professor in Sociology and Head of the Social Functioning Group of the Longitudinal Aging Study Amsterdam at the Vrije Universiteit Amsterdam in the Netherlands. Currently, her research projects encompass studies on the relationship between macro-level factors and loneliness, and optimizing interventions against loneliness for older migrants, based on co-created scientific mixed methods evidence.

George Pavlidis, PhD, is a lecturer in sociology at Karlstad University, Sweden, within the Institute for Social and Psychological Studies. He has studied a broad range of topics on ageing and adult development, focusing mainly on the social factors that influence the cognitive, mental, and social well-being of older persons. During his PhD and post-doctoral assignments, he focused on the intersecting risks of exclusion from social relations and loneliness later in life. His recent projects examine the link between the digital transformation of essential goods and services with the risks of social exclusion in older age.

Open Access This chapter is licensed under the terms of the Creative Commons Attribution 4.0 International License (http://creativecommons.org/licenses/by/4.0/), which permits use, sharing, adaptation, distribution and reproduction in any medium or format, as long as you give appropriate credit to the original author(s) and the source, provide a link to the Creative Commons license and indicate if changes were made.

The images or other third party material in this chapter are included in the chapter's Creative Commons license, unless indicated otherwise in a credit line to the material. If material is not included in the chapter's Creative Commons license and your intended use is not permitted by statutory regulation or exceeds the permitted use, you will need to obtain permission directly from the copyright holder.

Chapter 13
Policy Recommendations to Address Loneliness in Later Life

Mihaela Ghenţa and Aniela Matei

13.1 Loneliness in Older Age: The Role of Policy Interventions

The ageing of the population, changes in family structures and roles, urbanisation, and migration are among the societal trends that have reshaped the approach to life, values and relationships among people of all ages. These transformations of society led to the rise of isolation and loneliness among certain categories of the population and especially older people (Hwang et al., 2020). Even though loneliness (subjective feeling) and social isolation (lack or reduced social relationships) refer to different aspects and are recognised as distinct, most often they arise together (Hwang et al., 2020; World Health Organization, 2021); hence they are often used interchangeably (Cattan et al., 2005; Gardiner et al., 2018) or merged into a single concept (Collins, 2014).

The occurrence of loneliness and social isolation, as well as effects at the individual level have been researched during the last few decades (Flay et al., 2005). Recent global events such as the COVID-19 pandemic period have encouraged research aimed at understanding the mechanisms and impact of loneliness at the individual and societal levels (Becker et al., 2022, El-Osta et al., 2021; Hwang et al., 2020). In certain countries, loneliness and/or social isolation have become critical aspects of social and health policies (World Health Organization, 2021). Social isolation and loneliness have become significant not only at the individual level but also for governments, because of their effects on physical and mental health and related public costs for health and long-term care (Goldman et al., 2024; World Health Organization, 2021). Adequate support for quality social relationships

M. Ghenţa (✉) · A. Matei
National Scientific Research Institute for Labour and Social Protection (INCSMPS), Bucharest, Romania
e-mail: mihaela.ghenta@incsmps.ro

© The Author(s) 2025

M. Aartsen et al. (eds.), *Macro Social Influences on Loneliness in Later Life*, International Perspectives on Aging 47,
https://doi.org/10.1007/978-3-031-94565-6_13

affects the engagement of individuals in community life and society (World Health Organization, 2021). Loneliness and social isolation have proved to be risk factors for higher mortality (Yu et al., 2020). Pertaining the impact on mental health, several studies have pointed to increased depressive symptomatology (Lee et al., 2019), increased suicide risk (Fässberg et al., 2012), poor quality of life (Zebhauser et al., 2014), worsening of cognition (Hwang et al., 2020) and neurological decline (Kuiper et al., 2015). At the policy level, the reporting of social isolation and loneliness gradually raised awareness of these issues. It is important to maintain the distinction between the two terms, as they are addressed by different policy interventions (Holt-Lunstad et al., 2010).

Different policy responses have been designed either to raise awareness and acceptance of loneliness or to provide adequate support for social relationships and to increase the social inclusion of people affected by loneliness. Furthermore, Holt-Lunstad et al. (2010) proposed the inclusion of social isolation and loneliness in all relevant policy domains, but this requires increased awareness of the population and professionals in health and social care as well as national guidelines. Holt-Lunstad et al. (2010) noted the need to define national guidelines for social connection in order to fight loneliness that should be added to those designed for nutrition, physical activity, and sleep.

The aim of this chapter is to map policy interventions dedicated to loneliness in the EU during two strategic frameworks. Our goal is to understand the content and type of these interventions and whether progress has been made between the two timeframes in designing policy measures to tackle social isolation or loneliness.

13.2 Effectiveness of Loneliness Interventions for Older People

Numerous studies have evaluated the effectiveness of loneliness interventions using various research approaches, including qualitative study designs, cohort designs with and without control groups, cross-sectional designs (using surveys), single-group pre-post comparison designs, quasi-experimental study designs, and randomized controlled trials. These interventions target different mechanisms believed to influence loneliness, with psychological and sociological interventions being the most common.

In the scientific literature, different taxonomies have been developed for interventions to address loneliness. In a meta-analysis, Masi et al. (2011) identified four primary intervention strategies to mitigate this phenomenon among older people: 1) interventions that aim to improving social skills, 2) interventions that target enhancing social support, 3) interventions that increase opportunities for social contact, and 4) interventions that address maladaptive social cognition. They concluded that reducing maladaptive social cognitions had the greatest impact on loneliness. Mann et al. (2017) proposed a taxonomy that distinguishes between direct and indirect interventions. Indirect interventions are broader strategies focused on health or well-being and thus may indirectly affect loneliness, whereas direct interventions specifically address loneliness. They found that while cognitive interventions were the most promising, none of the four direct interventions had a robust evidence base. Gardiner et al. (2018) distinguished between social facilitation, psychological therapies, health and social care provision, animal interventions, befriending, and leisure/skill development. They concluded that most interventions showed some effectiveness in alleviating social isolation and loneliness, although the supporting evidence was typically of low quality. Cotterell et al. (2018) classified loneliness and social isolation interventions into individual, group (social, educational, or physical activity), service provision, technology-based, neighbourhood, and structural interventions. They noted that the impact of interventions was group-specific (e.g., only effective for older adults with chronic health conditions or specific ethnic minority groups). Additionally, educational programs focusing on social network maintenance and enhancement appear to be effective (Cohen-Mansfield & Perach, 2015). Interventions that target loneliness at all ages have a series of key elements that ensure their success: group interventions with an educational focus or specific support function, targeting a specific group, engaging the participants, utilizing existing services, and having a theoretical basis (Centre for Policy on Ageing, 2014). The World Health Organization (2021) classifies interventions to address social isolation and loneliness among older adults into three categories: (1) individual and relationship-level interventions that focus on maintaining and supporting people's relationships and changing how people think and feel about them; (2) community-level strategies that address infrastructures such as transportation, digital inclusion, and the built environment, and (3) societal-level strategies that include laws and policies.

Studies evaluating the effectiveness of interventions to reduce loneliness and social isolation have been criticized for poor study design, inadequate periods for measuring effectiveness, variability in definitions of isolation and loneliness, small sample sizes, and inconsistent research instrument reviews (National Academies of Sciences, Engineering, and Medicine et al., 2020). Nevertheless, some conclusions can be drawn, such as that the most successful interventions are those that include active participation of older adults, are group-based, emphasize the educational nature of the intervention, are tailored, and reduce maladaptive social cognitions. However, there is limited knowledge about how interventions developed for specific populations can be effective in other populations. To determine the transferability of certain interventions to other groups, additional qualitative, observational, and multilevel evaluations of loneliness interventions are needed.

13.3 Framework of Evaluation

As people age, the risk of experiencing chronic and multiple physical or mental diseases and cognitive limitations increases, leading to high need for formal or informal support. Long-term care services (in residential settings or at home) are designed to offer the necessary support for the older people. Loneliness in residential settings is often addressed in studies because social interactions are limited within this type of social services (Ghenţa et al., 2021), while a poor relationship with an informal carer is a determinant of feelings of loneliness and social inclusion in the case of home care services (Hajek et al., 2021). Long-term care regimes are built by taking into account factors that affect loneliness: family and family values regarding care and the availability of socio-medical services for older people.

The goal of this chapter (principal research question) was to map the policy response and progress considering the challenges in addressing loneliness in later life in European Union member states, considering two strategic time frameworks: 2014–2020 and 2020–2026. The documents analysed are national strategies and action plans, defined as public policy documents. The countries were grouped according to the *care regimes* using the typology of long-term care regimes as proposed by Lamura et al. (2007) and Schulmann et al. (2014). The care regime typology applies three factors (demand for care, provision of informal care, and provision of formal care) that allow the identification of the role and extent of social policy in ongoing care activities. The proposed typology includes the following clusters:

- Standard-care mix regime characterised by medium/high demand for care, medium/low provision of informal care and medium formal care. Examples are Germany, Austria, France, Luxembourg, and Belgium.
- Universal-Nordic regime characterised by medium demand for care, low provision of informal care and high formal care: Sweden, Denmark, The Netherlands, Iceland;
- Family based regime characterised by high demand for care, low provision of informal care and low formal care. Examples are Spain, Italy, Portugal, Ireland, Greece, Cyprus, and Malta.
- Transition regime characterised by low demand for care, high provision of informal care and medium/low formal care. Examples are Hungary, Poland, Czech Republic, Slovakia, Romania, Bulgaria, Estonia, Latvia, and Lithuania.

According to Schulmann et al. (2014), the characteristics of the care regimes evolve continuously in relation to the social, economic and health characteristics of the countries. In countries with a family-based care regime, the LTC systems rely mostly on informal care - family members and migrant carers. In recent years, the informal care provided by migrants has been transformed into a formal care workforce through policy measures (Leichsenring et al., 2013; Schulmann et al., 2014). Countries with a standard-care mix regime, assign the responsibility for care to family members, supported by services provided by religious and nongovernmental organisations (Lamura et al., 2008). Countries from the universal – Nordic cluster ensure access to formal solutions to cover the LTC demands, with a well-developed network of in-home/residential care (Lamura et al., 2008), and different funding mechanisms (Schulmann et al., 2014). Transition countries vary widely in terms of care provision and public expenditure for LTC (Lamura et al., 2008; Schulmann et al., 2014).

We applied document analysis, a qualitative research technique for reviewing or evaluating documents. Like other analytical methods in qualitative research, document analysis is performed to examine and interpret data in order to understand and develop empirical knowledge. In relation to other qualitative research methods, document analysis has both advantages and limitations. Among the strong advantages, we mention availability and lack of obtrusiveness and reactivity (unaffected by the research process). As main limitation, we consider the insufficient details and the biased selectivity. The policy response was defined in terms of the *national strategies* and *action plans* developed by the governments of the 27 EU Member States for the two policy cycles, and included Belgium (BE), Greece (EL), Lithuania (LT), Portugal (PT), Bulgaria (BG), Spain (ES), Luxembourg (LU), Romania (RO), Czechia (CZ), France (FR), Hungary (HU), Slovenia (SI), Denmark (DK), Croatia (HR), Malta (MT), Slovakia (SK), Germany (DE), Italy (IT), Netherlands (NL), Finland (FI) Estonia (EE), Cyprus (CY), Austria (AT), Sweden (SE), Ireland (IE), Latvia (LV), and Poland (PL). These policy documents mainly targeted not only *social inclusion* and *long-term care strategies/plans*, but also sustainable development strategies when the public resources could not be identified to support the nominated policy documents (see Table 13.1 for the references). In our research we decided to look for loneliness and social isolation, as they are recognised as separate but related concepts (Zólyomi, 2019).

13.3.1 Information Sources, Criteria for Selection, and the Process of Analysing Policy Documents

The main information sources were the European Social Policy Network (ESPN) *Thematic Reports on Challenges in long-term care* for 2018, the European Commission *Reports on the implementation of the Council Recommendation on access to affordable high-quality long-term care* for 2024, and the *technical reports* from governmental websites of relevant ministries and departments of the 27 selected countries (See Table 13.1). If information could not be identified in the documents defined as a source of information, we additionally used the Google search engine for all available national policies related to social isolation and loneliness. We focused on national level documents only (excluding any regional strategies).

We identified online documents in English and conducted document analysis using "*social isolation*" and "*loneliness*" as key words or related words (*lone, alone, isolation*). If no results were identified for a particular country, we searched for the

Table 13.1 Policy response and progress in addressing loneliness/social isolation in later life

Country	Document type	Source	Strategic frame 1 2014–2020			Strategic frame 2 2020–2027		
			Loneliness/ social isolation	Level of intervention	Type of intervention	Loneliness/ social isolation	Level of intervention	Type of intervention
Standard-care mix regimes (5)								
AT	Strategy on social inclusion /strategy on LTC	Federal Ministry Republic of Austria (2021), European Parliament, (2021), European Commission (2024a)	*Social isolation*	*Micro/meso*	*Responsive/ preventive*	*Loneliness/ social isolation*	*Micro, meso, macro*	*Responsive/ preventive*
BE	Strategy on social inclusion /strategy on LTC	European Commission (2019), European Parliament (2021)	*Social isolation*	*Micro, meso*	*Responsive/ preventive*	*Social isolation*	*Micro, meso*	*Responsive/ preventive*
FR	Strategy on social inclusion /strategy on LTC	European Commission (2018a, 2019, 2024b), European Parliament (2021)	*Social isolation*	*Micro, meso,macro*	*Responsive/ preventive/ partnership*	*Social isolation/ loneliness*	*Micro, meso, macro*	*Responsive/ preventive/ partnership*
DE	Strategy on social inclusion/strategy on LTC	European Parliament (2021)	*Social isolation*	*Micro/meso*	*Responsive/ preventive*	*Loneliness/ social isolation*	*Micro, meso, macro*	*Responsive/ preventive/ partnership*
LU	Strategy on social inclusion /strategy on LTC	Ministry of Family Affairs, Integration and the Greater Region (2019), European Commission (2024c)	*Social isolation*	*Micro/meso*	*Responsive/ preventive*	*Loneliness/ social isolation*	*Micro, meso*	*Responsive/ preventive*
Universal-Nordic regimes (4)								
DK	Strategy on LTC/ strategy on loneliness	European Commission (2018b), European Commission (2021)	*Social isolation/ loneliness*	*Micro, meso*	*Responsive/ preventive*	*Social isolation/ lonliness*	*Micro, meso, macro*	*Responsive/ preventive*

FI	Strategy on social inclusion/strategy on LTC	European Commission (2018c)	*Social isolation/ loneliness*	*Micro, meso*	*Responsive/ preventive*	*Loneliness/ social isolation*	*Micro, meso, macro*	*Responsive/ preventive/ partnership*
SE	Strategy on social inclusion/strategy on LTC	European Parliament (2021)	*Social isolation*	*Micro, meso*	*Responsive*	*Loneliness/ social isolation*	*Micro, meso, macro*	*Responsive/ preventive*
NL	Strategy on social inclusion/strategy on LTC	European Commission (2018d, 2019, 2021), European Parliament (2021)	*Social isolation*	*Micro, meso*	*Responsive/ preventive/ partnership*	*Loneliness/ social isolation*	*Micro, meso, macro*	*Responsive/ preventive/ partnership*
Family based regimes (7)								
CY	Strategy on social inclusion /strategy on LTC	Directorate General for European. Programmes, Coordination and Development (2021)	*Social isolation*	*Micro, mezo*	*Responsive*	*Social isolation*	*Micro, mezo*	*Responsive*
IE	Strategy on social inclusion/strategy on LTC	Department of Social Protection (2023), European Commission (2024d)	*Social isolation*	*Micro, meso*	*Responsive/ preventive*	*Loneliness/ social isolation*	*Micro, meso, macro*	*Responsive/ preventive*
IT	Strategy on social inclusion/strategy on LTC	European Parliament (2021), European Commission (2024e)	–	*Micro, mezo*	*Responsive*	*Social isolation*	*Micro, mezzo, macro*	*Responsive/ preventive*
EL	Strategy on social inclusion/strategy on LTC	European Commission (2018e), European Commission (2024f)	*Social isolation*	*Micro, mezo*	*Responsive*	*Loneliness/ social isolation*	*Micro, mezzo*	*Responsive/ preventive*
ES	Strategy on social inclusion/strategy on LTC	European Commission (2024g)	–	*Micro, mezo*	*Responsive*	*Social isolation*	*Micro, mezzo*	*Responsive/ preventive*

(continued)

Table 13.1 (continued)

Country	Document type	Source	Strategic frame 1 2014–2020			Strategic frame 2 2020–2027		
			Loneliness/ social isolation	Level of intervention	Type of intervention	Loneliness/ social isolation	Level of intervention	Type of intervention
MT	Strategy on social inclusion/strategy on LTC	Ministry for Health and Active Ageing (2022)	*Social isolation*	*Micro, mezo*	*Responsive*	*Loneliness/ social isolation*	*Micro, mezzo*	*Responsive/ preventive*
PT	Strategy on social inclusion/strategy on LTC	European Commission (2018f), European Commission (2024h)	*Social isolation*	*Micro, mezo*	*Responsive*	*Loneliness/ social isolation*	*Micro, mezzo*	*Responsive/ preventive/ partnership*
Transition regimes (11)								
BG	Strategy on social inclusion strategy on LTC, action plan on long-term care strategy	European Commission (2018g, 2019, 2021, 2024i), Ministry of Labour and Social Protection (2021)	*Social isolation*	*Micro, meso*	*Responsive*	*Loneliness, social isolation*	*Micro, mezzo*	*Responsive*
HR	Strategy on LTC	European Commission (2018h)	*Social isolation*	*Micro, meso*	*Responsive*	–	–	–
CZ	Strategy on social inclusion, strategy on LTC, action plan on social inclusion	Ministry of Labor and Social Affairs (2020, 2021)	–	–	–	*Loneliness, social isolation*	*Macro*	*Preventive/ responsive/ partnership*
EE	Strategy on LTC	Ministry of Social Affairs (2022a, 2022b)	–	–	–	*Social isolation*	*Micro, meso, macro*	*Preventive*
HU	Strategy on LTC, strategy on social inclusion	European Commission (2021)	–	–	–	*Social isolation*	*Micro, meso*	*Preventive*

LV	Strategy on LTC	European Commission (2018i), ISSA (2022)	*Social isolation*	*Micro, meso*	*Responsive*	*Social isolation*	*Micro, meso*	*Responsive*
LT	Strategy on LTC, strategy on social inclusion	No available data	–	–	–	–	–	–
PL	Strategy on LTC/ Programme	European Commission (2018j), Ministry of Family, Labor and Social Policy (2024), ISSA (2022), European Parliament (2021), Social Insurance Institution (2023)	*Social isolation*	*Micro, meso*	*Responsive*	*Social isolation*	*Micro, meso*	*Responsive*
SK	Strategy on LTC	World Health Organisation (2017)	*Social isolation*	*Micro, meso, macro*	*Preventive, partnership*	–	–	–
SI	Strategy on LTC	Government of the Republic of Slovenia (2017)	*Loneliness, social isolation*	*Micro*	*Preventive*	–	–	–
RO	Strategy on LTC, strategy on social inclusion	Ministry of Labor, Family, Social Protection and Elderly (2015), European Commission (2024j)	*Social isolation*	*Micro, meso*	*Responsive*	*Loneliness, social isolation*	*Micro, meso*	*Responsive*

Source: developed by authors

government website of that country using "*strategy/policy/plan on social isolation/loneliness*" to determine if governments published documents on loneliness and social isolation. Criteria for selection were type of document (strategy, policy, plans on social isolation/loneliness, technical reports from governmental websites of relevant ministries and departments), thematic subject of the policy document (social isolation and loneliness), and available language for the policy documents (English). All documents identified that did not meet the selection and analysis criteria were excluded from the analysis process. A total of 69 documents were consulted. The identification and analysis of the documents were carried out between 1st September 2024 and 1st October 2024.

13.3.2 Data Items and Data Charting Process

We applied the classification of interventions proposed by the World Health Organization (WHO) (2021) and an analysis matrix was defined for each strategic cycle taking into account three dimensions: (1) addressing the areas of *social isolation* and *loneliness* through policy documents; (2) *level of intervention* (*micro-* individual and relationship-level interventions; *meso*-community-level strategies; and *macro-* societal level strategies) and (3) *types of interventions* (responsive, preventive, based on a partnership).

13.4 Lessons from Policy Interventions

The strategic framework of 2014–2020 was characterised by a prevalence of policy responses targeted to reduce, in the majority of the cases, the social isolation experienced by older people (Table 13.1):

- In all five countries from the *standard-care mix regime* (AT, BE, FR, DE, and LU), in the documents analysed, there were references to the field of social isolation associated with measures and programmes implemented through public policies. Most countries reported the implementation of interventions at the micro and meso-levels, except for France where reports of macro level interventions were identified. Moreover, also in the case of France, all three types of interventions were identified: responsive/preventive/partnership. For countries belonging to this care regime, there is a concern for both preventive and responsive types of interventions. The demand for care in standard-care mix regime countries is medium/high, which is why preventive interventions have been the focus of the governments of these states, before 2020.
- In the case of European member states belonging to the *universal-Nordic regime* (DK, FI,SE, NL) characterised by high provision of formal care and medium demand for care, the concept of loneliness entered government discourse before

2020, being identified in countries such as Denmark and Finland, along with the concept of social isolation. However, our analysis did not identify macro-level interventions, only measures at the micro and meso levels. The types of interventions identified were predominantly reactive and preventive, apart from the Netherlands where partnership-type interventions were also identified.

- The countries that are part of the *family-based care regime* (CY, EL, ES, IE, IT, MT, and PT) have introduced the concept of social isolation to a lesser extent in the public policy documents before 2020, and the analysis identified this concept only in the case of five countries (CY, EL, MT, PT, and IE). All interventions identified were at the micro and meso-level, being responsive interventions for the strategic framework 2014–2020. This type of family-based care regime is characterised by low provision of formal care and high demand for care.
- Six countries (BG, HR, LV, PL, SK, and RO) from the *transition long-term care regime* were identified to have such references to social isolation and loneliness extracted from the European Social Policy Network thematic reports on long-term care, the WHO and national governmental documents. In five countries, strategies implemented interventions at the micro and meso-levels were identified, and the actions were taken to respond to the needs of older people living alone, while in SK preventive measures, based on partnership between different institutions and entities, were considered also at macro level. SI is the only country in this care regime that has mentioned preventive measures to address loneliness and social isolation among older people.

The strategic framework of 2020–2027 has been characterised by more interventions aimed at addressing both loneliness and social isolation among older people (Table 13.1):

- In the countries from the *standard-care mix regime* (AT, BE, FR, DE, and LU), the concepts of *social isolation* and *loneliness* have gained visibility in public policy documents (AT, FR, DE, and LU). The number of countries for which macro level interventions were identified in the analysed documents increased from 1 (FR) to 2 (FR, DE). Responsive/preventive interventions remained the majority for this strategic cycle, but the number of countries for which partnership interventions were identified increased (FR, DE).
- European member countries belonging to the *universal-Nordic regime* (DK, FI, SE, and NL) included the term "loneliness" in their public policy documents alongside that of social isolation. They have also moved to macro level interventions (strategies/programmes), while also maintaining micro and meso-level measures. The number of countries for which partnership interventions were identified increased (NL, FI).
- Additionally, in the countries that are part of the *family-based care regime* (CY, EL, ES, IT, IE, MT, and PT) the concept of social isolation was first visible in the public policy documents after 2020, and the analysis identified four countries that used the term (EL, IE, MT, and PT). With the exception of Italy and Ireland, where macro level interventions were identified, all interventions are maintained

at the micro and meso-level, being responsive/preventive, for the strategic framework 2024–2027.
- Three countries (BG, CZ, RO) from the *transition long-term care regime* implemented interventions to address loneliness and social isolation. These interventions were aimed to counteract the negative effects of both loneliness and social isolation. Preventive, responsive and partnership-based actions were implemented at the micro, meso- and macro levels. Policy documents from EE and HU proposed preventive actions, while PL and LV implemented responsive measures to address social isolation among older people. No data were found concerning the policy response to loneliness or social isolation in the cases of HR, LT, SK, and SI.

13.5 Implications and Further Directions

We analysed policy documents from two strategic frameworks to identify the public policy response aimed at reducing loneliness in old age in European countries within the care regime framework. We found differences between the considered strategic frameworks and between countries from different long-term care regimes.

13.5.1 Policy Initiatives and Implications

A common feature of all care regimes is related to the emphasis on the debate on loneliness during the COVID-19 pandemic. Countries with a *standard-care mix regime* were more advantaged by better management of this phenomenon from a public policy point of view, based on the experience gained in the area of social isolation before the COVID-19 pandemic. As an example, in France, the national programme MONALISA (MObilisation NAtionale contre L'Isolement des Agés – National mobilisation against the isolation of older people) started in 2013 with the purpose of reducing loneliness among older people (Box 13.1). Ten years later, after the COVID-19 pandemic period, the "Aging Well" Strategy (*macro-level initiative*), adopted in November 2023, proposes an interministerial approach with the implementation of 50 measures divided into four key areas, many measures contributing to reducing social isolation and intergenerational divides. In Germany one example of an initiative at the *meso-level* is that of the 540 multigenerational homes (Mehrgenerationenhäuser) which facilitates joint community activities and voluntary engagement for all age groups. In Austria, the "Long-term Care Task Force" (Taskforce Pflege), a working group (*partnership initiative*), was established in 2020 to draft a strategic plan for adjusting and expanding the care system. Reducing isolation and loneliness was one of the key requirements (Box 13.2). For countries coming from this care system, there is a current approach at the *micro, meso- and macro-levels* of *responsive, preventive, and partnership initiatives built* on the 2014–2020 implementation cycle.

Box 13.1 MONALISA (MObilisation NAtionale contre L'Isolement des Agés: National Mobilisation Against the Isolation of Older People (2012)
The French Minister in charge of older people and independent living with the support of AGE organisation "*Les Petits Frères des Pauvres*", developed a network aimed to bring together volunteers, non-profit associations and public institutions to fight older people's isolation. The program facilitates the mobilization of volunteers and implements 'citizen teams' (*équipes citoyennes*) to identify isolated older people and to provide appropriate support. During the COVID-19 pandemic, the MONALISA programme was adapted to the specific needs of the older peoples by introducing two additional activities: assistance to older individuals with increased fragility and online communication with isolated people.

Source: https://www.monalisa-asso.fr/

Box 13.2 Long-Term Care Task Force" (Taskforce Pflege) (2020)
In 2020, a reform of the LTC system, "Long-term Care Task Force" (*Taskforce Pflege*), was started to adjust and to expand the care system. A working group has started to work for a better governance of LTC service provision; better planning of needs and benefits, including minimum standards and data management within the system. The Austrian "Long-term Care Task Force" explicitly addressed the role of new technologies in promoting and financially supporting the assistive technologies, in advancing the research in the field of digital and assistive technologies, and in perceiving new technologies as a resource to support increased safety, a better quality of care and the promotion of social coherence and reduced loneliness.

Source: Trukeschitz, B., Österle, A. & Schneider, U. (2022)

Countries with a *universal-Nordic care regime* characterised by a high provision of formal care and medium demand for care also have extensive experience in managing the phenomena of social isolation and loneliness. The Netherlands has one of the best systems for older people's care (AARP International, 2018). The Dutch Ministry of Health, Welfare and Sport has developed a website that informs people how they can recognise the signs of loneliness, where to report it, and how to help combat it, for instance by joining neighbourhood initiatives. The Netherlands also has an action plan (initiative at the macro level) that targets loneliness: *One against loneliness. Action programme 2022–2025* (Partou, 2025). Another country from this care regime has, since 2023, a strategy/action plan (the Danish National Strategy

Against Loneliness/Danish Action Plan Against Loneliness) developed in partnership with two NGOs: the Ældre Sagen (The Elderly Association) and the General Red Cross (Box 13.3). The Circle of Friends (Ystäväpiiri) initiative from Finland focuses on older adults who feel lonely in their everyday lives. In Sweden, there are governmental grants for the development of interventions to target loneliness and new national guidelines on how to reduce loneliness in older adults.

Box 13.3 The National Partnership Against Loneliness (2023)
The National Partnership Against Loneliness is supported by the Danish government and brings together 115 stakeholders across municipalities, regions, companies, organizations, and civil society to propose Denmark's first strategy and action plan against loneliness. The main purpose of the Partnership is to develop a common strategy and action plan to reduce loneliness and reach the target of halving the prevalence of loneliness by 2040 among the adult Danish population.

Source: https://www.age-platform.eu/proposal-for-national-strategy-against-loneliness-in-denmark/

The analysis of public policies in countries that are part of the *family-based care regime* revealed that the concept of social isolation was introduced to a lesser extent in the public policy documents before 2020. The concept of social isolation began to be visible in the public policy documents after 2020. In Ireland, the Befriending Networks is a programme designed to support lonely and isolated older people through weekly volunteer visits (volunteers visit older people in their home once a week) and calls (each day to alleviate loneliness and provide support to coordinate various services they might need). In Spain, Open Protection Centers for older adults are structures that promote the social rights of elderly individuals, contributing to the prevention of health problems and social isolation among older people. Their goal is to prevent the emergence of psychological and social problems in old age, stimulating partnership initiatives between the non-governmental sector and government agencies specialised in older peoples' issues. In Italy, Legge 33/2023 (Decreto Anziani) aims to improve the quality of life for the older people by promoting accessibility to health care and reducing social isolation through coordinated efforts between health and social services. In the National Plan for Non-Self-Sufficiency 2022–2024, one of the key objectives is to encourage active participation in society to reduce isolation.

Based on our analysis, we argue that countries within the *transition regime* have registered limited progress between the strategic frameworks in terms of public recognition of loneliness, as only three out of eleven countries have been found to mention loneliness in their policy documents – BG, CZ and RO. These results highlight the need for in-depth research to investigate barriers to encourage progress and increased public awareness-raising. Policy documents in long-term care and social inclusion from transition countries propose solutions for social isolation as a result of the inability of older people or families to address the need for care. Even in countries that recognise loneliness in public long-term care/social inclusion policy documents, interventions are predominantly designed to respond to a public need. BG, PL and RO provide home and residential social services for people affected by social isolation (Ministry of Family, Labor and Social Policy, 2024; Ministry of Labour and Social Protection, 2021; European Parliament, 2021). For example, in Poland, in order to maintain services that have been seriously affected by the COVID-19 pandemic, virtual visits and meeting advisers via video link have been made accessible to older people, while in Latvia, Latvia's State Social Insurance Agency has mobilised, through local authorities, computer trainers (e-assistants) to inform users about online services (ISSA, 2022) (Box 13.4). Different programmes to support the alleviation of loneliness and social participation are taken into account at the Romanian level (European Commission, 2024j).

Box 13.4 E-assistant: Assistant in Receiving e-Services (2022)

In Latvia, in response to the challenges imposed by population ageing, the State Social Insurance Agency created an e-assistant on the public administration services portal. Within this initiative, the State Social Insurance Agency has deployed, through the unified customer service provided by local authorities, computer trainers (e-assistants) to familiarize users with online services. The service promotes customer digital skills and reduces the administrative burden related to the post-processing of applications received from local service centres.

Source: ISSA. (2022). Priorities for social security Trends, challenges and solutions

The importance of preventive measures in addressing either loneliness or social isolation among older people has been recognised in a limited number of transition countries (Ministry of Labour and Social Protection, 2021), and concrete measures have been developed only in the CZ, EE, and HU. For example, in the Czech Republic, macro level interventions address loneliness and social isolation as part of broader initiatives to reduce social exclusion. Regional and municipal authorities, as well as Czech regions will be involved in the implementation of a functional system aimed at preventing and weakening social exclusion processes and reducing the territorial concentration of social exclusion (Ministry of Labor and Social Affairs, 2020, 2021). In Estonia, policy documents for 2030, propose the creation of a network of older people's advocacy organisations to develop advocacy for older people, including social inclusion and any relevant aspect related to a preventive social work for older people, as well as the creation of awareness-raising measures (Ministry of Social Affairs, 2022a, 2022b). Preventative measures include preventative home visits and activities supporting good health in old age (European Commission, 2021).

13.5.2 Limitations

Our research has several limitations. First, we investigated only policy documents that were available in English, and we also limited our research to long-term care and social inclusion domains. National examples of interventions to address loneliness and social isolation were identified and presented to overcome this limitation. Secondly, because in very few cases we had access to public policy documents such as strategy/action plans in the English language, the classifications into types of interventions (preventive, responsive, and partnership) and levels of intervention (micro, meso, and macro) may be affected by classification bias made by researchers on the basis of the information resources available.

13.5.3 Further Directions

Our research reveals a heterogeneous adaptation of social policy responses to societal trends regarding social isolation and loneliness. Previous studies (Fakoya et al., 2020; Sandu et al., 2021) point to a multitude of factors (e.g. the variety of interventions, the characteristics of the target group population) that pose difficulties in designing policy recommendations that are able to address loneliness in later life. Based on our results we consider that policy response to loneliness in old age should consider the specific context, culture, traditions and models of care in place.

In the case of EU Member States with greater experience in the design of public policies to address the issue of social isolation and loneliness (the case of countries from the standard care mix regime and the universal-Nordic care regime), the emphasis will be placed to a greater extent on interventions that address loneliness in later life, taking into account the more pronounced demographic pressure in these countries and the care regimes they promote. Research in the field (Gardiner et al., 2020) indicates that the prevalence of loneliness among people living in long-term care institutions seems to be greater than that among those living in the community. Therefore, in countries with a *universal Nordic care regime*, characterised by a high demand for formal care, policies that address loneliness, including in later life, are more advanced in terms of strategies to address social isolation/loneliness. There are then countries from the *standard care mix regime*, where the demand for formal care is assessed as medium. Studies (Dickens et al., 2011) highlight that the problems of loneliness in later life will be reduced if interventions are implemented on a large scale in a multisectoral effort with multiple stakeholders. This trend is also observed in the case of countries in the *family-based care regime*.

In countries belonging to the *transitional regime*, we witness a reduced degree of acceptance of loneliness as a public, social and mental health issue. During the last decade, the policy response highlighted the interest in responding to limited social relationships (social isolation), rather than to loneliness. Further research should investigate if this is the result of cultural context (e.g. feeling ashamed to recognise that an individual is feeling alone), social policy, health care policy or a mixture of different individual and societal factors. Wide advocacy campaigns should encourage older people to recognise the signs of loneliness and social isolation and to seek adequate support from social and health care professionals. A policy action should value the role of new technologies to prevent and to counter loneliness and social isolation among older people from remote areas, affected by the migration of descendants, without social network. Access to new technologies and training in the use of digital devices should accompany the implementation of such measures.

Competing Interests The authors have no conflict of interest to declare that are relevant to the content of this chapter.

References

AARP International. (2018). *The Netherlands. The 2018 aging readiness & competitiveness report: Small innovative economies*. Retrieved March 10, 2025, from https://www.aarpinternational.org/file%20library/arc/countries/full%20reports/2018_netherlands.pdf.

Beckers, A., Buecker, S., Casabianca, E., & Nurminen, M. (2022, December 2). Effectiveness of interventions tackling loneliness. JRC Publications Repository. https://doi.org/10.2760/277109

Cattan, M., White, M., Bond, J., & Learmouth, A. (2005). Preventing social isolation and loneliness among older people: A systematic review of health promotion interventions. *Ageing & Society, 25*(1), 41–67.

Centre for Policy on Ageing. (2014). R*apid review: Loneliness—Evidence of the effectiveness of interventions*. Retrieved September 13, 2024, from http://www.cpa.org.uk/information/reviews/CPA-Rapid-Review-Loneliness.pdf.

Cohen-Mansfield, J., & Perach, R. (2015). Interventions for alleviating loneliness among older persons: A critical review. *American Journal of Health Promotion, 29*(3), e109–e125.

Collins, E. (2014). Preventing social isolation and loneliness in older people. https://www.iriss.org.uk/sites/default/files/iriss-insights-25.pdf.

Cotterell, N., Buffel, T., & Phillipson, C. (2018). Preventing social isolation in older people. *Maturitas, 113*, 80–84. https://doi.org/10.1016/j.maturitas.2018.04.014

Department of Social Protection (2023). *Roadmap for social inclusion 2020–2025 ambition, goals, commitments third progress report July 2022 to June 2023*. Retrieved September 13, 2024, from https://www.google.com/url?sa=i&url=https%3A%2F%2Fassets.gov.ie%2F285231%2Fd3ff6026-1031-4b08-85ef-59da90bdf0d3.pdf&psig=AOvVaw2IoH8UwYhmXc5Giu3KaSUJ&ust=1732701669509000&source=images&cd=vfe&opi=89978449&ved=0CAQQn5wMahcKEwjA7tbt3vmJAxUAAAAAHQAAAAAQBA.

Dickens, A. P., Richards, S. H., Greaves, C. J., & Campbell, J. L. (2011). Interventions targeting social isolation in older people: A systematic review. *BMC Public Health, 11*, 647.

Directorate General for European. Programmes, Coordination and Development, Republic of Cyprus. (2021). *Republic of Cyprus second voluntary national review Sustainable Development Goals (SDGs)*. Retrieved September 15, 2024, from https://sustainabledevelopment.un.org/content/documents/282512021_VNR_Report_Cyprus.pdf.

El-Osta, A., Alaa, A., Webber, I., Sasco, E. R., Bagkeris, E., Millar, H., Vidal-Hall, C., & Majeed, A. (2021). How is the COVID-19 lockdown impacting the mental health of parents of school-age children in the UK? A cross-sectional online survey. *BMJ Open, 11*(5), e043397. https://doi.org/10.1136/bmjopen-2020-043397

European Commission. (2018a). *ESPN Thematic Report on Challenges in long term care. France*. Retrieved October 29, 2024, from https://ec.europa.eu/social/main.jsp?pager.offset=0&advSe

archKey=espnltc_2018&mode=advancedSubmit&catId=22&policyArea=0&policyAreaSub=0&country=0&year=0.

European Commission. (2018b). *ESPN Thematic Report on Challenges in long term care. Denmark.* Retrieved October 29, 2024, from https://ec.europa.eu/social/main.jsp?pager.offset=0&advSearchKey=espnltc_2018&mode=advancedSubmit&catId=22&policyArea=0&policyAreaSub=0&country=0&year=0

European Commission. (2018c). *ESPN Thematic Report on Challenges in long term care. Finland.* Retrieved October 29, 2024, from https://ec.europa.eu/social/main.jsp?pager.offset=0&advSearchKey=espnltc_2018&mode=advancedSubmit&catId=22&policyArea=0&policyAreaSub=0&country=0&year=0

European Commission. (2018d). ESPN thematic report on challenges in long term care. The Netherlands. Retrieved October 29, 2024, from https://ec.europa.eu/social/main.jsp?pager.offset=0&advSearchKey=espnltc_2018&mode=advancedSubmit&catId=22&policyArea=0&policyAreaSub=0&country=0&year=0.

European Commission. (2018e). *ESPN thematic report on Challenges in long term care. Greece.* Retrieved October 29, 2024, from https://ec.europa.eu/social/main.jsp?pager.offset=0&advSearchKey=espnltc_2018&mode=advancedSubmit&catId=22&policyArea=0&policyAreaSub=0&country=0&year=0

European Commission (2018f). *ESPN thematic report on challenges in long term care. Portugal.* Retrieved October 29, 2024, from https://ec.europa.eu/social/main.jsp?pager.offset=0&advSearchKey=espnltc_2018&mode=advancedSubmit&catId=22&policyArea=0&policyAreaSub=0&country=0&year=0

European Commission. (2018g). *ESPN Thematic Report on Challenges in long term care. Bulgaria.* Retrieved October 29, 2024, from https://ec.europa.eu/social/main.jsp?pager.offset=0&advSearchKey=espnltc_2018&mode=advancedSubmit&catId=22&policyArea=0&policyAreaSub=0&country=0&year=0

European Commission. (2018h). *ESPN Thematic Report on Challenges in long term care. Croatia.* Retrieved October 29, 2024, from https://ec.europa.eu/social/main.jsp?pager.offset=0&advSearchKey=espnltc_2018&mode=advancedSubmit&catId=22&policyArea=0&policyAreaSub=0&country=0&year=0

European Commission. (2018i). *ESPN Thematic Report on Challenges in long term care. Latvia.* Retrieved October 29, 2024, from https://ec.europa.eu/social/main.jsp?pager.offset=0&advSearchKey=espnltc_2018&mode=advancedSubmit&catId=22&policyArea=0&policyAreaSub=0&country=0&year=0

European Commission. (2018j). *ESPN Thematic Report on Challenges in long term care. Poland.* Retrieved October 29, 2024, from https://ec.europa.eu/social/main.jsp?pager.offset=0&advSearchKey=espnltc_2018&mode=advancedSubmit&catId=22&policyArea=0&policyAreaSub=0&country=0&year=0

European Commission. (2019). *Joint report on health care and long-term care systems & fiscal sustainability.* Retrieved October 29, 2024, from https://www.sipotra.it/wp-content/uploads/2019/06/Joint-Report-on-Health-Care-and-Long-Term-Care-Systems-Fiscal-Sustainability.pdf.

European Commission. (2021). Long-term care report Trends, challenges and opportunities in an ageing society. *Volume II, Country profiles*. Retrieved October 27, 2024, from https://op.europa.eu/en/publication-detail/-/publication/b39728e3-cd83-11eb-ac72-01aa75ed71a1.

European Commission (2024a). *Report on the implementation of the Council Recommendation on access to affordable high-quality long-term care Austria.* Retrieved September 13, 2024, from https://ec.europa.eu/social/main.jsp?advSearchKey=lltimprep&mode=advancedSubmit&catId=22&doc_submit=&policyArea=0&policyAreaSub=0&country=0&year=0.

European Commission. (2024b). *Report on the implementation of the Council Recommendation on access to affordable high-quality long-term care France.* Retrieved September 27, 2024, from https://ec.europa.eu/social/main.jsp?advSearchKey=lltimprep&mode=advancedSubmit&catId=22&doc_submit=&policyArea=0&policyAreaSub=0&country=0&year=0.

European Commission. (2024c). *Report on the implementation of the Council Recommendation on access to affordable high-quality long-term care Luxembourg*. Retrieved September 27, 2024, from https://ec.europa.eu/social/main.jsp?advSearchKey=lltimprep&mode=advancedSubmit&catId=22&doc_submit=&policyArea=0&policyAreaSub=0&country=0&year=0.

European Commission. (2024d). *Report on the implementation of the Council Recommendation on access to affordable high-quality long-term care Ireland*. Retrieved September 27, 2024, from https://ec.europa.eu/social/main.jsp?advSearchKey=lltimprep&mode=advancedSubmit&catId=22&doc_submit=&policyArea=0&policyAreaSub=0&country=0&year=0

European Commission. (2024e). *Report on the implementation of the Council Recommendation on access to affordable high-quality long-term care Italy*. Retrieved September 27, 2024, from https://ec.europa.eu/social/main.jsp?advSearchKey=lltimprep&mode=advancedSubmit&catId=22&doc_submit=&policyArea=0&policyAreaSub=0&country=0&year=0.

European Commission. (2024f). *Report on the implementation of the Council Recommendation on access to affordable high-quality long-term care Greece*. Retrieved October 27, 2024, from https://ec.europa.eu/social/main.jsp?advSearchKey=lltimprep&mode=advancedSubmit&catId=22&doc_submit=&policyArea=0&policyAreaSub=0&country=0&year=0.

European Commission. (2024g). *Report on the implementation of the Council Recommendation on access to affordable high-quality long-term care Spain*. Retrieved September 27, 2024, from https://ec.europa.eu/social/main.jsp?advSearchKey=lltimprep&mode=advancedSubmit&catId=22&doc_submit=&policyArea=0&policyAreaSub=0&country=0&year=0

European Commission. (2024h). *Report on the implementation of the Council Recommendation on access to affordable high-quality long-term care Portugal*. Retrieved September 27, 2024, from https://ec.europa.eu/social/main.jsp?advSearchKey=lltimprep&mode=advancedSubmit&catId=22&doc_submit=&policyArea=0&policyAreaSub=0&country=0&year=0.

European Commission. (2024i). *Report on the implementation of the Council Recommendation on access to affordable high-quality long-term care Bulgaria*. Retrieved October 27, 2024, from https://ec.europa.eu/social/main.jsp?advSearchKey=lltimprep&mode=advancedSubmit&catId=22&doc_submit=&policyArea=0&policyAreaSub=0&country=0&year=0

European Commission. (2024j). *Report on the implementation of the Council Recommendation on access to affordable high-quality long-term care Romania*. Retrieved October 27, 2024, from https://ec.europa.eu/social/main.jsp?advSearchKey=lltimprep&mode=advancedSubmit&catId=22&doc_submit=&policyArea=0&policyAreaSub=0&country=0&year=0

European Parliament. EMPL Committee. (2021). *Ageing policies - access to services in different Member States*. Retrieved October 29, 2024, from https://www.europarl.europa.eu/RegData/etudes/STUD/2021/662940/IPOL_STU(2021)662940_EN.pdf

Fakoya, O. A., McCorry, N. K. & Donnelly, M. (2020). Loneliness and social isolation interventions for older adults: a scoping review of reviews. BMC Public Health 20, 129. https://doi.org/10.1186/s12889-020-8251-6.

Fässberg, M. M., van Orden, K. A., Duberstein, P., Erlangsen, A., Lapierre, S., Bodner, E., Canetto, S. S., De Leo, D., Szanto, K., & Waern, M. (2012). A systematic review of social factors and suicidal behavior in older adulthood. *Int J Environ Res Public Health, 9*(3), 722–745. https://doi.org/10.3390/ijerph9030722

Federal Ministry Republic of Austria (2021). *National Report Austria Fourth review and appraisal of the implementation of the Madrid International Plan of Action on Ageing 2002 and the Regional Implementation Strategy (MIPAA / RIS) 2018–2022*. Retrieved October 30, 2024, from https://unece.org/sites/default/files/2022-01/mipaa20-report-austria.pdf.

Flay, B. R., Biglan, A., Boruch, R. F., Castro, F. G., Gottfredson, D., Kellam, S., Mościcki, E. K., Schinke, S., Valentine, J. C., & Ji, P. (2005). Standards of evidence: Criteria for efficacy, effectiveness and dissemination. *Prevention Science, 6*(3), 151–175. https://doi.org/10.1007/s11121-005-5553-y

Gardiner, C., Geldenhuys, G., & Gott, M. (2018). Interventions to reduce social isolation and loneliness among older people: An integrative review. *Health and Social Care in the Community, 26*(2), 147–157. https://doi.org/10.1111/hsc.12367

Gardiner, C., Laud, P., Heaton, T., & Gott, M. (2020). What is the prevalence of loneliness amongst older people living in residential and nursing care homes? A systematic review and meta-analysis. *Age and Ageing, 49*(5), 748–757. https://doi.org/10.1093/ageing/afaa049

Ghenţa, M., Matei, A., Mladen-Macovei, L., Vasilescu, M. D., & Bobârnat, E.-S. (2021). Sustainable care and factors associated with quality of life among older beneficiaries of social services. *Sustainability, 13*(3), 1572. https://doi.org/10.3390/su13031572

Goldman, N., Khanna, D., El Asmar, M. L., Qualter, P., & El-Osta, A. (2024). Addressing loneliness and social isolation in 52 countries: A scoping review of National policies. *BMC Public Health, 24*, 1207. https://doi.org/10.1186/s12889-024-18370-8

Government of the Republic of Slovenia. (2017). *Active Ageing Strategy*. Retrieved October 30, 2024, from https://www.gov.si/assets/ministrstva/MSP/Direktorat-za-starejse-in-deinstitucionalizacijo/strategije/Active-Ageing-Strategy-2017.pdf.

Hajek, A., Kretzler, B., & König, H.-H. (2021). Informal caregiving, loneliness and social isolation: A systematic review. *International Journal of Environmental Research and Public Health, 18*(22), 12101. https://doi.org/10.3390/ijerph18221210

Holt-Lunstad, J., Smith, T. B., & Layton, J. B. (2010). Social relationships and mortality risk: A meta-analytic review. *PLoS Med, 7*(1), e1000316.

Hwang, T. J., Rabheru, K., Peisah, C., Reichman, W., & Ikeda, M. (2020). Loneliness and social isolation during the COVID-19 pandemic. *International Psychogeriatrics, 32*(10), 1217–1220. https://doi.org/10.1017/S1041610220000988

ISSA (2022). *Priorities for social security trends, challenges and solutions*. Retrieved October 30, 2024, from https://www.issa.int/sites/default/files/documents/2022-04/2-priorities-report-Europe-WEB.pdf.

Kuiper, J. S., Zuidersma, M., Oude Voshaar, R. C., Zuidema, S. U., van den Heuvel, E. R., Stolk, R. P., & Smidt, N. (2015). Social relationships and risk of dementia: A systematic review and meta-analysis of longitudinal cohort studies. *Ageing Research Reviews, 22*, 39–57. https://doi.org/10.1016/j.arr.2015.04.006

Lamura, G., Mnich, E., Bien, B., Krevers, B., McKee, K., Mestheneos, E., & Döhner, H. (2007). Dimensions of future social service provision in the ageing societies of Europe. *Advances in Gerontology, 20*(3), 13–30.

Lamura, G., Mnich, E., Nolan, M., Wojszel, B., Krevers, B., Mestheneos, L., Döhner, H., & EUROFAMCARE Group. (2008). Family carers' experiences using support services in Europe: Empirical evidence from the EUROFAMCARE study. *Gerontologist, 48*(6), 752–771. https://doi.org/10.1093/geront/48.6.752

Lee, E. E., Depp, C., Palmer, B. W., Glorioso, D., Daly, R., Liu, J., Tu, X. M., Kim, H.-C., Tarr, P., Yamada, Y., & Jeste, D. V. (2019). High prevalence and adverse health effects of loneliness in community-dwelling adults across the lifespan: Role of wisdom as a protective factor. *International Psychogeriatrics, 31*(10), 1447–1462. https://doi.org/10.1017/S1041610218002120

Leichsenring, K., Billings, J., & Nies, H. (Eds.). (2013). *Long-term care in Europe: Improving policy and practice*. Palgrave Macmillan.

Mann, F., Bone, J. K., Lloyd-Evans, B., Frerichs, J., Pinfold, V., Ma, R., Wang, J., & Johnson, S. (2017). A life less lonely: The state of the art in interventions to reduce loneliness in people with mental health problems. *Social Psychiatry and Psychiatric Epidemiology, 52*(6), 627–638. https://doi.org/10.1007/s00127-017-1392-y

Masi, C. M., Chen, H.-Y., Hawkley, L. C., & Cacioppo, J. T. (2011). A meta-analysis of interventions to reduce loneliness. *Personality and Social Psychology Review, 15*(3), 219–266.

Ministry for Health and Active Ageing. (2022). *A national health systems strategy for Malta 2023–2030 Investing successfully for a healthy future*. Retrieved October 30, 2024, from https://health.gov.mt/wp-content/uploads/2023/04/A_National_Health_Systems_Strategy_for_Malta_2023_-_2030_Investing_Successfully_for_a_Healthy_Future_EN.pdf.

Ministry of Family Affairs, Integration and the Greater Region. (2019). Practical guide for seniors. Retrieved April 30, 2025 from https://mfsva.gouvernement.lu/dam-assets/publications/guide-manuel/guide-pratique-pour-seniors/Guide-pratique-Seniors-EN.pdf.
Ministry of Family, Labor and Social Policy. (2024). *Care 75+ Program*. Retrieved October 30, 2024, from https://www.gov.pl/web/rodzina/program-opieka-75.
Ministry of Labor and Social Affairs. (2020). *Social inclusion strategy 2021–2030*. Retrieved October 30, 2024, from https://www.mpsv.cz/documents/20142/225517/Social+Inclusion+strategy+2021-2030.pdf/29e5f2c9-3894-6bf5-61ba-ca60ed6fd618.
Ministry of Labor and Social Affairs (2021). *Action Plan 2021–2023 for the Social Inclusion Strategy 2021–2030*. Retrieved October 30, 2024, from https://www.mpsv.cz/documents/20142/225517/Action+Plan+2021%E2%80%932023+for+the+Social+Inclusion+Strategy+2021%E2%80%932030.pdf/a829b513-2977-a23d-f3b9-5d81a93eede5
Ministry of Labor, Family, Social Protection and Elderly. (2015). *National strategy on social inclusion and poverty reduction 2015–2020*. Retrieved October 30, 2024, from https://www.mmuncii.ro/j33/images/Documente/Familie/2016/StrategyVol1EN_web.pdf.
Ministry of Labour and Social Protection. (2021). *Action plan for the period 2022–2027 for the implementation of the national strategy for long-term care*. Retrieved October 30, 2024, from https://www.mlsp.government.bg/uploads/40/sv/draft-action-plan-ltc-2022-2027-final-en.pdf.
Ministry of Social Affairs. (2022a). *Welfare development plan 2023–2030*. Retrieved October 30, 2024, from https://sm.ee/sites/default/files/documents/2023-05/Welfare%20Development%20Plan%202023-2030.pdf.
Ministry of Social Affairs. (2022b). *Annex to the welfare development plan 2023–2030*. Retrieved October 30, 2024, from https://sm.ee/sites/default/files/documents/2023-05/Annex%20to%20the%20Welfare%20Development%20Plan%202023-2030.pdf.
National Academies of Sciences, Engineering, and Medicine; Division of Behavioral and Social Sciences and Education; Health and Medicine Division; Board on Behavioral, Cognitive, and Sensory Sciences; Board on Health Sciences Policy; Committee on the Health and Medical Dimensions of Social Isolation and Loneliness in Older Adults. Social Isolation and Loneliness in Older Adults: Opportunities for the Health Care System. Washington (DC): National Academies Press (US); 2020 Feb 27. Retrieved October 30, 2024, from https://www.ncbi.nlm.nih.gov/books/NBK557974/. https://doi.org/10.17226/25663.
Partou. (2025). *Week against loneliness: Partou brings young and old together*. Retrieved October 30, 2024, from https://partou.nl/en/standing-together-against-loneliness/.
Sandu, V., Zólyomi, E., & Leichsenring, K. (2021). *Addressing loneliness and social isolation among older people in Europe* [Policy brief]. European Centre for Social Welfare Policy and Research. Retrieved October 10, 2024, from https://www.euro.centre.org/publications/detail/4127.
Schulmann, K., & Leichsenring, K. with contributions by Georgia Casanova, Vasilica Ciucă, Lăcrămioara Corcheş, Mihaela Ghenta, Žana Grigaliūnienė, Csaba Kucsera, Aniela Matei, Niku Määttänen, Gerhard Naegele, Gerli Paat-Ahi, Speranţa Pîrciog, Andrea Principi, Leonor Rodrigues, Ricardo Rodrigues, Bertha Sănduleasa, Sandra Schulze, Monika Reichert, Zsuzsa Szeman, Karin Wall. (2014). Social support and long-term care in EU care regimes. Framework conditions and initiatives of social innovation in an active ageing perspective. Retrieved October 30, 2024, from https://mopact.sites.sheffield.ac.uk/publications.
Social Insurance Institution. (2023). Social security in Poland. Retrieved October 30, 2024, from https://lang.zus.pl/documents/493369/574088/Social_security_in_Poland.pdf/8e1a8cad-f6ad-467a-8e81-1fedd2692082?t=1715335149681.
Trukeschitz, B., Österle, A., & Schneider, U. (2022). Austria's long-term care system: Challenges and policy responses. *Journal of LongTerm Care*, 88–101. https://doi.org/10.31389/jltc.112
World Health Organisation. (2017). *National active ageing 2014–2020 Slovak Republic*. Retrieved October 30, 2024, from https://extranet.who.int/countryplanningcycles/sites/default/files/planning_cycle_repository/slovakia/slovakia_en_google.pdf.

World Health Organization. (2021). *Advocacy brief: Social isolation and loneliness among older people.* Retrieved October 30, 2024, from https://iris.who.int/bitstream/handle/10665/343206/9789240030749-eng.pdf?sequence=1.

Yu, B., Steptoe, A., Chen, L.-J., Chen, Y.-H., Lin, C.-H., & Ku, P.-W. (2020). Social isolation, loneliness, and all-cause mortality in patients with cardiovascular disease: A 10-year follow-up study. *Psychosomatic Medicine, 82*(2), 208. https://doi.org/10.1097/PSY.0000000000000777

Zebhauser, A., Hofmann-Xu, L., Baumert, J., Häfner, S., Lacruz, M. E., Emeny, R. T., Döring, A., Grill, E., Huber, D., Peters, A., & Ladwig, K. H. (2014). How much does it hurt to be lonely? Mental and physical differences between older men and women in the KORA-age study. *International Journal of Geriatric Psychiatry, 29*(3), 245–252. https://doi.org/10.1002/gps.3998

Zólyomi, E. (2019). Peer review on "Strategies for supporting social inclusion at older age" [Discussion Paper]. European Commission.

Mihaela Ghenţa is a senior researcher at the National Scientific Institute for Labour and Social Protection (INCSMPS), economist specialised in social management and also a graduate of the Law Faculty of The University of Bucharest. She has extensive experience in social inclusion projects of disadvantaged population groups, labour market, migration, families, and social services for children and older persons. She has been involved in national and international projects in the field of social policies, social services, elderly population, and organisational management, as expert or project coordinator. She has (co)authored several articles/books and participated in numerous national and international conferences.

Aniela Matei is a sociologist, senior researcher within National Scientific Research Institute for Labour and Social Protection (INCSMPS) with a PhD degree in Sociology from the University of Bucharest. She has over 22 years of experience in implementing national and international research projects concerning social policies, including elderly persons (MoPAct- Mobilising the Potential of Acting Ageing in Europe – FP 7 project, Quality of life for Dependent Elderly in Romania and Methodology for continuous monitoring of the quality of care in the institutions providing long-term care services – projects financed by the Romanian Ministry of Labour and Social Protection).

Open Access This chapter is licensed under the terms of the Creative Commons Attribution 4.0 International License (http://creativecommons.org/licenses/by/4.0/), which permits use, sharing, adaptation, distribution and reproduction in any medium or format, as long as you give appropriate credit to the original author(s) and the source, provide a link to the Creative Commons license and indicate if changes were made.

The images or other third party material in this chapter are included in the chapter's Creative Commons license, unless indicated otherwise in a credit line to the material. If material is not included in the chapter's Creative Commons license and your intended use is not permitted by statutory regulation or exceeds the permitted use, you will need to obtain permission directly from the copyright holder.

Chapter 14
Linking Life Course Theory to Multi-Level Explanations of Loneliness: Towards a Sociology of Loneliness

Bianca Suanet and Marja Aartsen

14.1 Introduction

In recent years, there has been a notable surge in recognition of loneliness as a significant societal concern. This is evidenced by the World Health Organization's prioritization of loneliness and increased public discourse and media coverage. Loneliness, defined here as "the unpleasant experience that occurs when a person's network of social relationships is deficient in some important way, either quantitatively or qualitatively" (Perlman & Peplau, 1981, p. 31) is strongly linked to poor mental well-being (Beutel et al., 2017) and higher mortality rates (Wang et al., 2023). It imposes substantial economic burdens on welfare and medical systems (Meisters et al., 2021). Scholarly interest in loneliness has risen, with research output increasing significantly. Despite growing attention, our understanding of loneliness has suffered from "microfication" (Hagestad & Dannefer, 2001; Suanet & Pavlidis, 2025), or the tendency to focus on immediate aspects of everyday life while overlooking the broader, overarching aspects of the social context that define and set key parameters of daily experience. Theoretical and empirical frameworks addressing loneliness have emphasized the individual micro-level and ego-centric social network influences, often neglecting the local and national social context (Rapolienė & Aartsen, 2022; Suanet & van Tilburg, 2019). However, reciprocal interactions between the individual and their immediate and wider external environment, as described in Bronfenbrenner's socio-ecological model (1995), play a crucial role in loneliness prevalence (de Jong Gierveld & Tesch-Römer, 2012). Additionally, research has largely overlooked the impact of cumulative life course

B. Suanet (✉)
Amsterdam, The Netherlands
e-mail: biancasuanet@gmail.com

M. Aartsen
Norwegian Social Research (NOVA), Oslo Metropolitan University, Oslo, Norway

© The Author(s) 2025

M. Aartsen et al. (eds.), *Macro Social Influences on Loneliness in Later Life*, International Perspectives on Aging 47,
https://doi.org/10.1007/978-3-031-94565-6_14

advantage and disadvantage related to specific social categories on loneliness, even though recent studies have begun to adopt a life course perspective (e.g., Victor et al., 2022; Lam et al., 2022; Tiilikainen et al., 2024).

To address existing gaps and incorporate the impact of social context, we propose a Sociological Theory of Loneliness (SOLO). This theory integrates two paradigms of life course theory: the personological paradigm focusing on the individual life course, and the institutional paradigm, focusing on the life course as political construct (Dannefer & Settersten, 2010), while combining these two with Bronfenbrenner's socio-ecological model. SOLO delineates how an individual's later life is shaped by earlier experiences in the life course and the cohort in which one is born, as well as how it is constructed by socio-structural and socio-cultural factors at the meso- and macro-level and individual or micro-level. SOLO further acknowledges that multilevel factors can be linked with loneliness directly or in intersection, and that the impact on loneliness tends to accumulate over the life course. Finally, SOLO considers loneliness as a concept that is fundamentally about experiences in relation to others within a person's environment (Rapolienė & Aartsen, 2022; Suanet & van Tilburg, 2019).

Our objective with SOLO is to provide tools and inspiration for the sociological study of loneliness, thereby justifying our focus on theories within the sociological discipline. We believe that a comprehensive overview of relevant theories in sociology can inspire other scholars in the field to consider meso- and macro level correlates of loneliness to account for variations in loneliness that cannot be solely explained by micro-level factors. To accomplish this, we establish axioms – or basic assumptions - and propositions – or detailed hypotheses - derived from sociological theories and insights to outline a sociology of loneliness that is applicable to empirical research. Additionally, we discuss how SOLO can enhance future research and interventions aimed at alleviating loneliness by considering both the immediate and wider contexts of individuals.

14.2 Towards a Sociological Theory of Loneliness (SOLO)

SOLO integrates the main principles of life course theory and Bronfenbrenner's socio-ecological model to account for variations in loneliness that cannot be solely explained by micro-level factors. Life course theory is a well-established perspective, widely used across the social sciences (Mayer, 2009). Life course theory does not only see individuals as they are today but acknowledges that human development is a lifelong process, partly structured by policies, norms and values, and a person's network of relationships. Life course theory can take different perspectives, but an important distinction lies in the focus of the theory, which can be on the individual life course (the personological paradigm) or on the social and political context (the institutional paradigm) (Dannefer & Settersten, 2010). Within the personological paradigm several principles that shape the life course are distinguished: 1) life-span development, 2) human agency, 3) time and place, 4) timing and 5) linked lives (Elder et al., 2003; Elder, 1998). Applied to loneliness, this means that we see loneliness as a dynamic process that unfolds over the life course. Human agency refers to an individual's talents, choices, actions and skills, enabling them to actively shape their life within the opportunities and constraints provided by their context. Time and place (context) are about the historical time and place in which people live, which influences their current and future circumstances. Timing focuses on when events occur in a person's life course, shaping their experiences and outcomes. Linked lives refer to the networks of relationships that connect individuals to others, influencing their experiences and well-being (Elder et al., 2003).

The institutional paradigm focuses on the social and political structures that construct the life course (Dannefer & Settersten 2010). An important topic in this strand of reasoning is how age norms structure the activities that are appropriate for a certain age group. For example, it structures the timing of leaving the parental home, when one should marry and get children, and what an appropriate age for retirement is. In fact, age norms are seen as "social prescriptions" that will lead to standardized life courses. With respect to loneliness, it means that we acknowledge that the political and social structures of societies in which people live construct the norms about age-appropriateness which can impact loneliness by disturbing the balance between the ideal number and quality of social relations and the achieved number and quality of social relations.

Next to these two paradigms in life course theory, our theory also draws from Bronfenbrenner's socio-ecological model. Bronfenbrenner's model adds to the life course model a specific focus on the different multi-level layers of the context, the interaction between individual agency and this context, especially the structure of society, and it emphasizes the importance of change over historical time due to its focus on the chronosystem. Together, these provide an excellent basis for our theoretical model. In the socio-ecological model, originally focused on childhood development but applicable across the life course, Bronfenbrenner distinguishes between several layers of influence in the environment. In our sociological model of loneliness, we distinguish between four levels. The micro-level system pertains to the individual, including their agency and resources. The meso-system involves relationships with others and the local communities that people live in (linked lives and local community). The macro-system refers to cultural elements influencing loneliness, including cultural norms, standards for social relationships, welfare state regimes and the political context. Finally, and equivalent to Bronfenbrenner's chronosystem, the view of loneliness as a lifelong process that develops further over the life course with transitions and events is also part of our model.

Combining the life course approach with the simplified socio-ecological model of Bronfenbrenner, we argue that the immediate environment and society, intersecting with individual characteristics, exert direct and indirect influences on an individual's development in loneliness over the life course (Fig. 14.1). Our arguments feed into axioms and more concrete propositions for research (Table 14.1). For clarity and parsimony, we assign axioms and propositions to only one level of analysis (micro, meso, or macro), even though principles of intersectionality suggest that these distinctions can be somewhat arbitrary. For instance, the parental family is

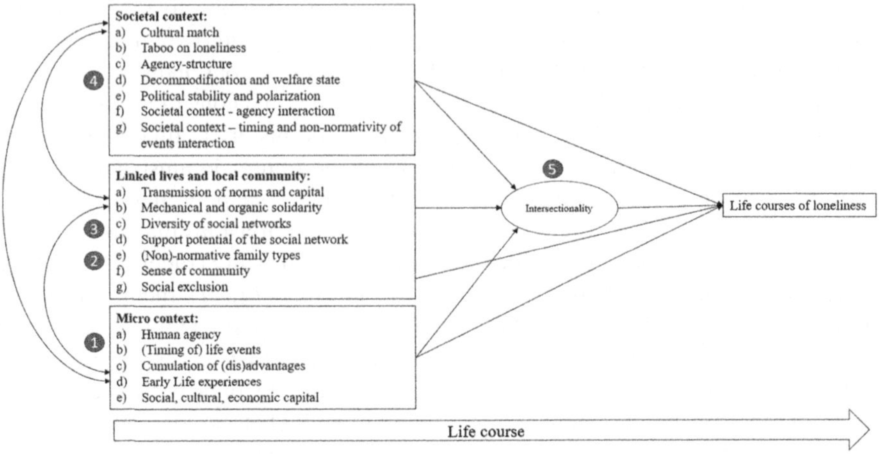

Fig. 14.1 Graphical representation of the various interacting systems contributing to experiences of loneliness across the life course of an individual

Table 14.1 Axioms and propositions for a sociological theory of loneliness

Axioms	Propositions
1. Loneliness trajectories unfold across the life course, and are shaped by human agency, timing of life events, earlier life experiences and the accumulation of disadvantage over time	a) Human agency plays a crucial role in determining individuals' opportunities to develop and maintain a satisfying network within any given context, as well as in bouncing back from negative experiences with loneliness *(agency proposition)* b) It is not what one has, but the comparison with what one had, that exerts the strongest effect on loneliness *(relative deprivation proposition)* c) Off-time and non-normative life events result in increased loneliness as they lead to social disapproval and fewer opportunities for social engagement, but what is considered off-time and non-normative is dependent on the meso and macro culture and structure *(non-normative and off-timing of life events proposition)* d) (Dis)advantages in (the causes) of loneliness tend to accumulate over the life course, resulting in larger intra-cohort variation over time *(cumulative disadvantage proposition)* e) Childhood and adolescent experiences of family and social relationships are important for understanding loneliness in adulthood, particularly concerning socialization, attachment styles, and social capital *(early life experiences proposition)* f) Having more social capital results in less loneliness through more social approval and social opportunities, and this also holds for cultural capital and economic capital that can be used to obtain social capital *(social capital proposition of loneliness)* g) The transmission of norms, values and amount and type of various forms of capital across generations significantly influences the individual's opportunity and agency for being less lonely later in life *(transmission of norms and capital proposition)*

(continued)

Table 14.1 (continued)

Axioms	Propositions
2. Loneliness is strongly influenced by the lives of other people to which they are linked	a) The mechanical solidarity proposition posits that in societies or groups with strong norms and values, those who are born into or belong to such societies or groups will experience higher levels of social integration and lower levels of loneliness. The organic solidarity proposition suggests that in societies with a high degree of labor division, social integration will be stronger, and loneliness will be less prevalent *(mechanical and organic solidarity proposition)* b) Social networks composed of both weak and strong ties play a crucial role in preventing loneliness *(network diversity proposition)* c) If the needs of a person exceed the level of support that is available in the social network, loneliness will increase (*social-convoy proposition)* d) Growing up in non-normative families will increase feelings of loneliness *(non-normative families proposition*)
3. Communities exert important influences on loneliness by providing a sense of community and opportunities for social integration	a) Lack of citizenship rights, insufficient means and inability to lead what is considered 'a normal life' (or a normative life) put people at a disadvantage when it comes to loneliness through anomie, alienation, and lack of opportunity (*Durkheimian sense of community proposition*) b) Disadvantage in loneliness may stem from processes operating at the intersection of micro and meso characteristics, by which people that are more disadvantaged in agency, timing and non-normativity are also more disadvantaged at the meso level of communities *(multi-level intersectionality proposition)*

(continued)

Table 14.1 (continued)

Axioms	Propositions
4. Loneliness derives from an interaction between the societal culture and structure, and the individual, in which the individual has certain opportunities but also standards for social relationships that are influenced strongly by the context	a) Cultural norms and values surrounding social relationships determine the standards that people have for their relationships and, therefore, how their social network impacts their loneliness *(cultural match proposition)* b) The more individualized and postmaterialist the lower the loneliness, as people have more relational freedom, have more emotional support and expression and attach more importance to high quality relationships (*individualization and postmaterialist values proposition*) c) The higher the cultural taboo on stigma and loneliness, the more likely that people become lonely and the less likely that loneliness can be solved effectively within a short time span (*Goffman's taboo and stigma proposition*) d) The stronger the societal ageism in a society, the more likely that older adults will experience loneliness in later life, due to exclusion, discrimination or internalization (*societal ageism proposition*) e) The likelihood of becoming lonely in old age is dependent on the strength and content of gender roles and attitudes, as well as gendered life courses within societies, which impact men and women differently across the life course (*gender role proposition*) f) Social structures and institutions, such as those related to education, work, and associations, are important channels that regulate loneliness through opportunities and constraints they provide to people *(Giddens agency-structure proposition)* g) Welfare states that have more universal rights, and are more generous, are likely to have lower loneliness, by elevating living conditions and reducing poverty which foster social participation and integration but also by making people feel more included and valued (*Esping Andersen's welfare state and de-commodification proposition*) h) Institutions play a role in producing loneliness in old age by policies and regulations that impact on the opportunity and resources to build a satisfying social network (*institutional framework proposition*) i) A political context characterized by political instability, high levels of polarization and low trust in political systems results in higher levels of loneliness as trust towards institutions and others is lower and people experience dividing cleavages in society constraining interactions and social ties (*political instability and polarization proposition*)
5. Loneliness is significantly shaped by overlapping social identities, such as gender, race, socioeconomic status, and disability	a) Agency is more important in cultural contexts that are more individualized, where social structures are more closed and where political systems are more volatile and unstable *(agency * societal context proposition)* b) Being off-time and non-normative in life events is more detrimental to loneliness in more collective cultures and are more strongly regulated socio-structurally *(timing and non-normativity of life events * societal context proposition)*

viewed as a micro factor by some and as a meso factor by others, but we assign it only to the meso-level. Furthermore, sociology as a discipline has a plurality in theoretical perspectives. We selected only those relevant for our SOLO model. This selection of theories is by no means meant to be complete, and there may be other theories that would support the parts of the model equally well. At a minimum, these theories serve as a foundation for scholars to adopt a sociological approach in the study of loneliness.

While Bronfenbrenner's socio-ecological model and life course theory have previously informed approaches to understanding loneliness, such as the HIDECO model (Drewelies et al., 2019) and Luhmann et al.'s model (2023), our approach is distinctive in that it combines the personological and institutional paradigm while considering the interplay between the multi-level factors. SOLO frames how these broader social and environmental factors interact with micro-level influences to explain variations in loneliness that cannot be fully accounted for by individual factors alone. In doing so, SOLO aims to contribute to a better understanding of the significant heterogeneity in late-life loneliness across European countries, shedding light on the paradoxical trend that loneliness is most prevalent in countries with a more collectivistic culture.

14.3 Axioms and Propositions for a Sociological Theory of Loneliness

14.3.1 Micro Context

Axiom 1 *Loneliness trajectories unfold across the life course, and are shaped by human agency, timing of life events, earlier life experiences, and the accumulation of disadvantage over time.*

To better understand the impact of life events and transitions, we need to shift from viewing loneliness as a static state to examining it as a dynamic trajectory, or 'life courses of loneliness'. Studies on loneliness trajectories reveal a diversity of stable and fluctuating patterns over the life course (e.g., Yang, 2018; Lam & Campbell, 2023). Identifying factors that trigger turning points in loneliness trajectories is crucial for developing strategies to reduce or prevent loneliness. However, implications of these patterns are not well-distinguished theoretically or empirically (Archer Lee et al., 2022). Chronic, intense loneliness rather than incidental feelings of loneliness can profoundly affect health and well-being, causing ongoing stress and hopelessness. Therefore, understanding how specific life course trajectories lead to prolonged loneliness, and why some individuals recover more quickly, is imperative.

Human agency is crucial in determining individuals' opportunities to develop and maintain a satisfying network within any given context, as well as in bouncing back from negative experiences with loneliness *(agency proposition)*. At the individual level, the first set of propositions revolves around agency of the individual itself: "Individuals construct their own life course through the choices and actions they take within the opportunities of history and social circumstance." (Elder et al., 2003, p.11). Agency is a very heterogeneous concept both in meaning and in measurement. It encompasses the resources, beliefs, and capacities that individuals possess (Hitlin & Johnson, 2015) and can be utilized to cultivate and sustain gratifying social relationships. Empirical evidence supporting this statement suggests that individuals with greater socio-economic and psychological resources, including mastery and self-efficacy, exhibit lower levels of loneliness (Suanet & van Tilburg, 2019). This correlation is attributable not only to enhanced opportunities for establishing a fulfilling network (Suanet & van Tilburg, 2019), but also to the adoption of more effective active coping strategies aimed at improving social connections, rather than resigning to the situation or rationalizing deficits (Schoenmakers et al., 2012).

Life events that are typically found to induce loneliness are the loss of loved ones, and loss of economic resources and health, rather than not having partner or being poor or in poor health (Aartsen & Jylhä, 2011). It is thus the situation, relative to what one recently had, that might exert the largest effects on loneliness *(relative deprivation proposition)*. The impact of live events on loneliness may also depend on the individual's age and the historical context (timing). According to the age normative perspective, loneliness tends to be lowest among individuals occupying socially expected roles for their age within a given society (Luhmann & Hawkley, 2016). For instance, never being married is associated with increased loneliness in mid and old age but not in young adulthood, where alternative sources of social connection may compensate for the lack of a partner (e.g. Luhmann & Hawkley, 2016). Similarly, employment status plays a crucial role in mitigating loneliness during mid-life, when individuals are expected to be employed, compared to young or old adulthood. The experience of loneliness linked to off-time transitions – for example family formation beyond the normative age – may stem from a decrease in opportunities for fulfilling adequate social ties, leading to a reduced sense of belonging or increased risk of social disapproval faced by those in the off-time or non-normative life states (Zoutewelle-Terovan & Liefbroer, 2018). Our postulate is that the impact of a loneliness-provoking event or transition depends on the individual's age and the historical time and place in which it occurs: off-time and non-normative life events result in increased loneliness due to social disapproval and fewer opportunities for social engagement (*non-normative and off-timing of life events proposition*). Losses of a partner are likely to be more strongly related to emotional loneliness, whereas life events that are non-normative in employment and other social contexts are more likely to impact on social loneliness, as these impact the opportunities for broader network engagement. However, what is considered off-time and non-normative is highly context-dependent. For example, in societies where higher value is placed on the family, off-time family formation will have a stronger impact on loneliness than in more individualistic societies.

Understanding the *dynamic* nature of loneliness requires focusing on cumulative (dis)advantage that enhance or protect against loneliness over the life course and the underlying processes leading to loneliness. According to the cumulative (dis)advantage perspective, an individual's experiences of loneliness are influenced by protecting or risk-full conditions earlier in life which tend to accumulate (Dannefer, 2020), leading to an increasing intra-cohort variation in loneliness over time *(cumulative disadvantage proposition).* A recent study showed that negative childhood experiences, such as the early death of parents or growing up in an apathetic family, lead to more severe loneliness trajectories in later life after the age of 65 (Tiilikainen et al., 2024). Recent qualitative research among older adults also suggests that family support earlier in life is crucial for later-life loneliness partly because of the support itself but also in creating a sense of belonging (Lam et al., 2022). Family support can thus accumulate social capital, akin to Kahn and Antonucci's 'support bank' idea, which emphasizes support given and received in close relationships over time (Antonucci et al., 2014). Hence, childhood and adolescent experiences of family and social relationships are crucial for understanding adult loneliness, particularly concerning socialization, sense of belonging, and attachment styles (*early life experiences proposition*). We expect these early life experiences to impact on both emotional and social loneliness, with attachment styles impacting on both emotional and social loneliness by setting patterns of interaction and emotional disclosure, whereas the social capital of parents might impact more on social loneliness due to building skills and opportunities for broader network engagement.

In line with the cumulative disadvantages proposition and the early life experiences proposition, social mobility scholars also argue that people's social background and the forms of capital owned by the family of origin account for much of a person's later capital through social reproduction, status attainment, and social mobility (e.g., Bourdieu & Passeron, 1990; Lee, 2025). In general, it can be expected that the more capital one gets from the family in which they are born, whether economic, cultural and social, the lower the loneliness will be, through more opportunities for social participation (*capital proposition of loneliness*). For example, economic resources stimulate active citizenship which increases opportunities for social contact, a good cultural understanding makes it easier to understand how and with whom to connect, and a lack of bridging and bonding (Granovetter, 1973) social capital hinders the making of new social connections. The impact of social mobility, on individual well-being or loneliness is however not so clear from the outset and needs to be examined more in-depth. On one hand, social mobility increases a person's agency, which is important for combating loneliness. On the other hand, social mobility can be disruptive, separating individuals from a sense of community and social support, a concept known as the dissociative hypothesis (Sorokin, 1959), though evidence for this hypothesis is weak (Chan, 2018).

14.3.2 Linked Lives

Axiom 2 *Loneliness is strongly influenced by the lives of other people to whom they are linked.*

In life course theory, the principle that networks of relationships influence an individual's experiences and well-being is known as the linked lives principle (Elder, 1998). Life does not unfold in a vacuum but rather an individual is embedded within a network of other people whose behaviors, resources, and health status can have profound impact on loneliness (Luo, 2023). The various types of capital discussed in the previous paragraph, possessed by, for example, the parents, influence their children's social capital by imparting socialization within their networks and teaching them social skills necessary for maintaining relationships. This is because various types of capital are transmitted across generations, reproducing societal inequalities. Bourdieu and Passeron (1990) described how individuals from families with greater cultural capital (institutionalized, embodied, and objectified forms like formal education, highbrow cultural participation, and cultural goods) are more likely to adopt socially desirable lifestyles. This leads to stronger connections with similar individuals and increased social approval. This process perpetuates social capital across generations. During socialization and attachment formation, initial interactions occur within the family unit. The *transmission proposition* holds that norms, values, attachment styles, and various forms of capital (economic, social, cultural) passed across generations significantly influence individuals' opportunities and ability to form satisfying social networks later in life.

The idea of linked lives is also central in the thinking of many great scholarly works such as in Durkheim's work on social integration and Antonucci's social convoy theory (2014), that focus on the division of labour and the interplay of personal and situational characteristics to understand what people's networks and support systems are. In Durkheim's work "the division of labor in society", the key mechanism for social integration is explained by two types of solidarity. Mechanical solidarity, as interpreted and discussed by Edles and Appelrouth (2010), stems from the collective norms and values of a society in which a person is born and raised. These norms and values are internalized by the individual and stimulate people to cooperate with other people of the same society. The second type is organic solidarity. Through the division of labor and the ongoing specialization of tasks, people become increasingly dependent on other people who can master crucial functions that are not mastered by the individual themselves (Edles & Appelrouth, 2010). With respect to loneliness, this work suggests at least two propositions. The *mechanical solidarity proposition* posits that in societies or groups with strong norms and values, people who share the same norms and values will experience higher levels of social integration and lower levels of loneliness. The *organic solidarity proposition* suggests that social integration can also be created by a high degree of interdependence for example, when there is an extensive specialization of labor. However, while a high degree of interdependence can foster social integration, it does not necessarily serve as a safeguard against loneliness. Loneliness emerges from a discrepancy between an individual's desired and actual state of social relationships. The relational connections established through an elevated division of labor may not fulfill an individual's requirements for social interaction.

In Granovetter's influential work on "The Strength of Weak Ties" (1973), the focus is on how information spreads through strong and weak ties. Weak ties, characterized by limited time investments and low levels of emotional intensity, intimacy, and reciprocity, can benefit individuals by serving as bridges to other social groups and networks, offering opportunities to form new friendships. Recent research by Lam et al. (2023) applies Granovetter's theory to understand variations in loneliness in relation to the number of strong and weak ties. They found that having more weak ties is associated with lower levels of loneliness, while a higher frequency of contact with strong ties, rather than the sheer number, is linked to reduced loneliness. This underscores the importance of both weak and strong ties in the social network combating loneliness, suggesting that a diverse network combining the two offers the best protection *(network diversity proposition)*. This aligns with Suanet and van Tilburg's (2019) findings that loneliness is lower in individuals with larger, more diverse social networks and active community participation. These network and tie factors are more likely to impact social loneliness, as they are about ties to and integration in the broader community.

In Antonucci's work on social relations, the focus is on how individuals are surrounded by other people who move with them through the life course as a convoy of social relations (e.g., Antouncci et al., 2014). This social convoy contributes to the individual's health and well-being through the provision of support. The interplay between personal characteristics (e.g., needs, gender, age) and situational characteristics (e.g., culture, norms, or context) defines the composition of the social network and support available in the network, which in turn leads to a chain of responses in the support potential of the network, the quality of relations and finally the individual's well-being and quality of life. Applied to the study of loneliness, our *social convoy proposition* states that if the needs of a person exceed the level of support that is available in the social network, loneliness will increase.

Families often form a secure base, and alongside the importance of parent-child relations for socialization (Axiom 1), the family as a whole is linked to later-life loneliness (Heshmati et al., 2021). Earlier, three-generation families and the later nuclear families with a father, mother, and children may have offered better protection against loneliness than the more diverse or hybrid family structures during times when extended families or nuclear families were the norm. However, changes in family formation due to increased divorce rates, remarriage creating blended families, and housing market issues forcing young adults to leave the family later complicate this picture. While the network diversity proposition implies that hybrid families might be more suited to protect against loneliness than traditional nuclear families, prevailing norms about the ideal family structure and loyalty conflicts with biological versus stepparents can create tensions that nullify the beneficial impact of a mixed family structure. Moreover, not all families provide a secure base; some can be dysfunctional, significantly affecting the well-being of those raised in such environments (Rokach & Chan, 2021). Non-traditional family structures might impact both emotional and social loneliness. Empirical research on family types and loneliness is scarce but crucial, given the family's role in shaping psychosocial skills, surpassing capital, and interactions with other social institutions. The suitability of extended, nuclear, or hybrid families in protecting against loneliness depends on the prevailing norms for family formation within a specific place and time and on the quality of the family relations *(non-normative families proposition).*

14.3.3 Local Communities

Axiom 3 *Communities exert important influences on loneliness by providing a sense of community and opportunities for social integration.*

While there is no unifying definition of communities, the basic understanding is that they involve people who interact and share the same values, behavior and beliefs, creating a sense of community that can be linked to loneliness (Prezza et al., 2001; Lim et al., 2021). We expect social loneliness to be more impacted by communities as they set the stage for how people can interact with their broader network. The local area and neighborhoods are types of communities that are important arenas for social integration because of their proximity. Neighbors can easily provide support and together with the built and natural environment, create a sense of community that often increases linearly with length of residency (Prezza et al., 2001). Communities can also be geographically dispersed such as with ethnic or professional communities, communities of volunteers, or internet communities, where the sense of community is based on shared values and beliefs, akin to mechanical solidarity. While communities are important for social integration, they are at the same time exclusionary, as communities draw lines between the members and non-members of the community (Etzioni, 2000). Only the members can profit from this sense of community and be protected against loneliness. Communities thus act as a 'double edged sword'; on the one hand creating the embeddedness of similar people while excluding those that are different. While the embeddedness in a community fulfills the desire for social connections and hence reduces loneliness, for those that are excluded, loneliness increases. Exclusion from communities can also result in what Durkheim terms anomie, the disconnection felt by the individual occurring when solidarity is threatened. As Abrutyn (2019) noted, anomie can result from three processes: dissolution, the breakdown of social bonds between individuals or between an individual and a group; dislocation, the detachment from one's physical and social environment, where identity is anchored; or disjunction, a mismatch between societal standards and an individual's values, achievements, and opportunities. *(Sense of community proposition).*

14.3.4 Social Context: Culture and Structure

Axiom 4 *Loneliness derives from an interaction between the societal culture and structure, and the individual, in which the individual has certain opportunities, but also standards for social relationships that are strongly influenced by the context.*

The third layer of Bronfenbrenner's model refers to the social context, which is similar to the institutional paradigm. We distinguish between culture and structure as two fundamentally different macro-sociological concepts and argue that both can shape loneliness in different ways. By culture, we mean the shared beliefs, values, and behaviors that provide a sense of identity and belonging, which are passed on to the next generations. Structure refers to the rules and institutions that guide social behavior, including norms, schools, workplaces, governments, political systems, and family formation. The relationship between structure and culture is interconnected and reciprocal. For example, institutions and organizations provide a framework for social interactions and shape the way people think, feel, and behave. At the same time, culture influences and shapes social structures, as shared beliefs and values can affect the way institutions are organized and maintained.

14.3.5 Culture

Culture profoundly influences loneliness by setting the standards for social relationships through shared norms and beliefs about what makes relationships meaningful. It dictates which types of relationships should offer specific kinds of social support and how individuals are integrated into social networks (Heu et al., 2021). The greater the alignment between social relationships and cultural ideals, the less loneliness is experienced *(the cultural match proposition)*. While existing research has predominantly focused on the individualism/collectivism continuum (Swader, 2019; Heu et al., 2021), studies suggest that individualized cultures in Northern and Western Europe, with reduced expectations regarding others and especially family members, contribute to lower rates of loneliness, termed the "cultural paradox" of loneliness (Heu et al., 2021). As indicated in Chap. 3 of this book by van Tilburg (2025), culture impacts loneliness via togetherness and individual standards, as well as autonomy and social norms that impact the personal network and then also loneliness.

Expanding cultural context studies to comprehend loneliness beyond the traditional individualism/collectivism framework is a crucial next step. One important and related aspect to individualism to consider is the prevalence of post-material values within a society (Inglehart, 2009). As individuals increasingly prioritize quality of life over material possessions, there's a potential for stronger social ties to develop. This shift in focus from material to immaterial aspects of relationships may lead to an emphasis on high-quality interactions, fostering deeper connections, but can also result in elevated standards. Furthermore, communication styles and goals within different cultures might play a significant role in influencing loneliness (Burleson, 2003). Some cultures prioritize affective communication, emphasizing emotional support exchange in relationships. In contrast, others may focus more on instrumental and transactional communication goals. In such cultures, where emotional disclosure is less prevalent, loneliness may originate and persist despite regular social contact. Cultures that endorse individualist and post-materialist mindsets may facilitate emotional support seeking more, as it's not perceived as disrupting the social environment (*individualization and post-material values proposition*).

Cultural taboos about loneliness are also known to vary across cultures, impacting loneliness prevalence and experience (Goffman, 1963; Pescosolido & Martin, 2015). In cultures where loneliness is taboo, discussing and seeking solutions may be less straightforward, potentially increasing loneliness. Coping strategies in these cultures might be more passive, rationalizing deficits rather than actively improving relationships, which is less effective in reducing loneliness (Schoenmakers et al.,

2012). Fear of the stigma of being seen as lonely reinforces this cycle, especially in collective cultures where 'loss of face' is a concern. Power distance, encompassing deference to higher status individuals, can also influence relationship formation and trust (Hofstede Insights, 2024).

A cultural aspect that is central in the institutional paradigm is age norms. Age norms prescribe what a person at a certain age is supposed to do, and violating the norm can be sanctioned (Dannefer & Settersten, 2010). In countries where age-normative systems are strong, societal ageism can occur, which refers to the systematic stereotyping and discrimination against individuals based on their age. Societal ageism can occur in all age groups, but it is most often discussed in relation to older adults (Ayalon & Tesch-Römer, 2017). Research has shown that ageism can increase social inequalities (Ayalon & Tesch-Römer, 2017) and lead to social isolation and reduced opportunities for engagement, contributing to feelings of loneliness among older individuals (Shiovitz-Ezra et al., 2018). As ageist attitudes are prevalent in media representations, workplace practices, and healthcare systems, older adults may internalize these stereotypes, further exacerbating their feelings of worthlessness and isolation. Additionally, social rejection can lead older adults to avoid and withdraw from social participation, increasing feelings of loneliness. Finally, discriminatory practices based on age can result in social exclusion, further heightening the risk of loneliness among older adults. Ultimately, the pervasive nature of ageism throughout the life course can hinder social connections and emotional well-being, making older adults particularly vulnerable to loneliness when ageism is stronger (*societal ageism proposition*).

Finally, within the broader framework of culture, gender roles and attitudes within a population are also likely to impact on loneliness. Gendered life courses, as described by Barbara Moen, refer to the distinct pathways that individuals experience throughout their lives based on their gender (2011). These pathways are shaped by societal norms, expectations, and roles associated with being male or female, influencing aspects such as education, career, family life, and retirement. The impact of gendered life courses on loneliness can be significant. For instance, traditional gender roles may lead women to prioritize caregiving and family responsibilities, potentially limiting their social interactions and leading to feelings of isolation if their roles shift, such as during retirement or after children leave home. Conversely, men might experience loneliness due to societal pressures to be self-reliant and avoid emotional expression, making it difficult for them to seek social support. Overall, the constraints of gendered life courses can affect individuals' social connections and emotional well-being, contributing to loneliness in various ways (*gender roles proposition*).

14.3.6 Structure

Structure refers to the formal and informal rules and norms as well as institutions, welfare systems and political systems that shape and constrain individual behavior. In his work on structuration theory, Giddens (1990) argued that people's behavior is not only the result of their own agency, but also of the institutions in society that have already set-up rules and systems that create or diminish opportunities and constraints for people's behavior, including socially. As such, we argue that social structures are important channels that regulate loneliness through the opportunities and constraints they provide to people to gain and maintain a supportive network *(agency-structure proposition)*.

The concept of the welfare state regime, first discussed by Esping-Andersen (1990), has been instrumental in understanding the macro structure's role in loneliness (e.g., Nyqvist et al., 2019). Welfare states with greater de-commodification by universality and generosity in social rights are likely to experience lower levels of loneliness (*welfare state and de-commodification proposition*). De-commodification refers to the degree to which individuals or families, can uphold a socially acceptable standard of living independently of market participation (Esping-Andersen, 1990). Such states improve living conditions, reduce poverty, and foster social participation and integration. Nyqvist et al. (2019) found the lowest loneliness rates in Nordic welfare regimes (e.g., Norway, Sweden), attributed to universal social rights, full employment, strong state intervention, and redistribution. Continental regimes (e.g., Germany, France) had slightly higher but still relatively low loneliness rates, prioritizing employment and family roles. The Anglo-Saxon regime (e.g., UK), despite limited service-provision, showed relatively low loneliness rates, possibly due to civil society associations and informal sociability compensating for limited state support. Southern and Eastern European states, with less developed welfare services, reported significantly higher loneliness rates among older adults. Focusing on the impact of specific welfare state policies and the intersection of welfare states with other macro-level factors such as cultural norms and political climate is needed for the future. In addition to the role of welfare states societal expectations and norms regarding age, employment, and familial responsibilities that are translated into structural policies and regulations concerning, for example, retirement age (sometimes varying by gender) and care obligations can create rigid pathways that limit personal agency and also have an impact on what their network looks like and how adequate they perceive their quantity and quality of ties to be. For example, heightening retirement ages can keep non-kin in the network longer but might give less time for familial roles, and it is yet unclear how these policies impact loneliness and via which mechanisms.

Finally, the broader political context is known to shape loneliness across the life course. An unstable, polarized political climate with low faith in the system intensifies loneliness due to diminishing trust in institutions and societal divisions limiting social interactions (*political instability and polarization proposition*). Rapolienė and Aartsen (2022) found increased loneliness in post-totalitarian Eastern Europe, attributed to lower general trust, likely rooted in historical violence and deportation experiences, which curtail social engagement. Loneliness and polarization might reciprocally affect each other, as loneliness can also lower trust in others (Langenkamp, 2023). High societal polarization potentially hampers the formation of quality relationships, erodes trust, and triggers interpersonal conflicts.

14.3.7 Intersectionality

Axiom 5 *Loneliness is significantly shaped by overlapping social identities, such as gender, race, socioeconomic status, and disability.*

Intersectionality, introduced by Crenshaw in the late 1980s, is widely used as a framework to understand how social identities such as race, gender or socio-economic status interact and create oppression and dissimilar access to resources (see also Chapters 2 and 6 of this book; Nyqvist et al., 2025; Lee, 2025). For instance, an older woman of color may face compounded stigma and social barriers, leading to greater isolation and loneliness than her peers. Additionally, these intersecting identities can influence access to resources and support networks, further exacerbating feelings of loneliness and social exclusion of those in disadvantaged positions. Consistent with this theoretical perspective and the idea of multi-level influences on loneliness, we contend that processes at one social level can alter the effects of processes at other levels, and that disadvantage on any of these levels can interact with other disadvantages to create a disadvantage that is larger than the sum of its parts. For example, older individuals or people with functional limitations (micro) may be more strongly affected by deprived neighborhoods (meso) due to their heightened reliance on local environments and restricted relocation opportunities (Scharf & de Jong Gierveld, 2008). Additionally, the macro cultural and structural influences likely moderate the relationship between agency and the timing of life events on loneliness. Agency is probably more significant in individualistic cultures with closed social structures, less generous welfare states, and volatile political systems, where personal actions are crucial for building satisfying social networks (*agency * societal context proposition*). In such contexts, active participation in shaping relationships is necessary and likely preferred (Allan, 2008). In more individualized cultures and less supportive welfare states, individuals must also compensate for weaker state support through personal actions in relationships. Moreover, being off-time or experiencing non-normative life events likely has a more detrimental effect on loneliness in more collective cultures, where socio-structural regulations are stricter and punishment for deviating from norms may be harsher, as well as in societies where welfare states have fewer universal rights and are less generous (*the timing and non-normativity of life events * societal context proposition*). For example, a late life-divorce as a non-normative life event would have more impact on the life chances and loneliness of those in less generous welfare states and the stigma would also be higher in more collectivistic cultures. Overall, exploring the intersections of culture, structure, individual agency, and life events could provide valuable insights into why certain individuals experience loneliness in specific macro contexts but not in others.

14.4 Implications for Future Research and Practice

In the above, we have described how the immediate environment and larger societal structures can both directly and indirectly affect an individual's trajectory in loneliness. This sociological approach to loneliness clarifies how loneliness is not only shaped by individual or micro-level conditions, but also socially constructed. This offers an important addition to the previously often individualistic or psychological approach to loneliness. In doing so, we aim to achieve a more comprehensive understanding of loneliness, which is informative for future research on loneliness, and for more effective, systemic strategies for prevention and reduction. In this section, summarized in Table 14.2, we discuss the implications of this sociological approach for research and practice.

The first implication of a sociological approach to loneliness is that for a better understanding of the origins of loneliness, research should focus on cross-level

Table 14.2 Implications for future research and practice

1. Research on loneliness should look at the interaction between micro- meso- and macro- factors in loneliness trajectories of people and focus on diversity in trajectories for different people	a) Rather than looking at average levels and change of loneliness, we need to investigate subgroup differences in loneliness trajectories to determine how the context has a different impact for different social groups *(diversity in loneliness trajectories across time and space focus)* b) Rather than taking only the individual as the unit of analysis, cross-level interactions between individual characteristics and meso- and macro-factors should be investigated to better understand the origins of loneliness *(cross-level interaction focus)* c) We need to move towards a harmonization of (international, national and regional) data sources in order to be able to compare different contexts and groups to each other, to get a tighter grip on explanations for variations. *(comparative contextual loneliness research focus)*
2. Interventions to counter loneliness will become more effective if they consider the meso and macro-context that can be used to prevent and cure loneliness rather than only focusing on 'curing' the lonely individual	a) By shifting the focus on prevention and curing of loneliness by communities and societies we acknowledge that loneliness is in its core a relational concept *(need for prevention and curation of loneliness by communities and society focus)* b) By focusing on societal frames in policies and interventions to lower loneliness, we lower taboo and stigma on loneliness as we make it a shared issue that we discuss within society *(taboo and stigma intervention focus)* c) Rather than taking a one size fits all approach, we need to tailor interventions for loneliness to the wishes, norms and values of the people that are being targeted *(need for culturally sensitive interventions)*

interactions between individual characteristics and societal factors. Intersectionality factors like gender, age, and ethnicity are crucial in understanding why some individuals face lifelong loneliness while others do not (Burholt & Aartsen, 2021). Research should explore subgroup and individual variation in loneliness trajectories, focusing on cumulative disadvantages across the life course and generations. This approach can reveal how some experience persistent loneliness due to accumulated disadvantages, while others may find personal growth through solitude (Archer Lee et al., 2022). The adverse effects of loneliness on health and well-being are likely to be more pronounced among those experiencing it intensely over a longer period with limited options for network activation (Shiovitz-Ezra & Ayalon, 2010). This also demonstrates how different social groups within a context may be advantaged in becoming and recovering from loneliness.

Another implication of a sociology of loneliness is that it informs the development of effective interventions and assigns broader responsibility for addressing loneliness. Current interventions, such as offering social activities and improving social skills, vary substantially in their effectiveness (Hickin et al., 2021). Recognizing loneliness as arising from interactions between individuals and their contexts, interventions should also focus on creating inclusive societies and institutions that promote high-quality social interactions and provide a sense of purpose and meaning in relationships (see also Chap. 13 of this book on interventions; Ghenta & Matei, 2025). Chater and Loewenstein (2023) recently argued that public policy and interventions for social issues should focus more on systemic solutions (S-frame) rather than only focus on an individual frame (I-frame). Such a view resonates with framing loneliness as a social justice issue as well (Barreto et al., 2024). Hence, a focus on 'curing' loneliness among individuals needs to be complemented with a dual strategy that includes establishing communities and societies that integrate people more strongly and make them more resilient to and prevent long-lasting and intense loneliness, as well as early life course interventions to ensure that people develop satisfying networks capable of coping with inevitable losses associated with aging, especially towards the end of life. In such a strategy, social integration of individuals would be actively promoted and enhanced by the cultural and structural elements of the context, such as workplaces, education, neighborhood associations, cultural norms and social policies. Rather than adopting a one-size-fits-all approach imposed by scholars and policymakers, interventions for loneliness need to be tailored to the wishes, norms, and values of the people being targeted, to obtain culturally sensitive interventions based on lived experience.

14.5 To Conclude

While a sociological theory of loneliness is an important step in our further understanding of loneliness, it is by no means a grand theory of loneliness that makes all other theories obsolete. On the contrary, addressing loneliness effectively requires a holistic and interdisciplinary approach. Sociological theories should be complemented with psychological theories, such as attachment and resource allocation models (Huxhold et al., 2022), and public health perspectives that view loneliness as social pain (Cacioppo & Cacioppo, 2018). As research on loneliness is quickly expanding worldwide, it's crucial to recognize that our views are often shaped by a (neo-liberal) policy context that emphasizes individual responsibility for loneliness, rather than framing it as a societal issue. We posit that a sociological perspective incorporating life course principles, such as cumulative disadvantage and linked lives, along with consideration of the meso- and macro-contexts influencing individuals (structure), can enhance our understanding of loneliness. Furthermore, exploring how individuals reciprocally impact these contexts (agency) provides additional insight. This comprehensive approach allows us to view loneliness not merely as an abstract phenomenon, but fundamentally as individuals' subjective experiences of their relationships with others. A sociological approach to loneliness can also contribute to more inclusive and just societies, benefiting not only those with advantageous life courses but everyone. Unlocking this yet under-explored potential can contribute to better mitigating loneliness in our populations.

Competing Interests The authors have no conflict of interest to declare that are relevant to the content of this chapter.

References

Aartsen, M., & Jylhä, M. (2011). Onset of loneliness in older adults: Results of a 28 year prospective study. *European Journal of Ageing, 8*(1), 31–38. https://doi.org/10.1007/s10433-011-0175-7

Abrutyn, S. (2019). Toward a general theory of anomie: The social psychology of disintegration. *European Journal of Sociology, 60*(1), 109–136. https://doi.org/10.1017/S0003975619000043

Allan, G. (2008). Flexibility, friendship, and family. *Personal Relationships, 15*(1), 1–16. https://doi.org/10.1111/j.1475-6811.2007.00181.x

Antonucci, T. C., Ajrouch, K. J., & Birditt, K. S. (2014). The convoy model: Explaining social relations from a multidisciplinary perspective. *The Gerontologist, 54*(1), 82–92. https://doi.org/10.1093/geront/gnt118

Archer Lee, Y., Lay, J. C., Pauly, T., Graf, P., & Hoppmann, C. A. (2022). The differential roles of chronic and transient loneliness in daily prosocial behavior. *Psychology and Aging, 37*(5), 614–625. https://doi.org/10.1037/pag0000681

Ayalon, L., & Tesch-Römer, C. (2017). Taking a closer look at ageism: self- and other-directed ageist attitudes and discrimination. European Journal of Ageing, 14(1), 1–4

Barreto, M., Doyle, D. M., & Qualter, P. (2024). Changing the narrative: Loneliness as a social justice issue. *Advances in Political Psychology, 45*(51), 157–181. https://doi.org/10.1111/pops.12965

Beutel, M. E., Klein, E. M., Brähler, E., et al. (2017). Loneliness in the general population: Prevalence, determinants and relations to mental health. *BMC Psychiatry, 17*, 97. https://doi.org/10.1186/s12888-017-1262-x

Bourdieu, P., & Passeron, C. (1990). *Reproduction in education, society and culture*. Sage.

Bronfenbrenner, U. (1995). Developmental ecology through space and time: A future perspective. In P. Moen, G. H. Elder Jr., & K. Lüscher (Eds.), *Examining lives in context: Perspectives on the ecology of human development* (pp. 619–647). American Psychological Association. https://doi.org/10.1037/10176-018

Burholt, V., & Aartsen, M. (2021). Introduction: Framing exclusion from social relations. In K. Walsh et al. (Eds.), *Social exclusion in later life, international perspectives on aging* (Vol. 28). https://doi.org/10.1007/978-3-030-51406-8_6

Burleson, B. R. (2003). The experience and effects of emotional support: What the study of cultural and gender differences can tell us about close relationships, emotion, and interpersonal communication. *Personal Relationships, 10*(1), 1–23. https://doi.org/10.1111/1475-6811.00033

Cacioppo, J. L., & Cacioppo, S. (2018). Loneliness in the modern age: An evolutionary theory of loneliness (ETL). *Advances in Experimental Social Psychology, 59*, 127–197. https://doi.org/10.1016/bs.aesp.2018.03.003

Chan, T. W. (2018). Social mobility and the well-being of individuals. *British Journal of Sociology, 69*(1), 183–206. https://doi.org/10.1111/1468-4446.12285

Chater, N., & Loewenstein, G. (2023). The i-frame and the s-frame: How focusing on individual-level solutions has led behavioral public policy astray. *Behavioral and Brain Sciences, 46*, e147. https://doi.org/10.1017/S0140525X22002023

Dannefer, D. (2020). Systemic and reflexive: Foundations of cumulative dis/advantage and life-course processes. *The Journals of Gerontology. Series B, Psychological Sciences and Social Sciences, 75*(6), 1249–1263. https://doi.org/10.1093/geronb/gby118

Dannefer, D., & Settersten, R. A., Jr. (2010). The study of the life course: Implications for social gerontology. In D. Dannefer & C. Phillipson (Eds.), The SAGE handbook of social gerontology (pp. 3–19). SAGE Publications.

De Jong Gierveld, J., & Tesch-Römer, C. (2012). Loneliness in old age in eastern and Western European societies: Theoretical perspectives. *European Journal of Ageing, 9*(4), 285–295. https://doi.org/10.1007/s10433-012-0248-2

Drewelies, J., Huxhold, O., & Gerstorf, D. (2019). The role of historical change for adult development and aging: Towards a theoretical framework about the how and the why. *Psychology and Aging, 34*(8), 1021–1039. https://doi.org/10.1037/pag0000423

Edles, L. D., & Appelrouth, S. (2010). *Sociological theory in the classical era. Text and readings*. California State University, Pine Forge Press.

Elder, G. H. (1998). The life course as developmental theory. *Child Development, 69*(1), 1–12. https://doi.org/10.2307/1132065

Elder, G. H., Johnson, M. K., & Crosnoe, R. (2003). The emergence and development of life course theory. In J. T. Mortimer & M. J. Shanahan (Eds.), *Handbook of the life course. Handbooks of sociology and social research*. Springer. https://doi.org/10.1007/978-0-306-48247-2_1

Esping-Andersen, G. (1990). The three political economies of the welfare state. *International Journal of Sociology, 20*(3), 92–123. http://www.jstor.org/stable/20630041

Etzioni, A. (2000). Creating good communities and good societies. *Contemporary Sociology, 29*(1), 188–195. https://doi.org/10.2307/2654943

Ghența, M., & Matei, A. (2025). Policy recommendations to address loneliness in later life. In M. Aartsen, I. Precupetu, & B. Suanet (Eds.), *Macro social influences on loneliness in later life: Towards a better understanding of the loneliness paradox in later life*. Springer.

Giddens, A. (1990). *The consequences of modernity*. Polity Press.

Goffman, E. (1963). *Stigma. Notes on the Management of Spoiled Identity*. Penguin Books.

Granovetter, M. S. (1973). The strength of weak ties. *American Journal of Sociology, 78*(6), 1360–1380. https://www.jstor.org/stable/2776392.

Hagestad, G. O., & Dannefer, D. (2001). Concepts and theories of aging: Beyond microfication in social science approaches. In R. Binstock & L. George (Eds.), *Handbook of aging and the social sciences* (2nd ed.). Academic.

Heshmati, S., Blackard, M. B., Beckmann, B., & Chipidza, W. (2021). Family relationships and adolescent loneliness: An application of social network analysis in family studies. *Journal of Family Psychology, 35*(2), 182–191. https://doi.org/10.1037/fam0000660

Heu, L. C., van Zomeren, M., & Hansen, N. (2021). Does loneliness thrive in relational freedom or restriction? The culture-loneliness framework. *Review of General Psychology, 25*(1), 60–72. https://doi.org/10.1177/1089268020959033

Hickin, N., Käll, A., Shafran, R., Sutcliffe, S., Manzotti, G., & Langan, D. (2021). The effectiveness of psychological interventions for loneliness: A systematic review and meta-analysis. *Clinical Psychology Review, 88*, 102066. https://doi.org/10.1016/j.cpr.2021.102066

Hitlin, S., & Johnson, M. K. (2015). Reconceptualizing agency within the life course: The Power of looking ahead. *American Journal of Sociology, 120*(5), 1429–1472. https://doi.org/10.1086/681216

Hofstede Insights. (2024). *Country Scores*. Available online at: https://www.hofstede-insights.com/product/compare-countries/. Accessed May 30, 2024.

Huxhold, O., Fiori, K. L., & Windsor, T. (2022). Rethinking social relationships in adulthood: The differential investment of resources model. *Personality and Social Psychology Review, 26*(1), 57–82. https://doi.org/10.1177/10888683211067035

Inglehart, R. (2009). Postmaterialist values and the shift from survival to self-expression values. In R. J. Dalton & H.-D. Klingemann (Eds.), *The Oxford handbook of political behavior* (online ed.). Oxford Academic. https://doi.org/10.1093/oxfordhb/9780199270125.003.0012

Lam, J., Broccatelli, C., & Baxter, J. (2023). Diversity of strong and weak ties and loneliness in older adults. *Journal of Aging Studies, 64*, 101097. https://doi.org/10.1016/j.jaging.2022.101097

Lam, J., Dickson, C., & Baxter, J. (2022). Ageing and loneliness: A life course and cumulative disadvantage approach. In J. Baxter, J. Lam, J. Povey, R. Lee, & S. R. Zubrick (Eds.), *Family dynamics over the life course: Foundations, turning points and outcomes* (pp. 279–296). Springer. https://doi.org/10.1007/978-3-031-12224-8_13

Lam, J., & Campbell, A. (2023). Trajectories of loneliness among older women and men: Variation by sexual identity? *The Gerontologist, 63*(2), 328–337. https://doi.org/10.1093/geront/gnac058

Langenkamp, A. (2023). The influence of loneliness on perceived connectedness and trust beliefs—longitudinal evidence from The Netherlands. *Journal of Social and Personal Relationships, 40*(7), 2298–2322. https://doi.org/10.1177/02654075221144716

Lee, S. (2025). Understanding late-life loneliness: Micro and meso-level determinants. In M. Aartsen, I. Precupetu, & B. Suanet (Eds.), *Macro social influences on loneliness in later life: Towards a better understanding of the loneliness paradox in later life*. Springer.

Lim, M. H., Allen, K. A., Furlong, M. J., Craig, H., & Smith, D. C. (2021). Introducing a dual continuum model of belonging and loneliness. *Australian Journal of Psychology, 73*(1), 81–86. https://doi.org/10.1080/00049530.2021.1883411

Luhmann, M., & Hawkley, L. (2016). Age differences in loneliness from late adolescence to oldest old age. *Developmental Psychology, 52*(6), 943–959. https://doi.org/10.1037/dev0000117

Luhmann, M., Buecker, S., & Rüsberg, M. (2023). Loneliness across time and space. *Nature Review Psychology, 2*, 9–23. https://doi.org/10.1038/s44159-022-00124-1

Luo, Y. (2023). Own health, spousal health and transitions in loneliness among middle-aged and older adults in China. *Ageing & Society, 43*(7), 1576–1602. https://doi.org/10.1017/S0144686X21001264

Mayer, K. U. (2009). New directions in life course research. *Annual Review of Sociology, 35*, 413–433. https://doi.org/10.1146/annurev.soc.34.040507.134619

Meisters, R., Westra, D., Putrik, P., Bosma, H., Ruwaard, D., & Jansen, M. (2021). Does loneliness have a cost? A population-wide study of the association between loneliness and healthcare expenditure. *International Journal of Public Health, 66*(2), 581286. https://doi.org/10.3389/ijph.2021.581286

Moen, P. (2011). From 'work-family' to the 'gendered life course' and 'fit': Five challenges to the field. *Community, Work & Family, 14*(1), 81–96. https://doi.org/10.1080/13668803.2010.532661

Nyqvist, F., Nygård, M., & Scharf, T. (2019). Loneliness amongst older people in Europe: A comparative study of welfare regimes. European Journal of Ageing, 16(2), 133–143. https://doi.org/10.1007/s10433-018-0487-y

Nyqvist, F., McHugh Power, J., & Coll-Planas, L. (2025). Theorizing loneliness in later life: Micro, meso, and macro perspectives. In M. Aartsen, I. Precupetu, & B. Suanet (Eds.), *Macro social influences on loneliness in later life: Towards a better understanding of the loneliness paradox in later life*. Springer.

Perlman, D., & Peplau, L. A. (1981). Toward a social psychology of loneliness. In R. Gilmour & S. Duck (Eds.), *Personal relationships: 3. Relationships in disorder* (pp. 31–56). Academic Press.

Pescosolido, B. A., & Martin, J. K. (2015). The stigma complex. *Annual Review of Sociology, 41*, 87–116. https://doi.org/10.1146/annurev-soc-071312-145702

Prezza, M., Amici, M., Roberti, T., & Tedeschi, G. (2001). Sense of community referred to the whole town: Its relations with neighboring, loneliness, life satisfaction, and area of residence. *Journal of Community Psychology, 29*(1), 29–52. https://doi.org/10.1002/1520-6629(200101)29:1<29::AID-JCOP3>3.0.CO;2-C

Rapolienė, G., & Aartsen, M. (2022). Lonely societies: Low trust societies? Further explanations for national variations in loneliness among older Europeans. *European Journal of Ageing, 19*(3), 485–494. https://doi.org/10.1007/s10433-021-00649-z

Rokach, A., & Chan, S. (2021). The many faces of child emotional maltreatment. *Journal of Psychiatry Research Reviews & Reports, 3*, 127. https://doi.org/10.47363/JPSRR/2021(3)127

Scharf, T., & de Jong Gierveld, J. (2008). Loneliness in urban neighbourhoods: An Anglo-Dutch comparison. *European Journal of Ageing, 5*(2), 103–115. https://doi.org/10.1007/s10433-008-0080-x

Schoenmakers, E. C., Van Tilburg, T. G., & Fokkema, T. (2012). Coping with loneliness: What do older adults suggest? *Aging & Mental Health, 16*(3), 353–360. https://doi.org/10.1080/13607863.2011.630373

Shiovitz-Ezra, S., & Ayalon, L. (2010). Situational versus chronic loneliness as risk factors for all-cause mortality. *International Psychogeriatrics, 22*(3), 455–462. https://doi.org/10.1017/S1041610209991426

Shiovitz-Ezra, S., Shemesh, J., & McDonnell-Naughton, M. (2018). Pathways from ageism to loneliness. In L. Ayalon & C. Tesch-Römer (Eds.), Contemporary perspectives on ageism (pp. 93–106). Springer. https://doi.org/10.1007/978-3-319-73820-8_9

Sorokin, P. A. (1959). *Social and cultural mobility*. Free Press.

Suanet, B., & van Tilburg, T. G. (2019). Loneliness declines across birth cohorts: The impact of mastery and self-efficacy. *Psychology and Aging, 34*(8), 1134–1143. https://doi.org/10.1037/pag0000357

Suanet, B., & Pavlidis, G. (2025). And, you know: There's such a thing as society: Towards a clarification of the 'loneliness paradox' by a macrofication of loneliness studies. In M. Aartsen, I. Precupetu, & B. Suanet (Eds.), *Macro social influences on loneliness in later life: Towards a better understanding of the loneliness paradox in later life*. Springer.

Swader, C. S. (2019). Loneliness in Europe: Personal and societal individualism-collectivism and their connection to social isolation. *Social Forces, 97*(3), 1307–1336. https://doi.org/10.1093/sf/soy088

Tiilikainen, E., Aartsen, M., & Kraav, S.-L. (2024). Early-life circumstances and late life loneliness trajectories among Finnish older adults. *BMC Geriatrics, 24*, 459. https://doi.org/10.1186/s12877-024-04967-6

van Tilburg, T. G. (2025). Unravelling the socio-cultural influence on loneliness. In M. Aartsen, I. Precupetu, & B. Suanet (Eds.), *Macro social influences on loneliness in later life: Towards a better understanding of the loneliness paradox in later life*. Springer.

Victor, C., Rippon, I., Barreto, M., Hammond, C., & Qualter, P. (2022). Older adults' experiences of loneliness over the lifecourse: An exploratory study using the BBC loneliness experiment. *Archives of Gerontology and Geriatrics, 102*, 104740. https://doi.org/10.1016/j.archger.2022.104740

Wang, F., Gao, Y., Han, Z., Yu, Y., Long, Z., Jiang, X., Wu, Y., Pei, B., Cao, Y., Ye, J., Wang, M., & Zhao, Y. (2023). A systematic review and meta-analysis of 90 cohort studies of social isolation, loneliness and mortality. *Nature Human Behaviour, 7*(8), 1307–1319. https://doi.org/10.1038/s41562-023-01617-6

Yang, K. (2018). Longitudinal loneliness and its risk factors among older people in England. *Canadian Journal on Aging / La Revue Canadienne Du Vieillissement, 37*(1), 12–21. https://doi.org/10.1017/S0714980817000526

Zoutewelle-Terovan, M., & Liefbroer, A. C. (2018). Swimming against the stream: Non-normative family transitions and loneliness in later life across 12 nations. The Gerontologist, 58(6), 1096–1108. https://doi.org/10.1093/geront/gnx184

Bianca Suanet, PhD, is a sociologist, specializing in loneliness, social relations, and care use among older adults, especially in relation to the impact of societal and policy changes. She was formerly Professor of Ageing and Social Change at the Linköping University in Sweden and Associate Professor in Sociology and Head of the Social Functioning Group of the Longitudinal Aging Study Amsterdam at the Vrije Universiteit Amsterdam in the Netherlands. Currently, her research projects encompass studies on the relationship between macro-level factors and loneliness, and optimizing interventions against loneliness based on scientific evidence for older migrants.

Marja Aartsen, PhD, is currently research professor and social gerontologist at NOVA – Norwegian Social Research at OsloMet. She specializes in longitudinal research on social relations, social exclusion, loneliness, and cognitive functioning in the second half of life. She is interested in social issues related to aging in place and active or successful ageing. Resent research projects and collaborations include gendered pathways to exclusion from social relations (GENPATH), reducing old-age social exclusion (ROSENET) and a multidimensional approach to social exclusion and its health consequences (AMASE). She was editor of the European Journal of Ageing from 2017 until summer 2022.

Open Access This chapter is licensed under the terms of the Creative Commons Attribution 4.0 International License (http://creativecommons.org/licenses/by/4.0/), which permits use, sharing, adaptation, distribution and reproduction in any medium or format, as long as you give appropriate credit to the original author(s) and the source, provide a link to the Creative Commons license and indicate if changes were made.

The images or other third party material in this chapter are included in the chapter's Creative Commons license, unless indicated otherwise in a credit line to the material. If material is not included in the chapter's Creative Commons license and your intended use is not permitted by statutory regulation or exceeds the permitted use, you will need to obtain permission directly from the copyright holder.

Chapter 15
Loneliness Re-Examined: Societal Influences and Future Research Directions

Marja Aartsen, Bianca Suanet, Thomas Hansen, and Iuliana Precupetu

15.1 Introduction

By adopting a macro-social lens, this book presents the first contours of how societal, cultural, and policy-related factors influence loneliness. It outlines the broader conditions that shape experiences of loneliness. With this edited book, we hope to inspire researchers to further explore this important yet understudied theme in their future work and to provide perspectives and pathways for doing so.

In the second part of the book, Nyqvist and others charted the main theories relevant to older adults, including biological, developmental, cognitive, personality, and existential theories at the micro-level, interpersonal networks and relationships at the meso-level, and structural and cultural factors at the macro-level (Chap. 2; Nyqvist et al., 2025). This comprehensive theoretical review underscored the interconnectedness of multiple levels of analysis, providing a robust foundation to address the complex nature of loneliness in later life. Van Tilburg theoretically unraveled some socio-cultural influences on loneliness, focusing on societal values and norms surrounding individualism and collectivism. By going beyond the mere assumption that people in individual countries value independence more than

M. Aartsen (✉)
Norwegian Social Research (NOVA), Oslo Metropolitan University, Oslo, Norway
e-mail: maraar@oslomet.no

B. Suanet
Amstelveen, The Netherlands

T. Hansen
Norwegian Institute of Public Health, Oslo, Norway

I. Precupetu
Research Institute for Quality of Life, Romanian Academy, Bucharest, Romania

Research Institute of the University of Bucharest, Bucharest, Romania

© The Author(s) 2025

M. Aartsen et al. (eds.), *Macro Social Influences on Loneliness in Later Life*,
International Perspectives on Aging 47,
https://doi.org/10.1007/978-3-031-94565-6_15

people in collectivistic countries and are therefore less lonely, van Tilburg presented a model with four paths of influence to explain how individualistic and collectivistic values and norms shape people's relationship standards and their likelihood of experiencing loneliness. Each path is supported by research evidence (Chap. 3; van Tilburg, 2025). Van Regenmortel and other colleagues addressed the more macro-structural aspects of societies that can impact loneliness by adopting a social exclusionary perspective. They examined the disadvantages across multiple domains, such as neighborhoods, services, finances, social interactions, civic engagement, and socio-cultural aspects, and highlighted the connection between old-age social exclusion and loneliness (Chap. 4; Van Regenmortel et al., 2025).

The third part shifted focus to empirical evidence, and Vasile and Aartsen provided an updated overview of the prevalence of old-age loneliness in Europe to debunk the myth that there is a loneliness-epidemic (Chap. 5; Vasile & Aartsen, 2025). Similar to what Yang and Victor published in 2011, they provided loneliness prevalence in different age groups in Europe in 2014 and 2023, based on data from the European Social Survey. The comparison of loneliness prevalence in 2014 and 2023 did not support the idea of a loneliness pandemic. However, loneliness remains prevalent, particularly among the youngest (15–19) and oldest (80+) age groups. Lee, in another empirical chapter, provided a state-of-the-art overview of evidence-based micro- and meso-level determinants of loneliness, addressing the relevance and significance of individual characteristics, community dynamics, and their cumulative impacts on late-life loneliness (Chap. 6; Lee, 2025). In the next chapter, Tufă employed a systematic review of literature on macro factors with the aim to create a comprehensive picture of current research evidence. Macro factors typically related to loneliness are cultural values and norms in society, migration patterns, and welfare generosity. Other factors for which growing evidence emerge are religiosity and societal trust. Finding the proper data to study these societal factors, however, remains a challenge (see Chap. 7; Tufa, 2025).

The book then moves to recent developments in loneliness research (part four) and discusses several contemporary societal changes and conditions likely to impact loneliness, drawing on Bronfenbrenner's (1995) concept of the chronosystem, the outermost layer of contextual influences surrounding an individual that may affect loneliness. The chapters described the impact of current mega-societal trends, such as digitalization, climate change, and societal crises on loneliness. Seifert (Chap. 8; Seifert, 2025) discussed the two faces of ICT and the links with loneliness. He finds that ICT can act as a protective factor against loneliness, while at the same time it can be a potential risk factor for exclusion and loneliness. Ayalon, in the next chapter (Chap. 9; Ayalon, 2025), discussed how climate change can be linked to loneliness, and how climate change outcomes at the micro-, meso-, and macro-levels can mediate the relationship between climate change and loneliness. Finally, Klasen and colleagues (Chap. 10; Klasen et al., 2025) concluded with an examination of various societal crises and how that relates to social integration and loneliness. They proposed that societal crises disrupt various facets of social integration, thereby contributing to loneliness.

In the last section (part 5), authors explore some novel empirical and theoretical ways to approach studying macro level factors in loneliness. Precupetu and others introduced a promising new method derived from political sciences to differentiate between the wide range of macro-social factors that have been discussed in the book and elsewhere which can explain variations in loneliness prevalence. This so-called qualitative comparative analysis (QCA) can help to define the necessary and sufficient macro-conditions that explain country-level variations in loneliness (Chap. 11; Precupetu et al., 2025). Suanet and Pavlidis attempted to solve the loneliness paradox by advocating for a greater emphasis on macro-level influences (Chap. 12; Suanet & Pavlidis, 2025). They explored the interplay between societal structures, cultural values, and individual experiences of loneliness, and proposed methodological advancements to uncover the complex dynamics between macro- and micro-level factors. Ghenţa and Matei (Chap. 13; Ghenţa & Matei, 2025) analyzed policy documents and interventions at micro-, meso-, and macro levels to better understand the current policy landscape regarding loneliness in various European countries and trends therein, and to identify gaps and opportunities for enhancing support systems for older adults. In the last contributed chapter, Suanet and Aartsen presented the SOLO model of loneliness, combining the life course framework with Bronfenbrenner's socio-ecological model (Chap. 14; Suanet & Aartsen, 2025). They discussed how loneliness comes about as an interaction between the individual and context by drawing on sociological perspectives. In this chapter, the authors hoped to inspire others to pursue a 'sociology of loneliness', by citing relevant sociological perspectives to the study of loneliness from a micro-, meso-, and macro-level framework.

In the remainder of this chapter, we explore three societal developments that have not been discussed in detail in the contributed chapters but that may also be linked to loneliness: loneliness among older migrants as an example of a structurally disadvantaged group, the growth of populist parties and loneliness, and the potential impact of the increased use of artificial intelligence in society on loneliness. Next, we summarize the results of a more rigorous approach to evaluate the effectiveness of loneliness interventions to better guide policy decisions regarding the implementation of efficacious and scalable interventions. We conclude with describing how the book has hopefully transformed our understanding of loneliness.

15.2 New Research Directions on Societal Developments

Over the past few years, studies on the macro-level influences on loneliness have started to emerge, as evidenced in this edited book. Additionally, theoretical advancements have contributed to new ways of conceptualizing and explaining loneliness. However, despite the rapid growth of the field, many questions remain, as we are only beginning to uncover how context influences loneliness. Through this discussion, we aim to provide suggestions for future research directions and advance the study of macro-level influences on loneliness.

15.2.1 Non-Western Migrants and Loneliness

Loneliness among older non-Western migrants is influenced not only by individual circumstances and social networks but also by broader societal structures, policies, and cultural norms. Research shows that loneliness rates among older migrants, particularly in Europe, are up to twice as high as those of native populations (Fokkema & Naderi, 2013; Ten Kate et al., 2020; Wu & Penning, 2015). While studies often focus on general, individual risk factors, macro-level influences, such as welfare policies, economic conditions, and cultural expectations, play a crucial role in shaping loneliness among this group. Older migrants face double vulnerability, or even triple jeopardy (Norman, 1985), due to migration as a disruptive life event, their ageing process, and their ties to both host and home societies.

Van Tilburg and Fokkema (2021) explain that loneliness among older migrants results from a combination of individual disadvantages (e.g., health and financial difficulties), social network characteristics (e.g., family-centered but homogeneous ties), and structural inequalities (e.g., discrimination and cultural differences). They highlight that while older migrants often have frequent social contact, its protective effect depends on factors such as relationship quality, cultural expectations, and social integration. The SOLO model of Suanet and Aartsen (2025) reinforces this perspective by emphasizing the dynamic interplay between different levels and life-course influences. So, while personal relationships remain central, macro-level factors—such as welfare policies, migration history, labor market structures, and cultural attitudes—shape the conditions that mitigate or exacerbate loneliness. For instance, older migrants may have strong family ties, but if their broader social participation is limited due to structural barriers, they remain vulnerable to loneliness. Moreover, the model and findings suggest that loneliness should not only be analyzed in terms of network size or contact frequency but also through a lifelong accumulation of disadvantages and opportunities, affecting social inclusion and belonging at different stages of life. Notably, many studies show that older migrants often have large networks and do not age alone, even compared to native populations (Fokkema & Ciobanu, 2021). Thus, loneliness in this group should be explored beyond conventional structural network measures, focusing instead on relationship quality, social support, and sense of belonging at multiple levels (Klok et al., 2017), and how their cultural and structural context evolves over time.

One of the key macro-level factors influencing loneliness among older migrants is the welfare system and its policies. Access to pensions, healthcare, and social services varies across countries, shaping their ability to engage socially. Welfare states with universal benefits, financial security and healthcare reduce stressors linked to the relatively isolated situation of older migrants (Joshi et al., 2024a, 2024b). In contrast, where benefits depend on employment history or citizenship, many older migrants, having worked in informal or low-wage jobs, may lack financial stability and resources for social participation (Dwyer & Papadimitriou, 2007; Ciobanu et al., 2017). Economic insecurity often leads to social withdrawal and exclusion (Huxhold et al., 2022), while financial precarity further limits the ability to maintain relationships, reinforcing loneliness.

Cultural norms, values, and mismatches in expectations significantly influence loneliness among older migrants. Moving between collectivistic and individualistic societies can cause culture shocks, and large generational differences in caregiving expectations. In many cultures, older adults rely on family support, but migration often disrupts these structures (Hansen, 2013). Adult children may be unable to provide expected care, creating experiences of loneliness. In more individualistic societies in Europe, state-provided care for older adults may not accommodate the cultural or linguistic needs of older migrants, making this alternative support harder to establish and, as a result, it tends to be underused by older migrants (Chiarenza et al., 2019; Hansen, 2013). Additionally, stigma and likely also taboo around loneliness are often stronger in collectivistic cultures (Barreto et al., 2024), discouraging open discussions about expectations for the relationships. Understanding how differences in cultural norms—both between generations and between home and host societies—shape expectations and interactions is crucial. Migrants often navigate conflicting expectations: older generations may hold traditional views on family obligations and caregiving, while younger generations, influenced by the host society's values, may adopt more individualistic attitudes (Hansen, 2013). Similarly, the norms and support structures in the country of origin may differ significantly from those in the host country, creating mismatches in how care and social roles are perceived. These discrepancies can lead to misunderstandings, unmet expectations, and feelings of loneliness, particularly when older migrants expect family members to provide care that they are unable or unwilling to give, or when state-provided care does not align with their cultural and linguistic needs (Chiarenza et al., 2019). Bridging these gaps across generations and societies requires a deeper understanding and development of culturally sensitive services and tailored loneliness interventions for older migrants that help them and society to navigate these cultural aspects better.

Furthermore, many older migrants live in ethnic enclaves, which can provide strong community networks but also reinforce segregation from the native population (Borjas, 2000; Klaesson & Öner, 2021). In Sweden, as well as countries like France, discussions have arisen about the existence and impact of 'parallel societies' that have fewer ties to the general society and operate more independently affecting many social outcomes and residents' perspectives on belonging and social order (Esaiasson & Sohlberg, 2024). The segregation processes are partly structured by housing policies and the availability of affordable housing (Klaesson & Öner, 2021). Furthermore, if these neighborhoods lack accessible public spaces, community centers, or transport options, opportunities for social participation may be limited and the resources for creating a cohesive community might be harder to mobilize than in more advantaged areas. Urban planning that encourages interaction, such as intergenerational meeting spaces and inclusive community centers while also providing these neighborhoods with sufficient resources to maintain social order and good transportation links to networks and labor markets outside the neighborhoods can help foster connections between migrants and native-born populations, reducing loneliness and creating a sense of belonging to the host country as well.

Future research on loneliness among older migrants could benefit from an interdisciplinary approach, integrating sociological, psychological, and policy perspectives to understand structural and social determinants. Comparative studies using macro-level indicators, alongside meso- and micro-level factors, are needed to examine how welfare regimes and integration policies shape loneliness among older migrants across countries. More research is also needed on the taboo and stigma surrounding loneliness in migrant communities and its impact on older migrants. This applies not only to the conceptualization of these concepts of taboo and stigma, but also to understanding the main causes among migrants and which measures should be taken to ensure that talking about loneliness becomes easier. To reduce migrant loneliness, efforts should focus on effective interventions at multiple levels, from policy reforms ensuring equitable access to services to local initiatives fostering intergenerational and intercultural connections. Finally, fostering more structured dialogue between researchers, policymakers, and civil society will help translate findings into practical solutions. By taking these steps, research and policy can contribute to a more inclusive society that recognizes not only the vulnerabilities but also the social, economic, and cultural contributions of older migrants.

15.2.2 Populist Parties and Loneliness

Populist parties, right- and left-wing, have been on the rise in European countries. While in 1990 they received around 10% of the vote in democracies, in 2016 they obtained about 25% of the votes (Stoetzer et al., 2021). Recent trends show an increasing electoral strength of these parties, with countries in Europe experiencing populists surging to power and others where they have grown substantially in the latest elections (Pew Research Center, 2022). Even when populist parties are not in power, they have the capacity to attract individuals away from mainstream politics and influence party dynamics and public policy in their countries, thus affecting the lives of a considerable number of people (Gidron & Hall, 2017).

Increasing income inequality has been a major driver of support for populist parties, particularly those on the right (Han, 2016), mainly through growing economic insecurities, especially for those at the lower end of the economic ladder, and the erosion of political trust (Stoetzer et al., 2021). Significant economic and cultural changes in societies have also played a role in growing support for populist parties by influencing social integration. Technological changes favoring skilled labour and global outsourcing in Western countries (Colantone & Stanig, 2018) have particularly affected people facing economic disadvantages, contributing to increasing feelings of marginalization and displacement (Gidron & Hall, 2020). In Eastern countries, persistent poverty and social exclusion decades after the fall of communist regimes have left large groups of population isolated from the mainstream society and feeling as though they do not have access to the gains and benefits of a free-market economy and democracy. Moreover, changes in cultural frameworks towards post-materialist and multicultural values in the Western world have prompted reactions from individuals holding with more traditional beliefs, particularly among older and less secure groups who feel threatened by the erosion of familiar traditional values, leading them to feel increasingly disconnected from their societies (Norris & Inglehart, 2019; Gidron & Hall, 2020).

Populist parties are not business as usual. They use an ingroup–outgroup rationale that emphasises the difference between *them*, a corrupt or incompetent elite, and *us*, a moral but ignored population, using existing divisions in society, or further accentuating them (Rooduijn et al., 2021). Right-wing parties tend to maintain that the native population can be under threat from non-native ideas and groups (e.g. refugees, ethnic minorities) and design their programs based on nationalism, authoritarianism, and cultural conflicts, whereas left-wing parties focus on economic justice and inequalities, emphasizing the needs of those left behind (Mudde & Kaltwasser, 2018). The populist narratives stress a sense of belonging to a certain community, appealing thus to those who feel overlooked, isolated, and disconnected from mainstream politics.

There is little knowledge about the potential link between loneliness and support for populist parties. Previous research has shown that loneliness is associated with political disengagement, as people who are lonely are less likely to participate in political activities such as voting, contacting a politician or signing a petition (Langenkamp, 2021a, 2021b). Petersen et al. (2023) recently showed that in some countries there is a positive association between loneliness and populist radical right support. While it is not clear yet if loneliness in itself can lead to support for populism, it is likely that social exclusion, involving isolation from mainstream society and the consequent feelings of marginalization, which highly associate with loneliness to drive support for populist parties. Individuals experiencing social marginalization – due to weakened attachments to societal norms, lower social engagement, or a diminished sense of social respect – tend to feel alienated from mainstream politics and support radical parties (Gidron & Hall, 2020; Langenkamp & Bienstman, 2022).

The increasing prominence of populist parties in the current political environment can drive higher levels of loneliness through various mechanisms at play. Populism and political extremism often result in heightened social polarization, which can alienate individuals from those with differing views. This polarization can create an environment where people feel isolated from broader social networks, potentially leading to intensified feelings of loneliness. Moreover, populist parties often use new media technologies to create and reinforce echo chambers – groups where individuals are exposed predominantly to like-minded views and where dissenting opinions are excluded (Rietdijk, 2021). While these groups may provide a sense of belonging to their members, they also isolate people from diverse perspectives and broader social interactions, which can lead to or enhance loneliness when they encounter opposing views. Furthermore, stigmatization of individuals adhering to populist parties by mainstream society (Gest et al., 2018) can lead to social withdrawal and feelings of loneliness as people may become reluctant to engage with others who hold different beliefs. Finally, it is worth mentioning that maintaining and fostering a persistent conflictual atmosphere and political polarization can have a bearing on emotional well-being, including feelings of anxiety and ultimately loneliness (Smith et al., 2023).

The current political landscape in Europe, marked by the rise of populist and right-wing movements, adds even more complexity to loneliness among older people, some of whom are particularly vulnerable. For example, increasing polarization around migration and integration in European societies likely affects older migrants' sense of belonging and identity, and shapes public perceptions of ageing migrant populations among native populations, likely creating more issues in relationships and contributing to loneliness due to the perception of these relationships. Exclusionary policy and discourse narratives risk further limiting their opportunities for and experiences of social connection for older migrants in the coming years.

To unravel the role of populist parties in loneliness, more theoretical and empirical research is needed. Claiming there is a bidirectional relationship between populist parties and loneliness would be oversimplifying. As loneliness is shaped by the social–cultural and historical–political characteristics of various societies (Rapolienė & Aartsen, 2022), political contexts should receive increasing attention as key macro factors in explaining loneliness, while considering the synergic effects of social polarization, erosion of trust and social integration.

15.2.3 AI and Loneliness

We stand on the brink of a society where artificial intelligence (AI) shapes our daily lives and even political opinions (Auliya et al., 2024), yet its implications for loneliness remain difficult to foresee. Movies or TV-series such as "Her" (2014), "Ex Machina" (2015) and "Äkte människor (Real humans)" (2014–2016) envision that romantic relations can exist between real people and virtual entities or AI-powered humanoid robots. In addition to cineasts, some scholars also claim that romantic relations are possible with AI-powered entities (Song et al., 2022), but overall, the empirical support for a beneficial effect on loneliness is at best weak, partly because older adults do not feel comfortable with humanoid robots helping to reduce loneliness (Berridge et al., 2023). Envisioning humanoid robot-human interactions as a substitute for human-human interaction is a distant dream—or perhaps nightmare—if it is even possible. However, AI is much more than only humanoid robots. For this chapter, we refer to the Merriam-Webster dictionary where AI is defined as "the capability of computer systems or algorithms to imitate intelligent human behavior" (see Wang, 2019; Stone, 2020 for more thoughtful definitions). Generative chatbots such as ChatGPT are computer programs that are designed to converse with human beings, and as such imitate intelligent human behavior.

Generative chatbots use algorithms, machine learning techniques and Large Language Models (LLMs) to generate responses to the questions that a user of the chatbot asks. There are all kinds of chatbots, but the most relevant in relation to loneliness are chatbots that are developed to improve mental health and reduce loneliness by providing companionship. Examples of such chatbots are Replika (www.replika.com) with currently more than 2,5 million active users worldwide (De Freitas et al., 2024) and Woebot (woebothealth.com), the latter of which is especially developed to advise on mental health issues. Preliminary results derived from various qualitative and mixed methods studies suggest some positive results in improving mental health (Boucher et al., 2021) and reducing loneliness (Kim et al., 2025; Maples et al., 2024). In a working paper, De Freitas and colleagues explain how AI companionships can reduce loneliness (De Freitas et al., 2024). They argue that AI does not only mimic conversation, but by keeping track of cues and information that the user provides, AI can synthesize advice and refer back to earlier comments which makes people feel heard. Feeling heard, they argue, involves empathy and creates trust and sympathy, which is essential in alleviating loneliness. The first studies on AI chatbots suggest that they might work well as companions and advisors, at least among students (Maples et al., 2024), but it is too early to draw robust conclusions.

Despite certain potentials to reduce loneliness, there are also caveats to the use and further penetration of AI in our daily lives. Obviously, and as it stands now, the type of support that AI-entities and chatbots provide is limited to one type of support, i.e., emotional support. If in-person contact is replaced by online contact opportunities for providing practical support and help with tasks in and around the house for example will be reduced, potentially leading to support deficiencies. Although not yet supported with robust empirical evidence, there are concerns about potential harm that can be caused by the over reliance on chatbots as communicated in the media and by organizations overseeing privacy laws, in particular with respect to an increased risk of suicide in people using chatbots as therapeutic agents (Abrams, 2025).

Less obvious but no less influential is how AI influences and even intentionally steers opinions of individuals towards specific directions (Auliya et al., 2024). This process can be reinforced by AI-driven social media platforms that drive people into echo chambers where exposure to different and more nuanced perspectives is limited (Cinelli et al., 2021). Consequently, people easily become alienated or excluded from wider society with negative consequences for feelings of loneliness. Loneliness, in turn, may not only fuel the rise of populist parties but also propel the creation of conspiracy theories (Bierwiaczonek et al., 2024). Since it is the already lonely person who engages more frequently with AI chatbots (Pani et al., 2024) the potential advantages and disadvantages are likely to be unequally distributed across social groups.

In sum, research on how AI and algorithms steer the development or erosion of social networks is essential to understand future developments in the etiology and prevalence of loneliness. AI chatbots designed for companionship and mental health support show promise in reducing loneliness, but there are significant caveats. We need more robust research designs and longitudinal studies to understand the nuanced causal relationship between AI and loneliness across different demographics and cultural groups. Particular attention is needed for vulnerable groups such as lonely people, and people at risk of suicide to ensure they receive the necessary support and are not disproportionately affected by the negative aspects of AI. Additionally, stronger evidence is required to substantiate claims that steering individuals into echo chambers exacerbates feelings of loneliness.

15.3 Existing loneliness Interventions

With growing popular, scholarly, and policy interest in loneliness and its individual and societal costs, there has been an increasing focus on identifying effective interventions. A rising number of primary studies, systematic reviews, and even umbrella reviews—which synthesize systematic reviews—have explored a wide range of interventions. In a recent umbrella review, Hansen et al. (2024) synthesized findings from 29 systematic reviews, focusing exclusively on results from randomized controlled trials (RCTs)—the gold standard for evaluating intervention efficacy. The review also addressed social isolation, defined as an objective lack of social contacts or interactions, which has comparable health impacts to loneliness (Steptoe et al., 2013).

The included systematic reviews assessed a wide range of interventions, and most of the evidence was derived from older adults. The most promising and consistent results have been shown for psychological interventions (e.g., cognitive-behavioral therapy, psychoeducation, social skills training) (Hansen et al., 2024). These approaches target maladaptive social cognitions, emotional responses, and behavioral barriers that contribute to loneliness. The moderate to large positive effects often exhibited may reflect that they address the cognitive-behavioral underlying roots of loneliness, such as cognitive biases, social withdrawal, low self-worth, anxiety, and depressive mood.

By contrast, social interventions (e.g., structured social contact, group activities, befriending programs) show weak and inconsistent effects on loneliness but benefits for social isolation. While some well-powered meta-analyses report small positive effects (e.g., Lasgaard, 2022), overall evidence remains inconsistent, suggesting a limited and uncertain impact on loneliness. This uncertainty indicates that increasing social contact alone may not alleviate loneliness without psychological change. Factors like mistrust, negative self-beliefs, hypersensitivity to rejection, and social anxiety often underpin loneliness, hindering meaningful relationships. The evidence for the effects from other types of interventions was small and inconsistent. For instance, the few systematic reviews centered on physical activities, learning new hobbies, and health and social care services reported inconsistent or no evidence of effect.

The rise of digital communication technologies, from social media to mobile apps, has created new ways to address loneliness. Compared to traditional approaches, digital interventions offer advantages such as reaching individuals facing stigma or logistical barriers, providing flexible access, and scaling cost-effectively. Additionally, digital tools enable personalized, tailored interventions, which are key to improving effectiveness (Hansen et al., 2024; Morrish et al., 2023). However, concerns remain about whether digital interactions can truly replace in-person relationships. One should be mindful, also, that while older adults are becoming more tech-savvy, many still struggle with digital platforms (Sha et al., 2024).

As shown in the umbrella review and a recent systematic review of 40 RCTs on digital interventions, effects are mixed (Hansen et al., 2024, 2025). Psychological interventions, particularly those with group-based interaction, showed the strongest effects, while social interventions had uncertain outcomes. Robotic pets reduced loneliness, but conversational robots had little impact. Training in communication technology for older adults showed modest effects. Activity-based interventions were more effective in group settings, reinforcing the role of social engagement. Overall, and as evidenced by others (Lasgaard, 2022), digital interventions appear to have effects comparable to non-digital ones.

Moving forward, it is critical to improve intervention design and efficacy by addressing and improving many of the limitations in the literature. First, the methodological quality of interventions and evaluations varies greatly, with issues such as small sample sizes, high attrition rates, lack of adequate control groups, and inconsistent outcome measures. Specifically, there is a pressing need for more high-quality, well-powered RCTs. Second, many trials lack clear theoretical bases, making it difficult to identify key mechanisms and understand how interventions are expected to have an impact. It remains unclear whether interventions target lonely individuals, those at risk, or the general population, highlighting the need for greater clarity in future design and evaluation. Third, long-term follow-up data is scarce, limiting insights into sustained effects. Fourth, integrating elements from different approaches to treat individuals holistically and individually is another avenue for future research. Given the heterogeneous nature of loneliness, interventions should shift from one-size-fits-all to targeting specific risk groups and triggers (Barbosa Neves et al., 2023). Digital platforms could serve as a valuable facilitator for these tailored interventions.

Moreover, while the field has primarily focused on micro-level interventions targeting lonely or at-risk individuals, it is essential to consider broader meso- and macro-level strategies to prevent or reduce loneliness (Barreto et al., 2024). Community (meso) and societal (macro) level interventions to reduce loneliness aim to address the broader social, environmental, and policy contexts that shape individuals' experiences of social connection. Community or local-level interventions typically include initiatives that improve opportunities for social participation, foster neighborhood engagement, and promote access to shared public spaces or services. Structural or societal-level approaches involve broader policies and governance efforts, such as national strategies or action plans, funding for social care systems, or public campaigns—most notably, the UK's appointment of a Minister for Loneliness in 2018 and the nationwide Campaign to End Loneliness.

Despite the growing recognition of loneliness as a public health concern and the emergence of such initiatives, the research into their effectiveness remains limited (Hansen et al., 2024; Crowe et al., 2024). Evidence from the UK shows that while some local interventions (e.g., targeted programs among specific groups) may yield modest improvements, these effects do not translate into significant population-level changes in loneliness or mental health outcomes. For example, a recent evaluation of the UK's Campaign to End Loneliness found no statistically significant overall impact on loneliness or depressive symptoms among older adults, even in areas with high levels of local implementation. However, the study did detect modest benefits in certain subgroups, particularly among well-educated and higher-income individuals, suggesting that while localized or targeted interventions may offer benefits, these do not necessarily scale into significant population-wide change (Li et al., 2024). Similarly, EU policy analysis shows growing attention to loneliness in national strategies, yet most interventions remain micro- or meso-level in scope, and their actual impact on reducing loneliness remains poorly understood (see Chap. 13 of this book; Ghența & Matei, 2025). This suggests that while well-intentioned and sometimes impactful at the community level, these efforts have not yet produced systemic shifts in loneliness prevalence, highlighting the need for more robust, long-term, and integrative approaches.

Beyond structural interventions, other types of interventions should be explored in future RCTs. For instance, "social prescribing" interventions, which have shown promise in non-RCT trials (Reinhardt et al., 2021; Vidovic et al., 2021), could offer valuable insights into tackling social isolation and loneliness. Additionally, the effectiveness of giving support in addressing social disconnection is worth noting (Hansen et al., 2024). Positive psychology interventions have long emphasized that acts of generosity and prosocial behavior can be more impactful than receiving support, challenging the notion that individuals must always be passive recipients of interventions to address loneliness. Volunteering and digital interventions, particularly through group interactions and online forums, provide flexible opportunities for reciprocal support, fostering meaningful connections and strengthening social bonds.

Finally, to our knowledge, no RCT-based studies have examined AI-driven social chatbots such as Replika. These chatbots use LLMs to generate personalized, open-ended conversations, often indistinguishable from human speech. While currently app-based, future iterations may incorporate voice and embodied features (e.g., humanoid or animal-like robots) for more lifelike interactions. Early data suggest users form non-judgmental, supportive relationships with these agents (Skjuve et al., 2021; Xie & Pentina, 2022). Risks such as addiction, emotional dependence, and withdrawal from human interaction must, however, be considered and measures should be included. Still, AI holds promise as a supplement to human contact, providing a safe space for self-expression and connection, particularly for individuals experiencing social anxiety, shyness, or loneliness (Allen et al., 2024). Relatedly, future research should explore how digital platforms can facilitate real-world, in-person connections to combat loneliness. This could involve digital signposting interventions, directing individuals to community services and social activities tailored to their interests and needs, like social prescribing models. These online platforms already exist in many countries to connect individuals with local events, activities, and social opportunities, helping them engage with their community and combat loneliness.

15.4 A Look Under the Hood of Perlman and Peplau's Cognitive Approach to Loneliness

Now that the wide range of micro-, meso-, and macro level conditions are distinguished and integrative theories and perspectives on the etiology of loneliness are discussed, the next step is to delineate how mechanisms linking the multilevel conditions to loneliness can be quantified and empirically measured. A more detailed look "under the hood" of the cognitive approach to loneliness might be helpful in that respect. This approach is central in the book and in most contemporary research on loneliness. It defines loneliness as "an unpleasant experience that occurs when a person's network of social relations is deficient in some important way, either quantitatively or qualitatively" (Perlman & Peplau, 1981, p. 31). Stated differently, when the status quo of the achieved quality or quantity of social relations changes, loneliness occurs unless the ideal quality of quantity of social relations is also changed to restore the balance. At the same time, if the ideal quality or quantity of social relations changes, loneliness occurs unless the achieved social relations are also changed to restore the balance. For example, losing a spouse leads to a reduction in the achieved quality of social relations and, if the person does not adjust their perception of the ideal quality of social relations, they feel lonely. Similarly, if the society in which people live changes the conditions for meeting other people, as happened during the COVID-19 pandemic, people feel lonely if they do not adjust their ideas about the ideal level of contacts (Fig. 15.1).

The impact of multilevel conditions and their interactions leading to loneliness is not necessarily equal across the four components. For example, life transitions such as retirement may affect the quantity of social relations, as people lose daily contact with colleagues, while the quality of social relations remains unaffected. Conversely, losing a close friend or partner may significantly impact the quality of social relations but not the quantity. Similarly, some macro-social conditions may influence the quantity of social relations, while others affect their quality. *Structural conditions* of a society, such as wealth, infrastructure, and income (see Chap. 12; Suanet & Pavlidis, 2025), may be more crucial for maintaining or restoring the quantity of social relations after a loss. However, restoring the quality of social relations, for instance, after bereavement, may not be easily achieved through wealth and income alone. *Cultural conditions*, including norms and values, can shape the ideal number and quality of social relations. In individualistic societies, autonomy and choice in social relations may therefore have greater implications for well-being than in collectivistic societies, where traditional social bonds are more significant (Lykes & Kemmelmeier, 2014; van Tilburg, 2025).

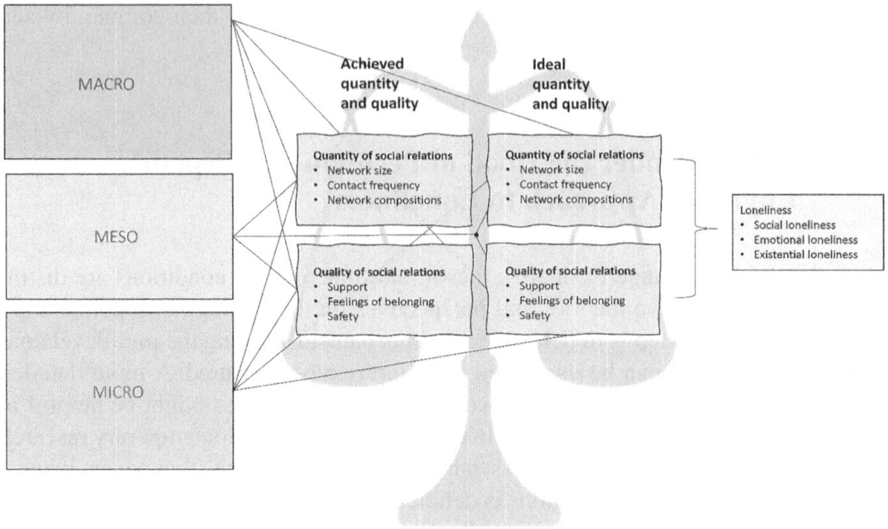

Fig. 15.1 Schematic representation of the multi-level influences on the balance between achieved and ideal quality and quality of social relations leading to different types of loneliness

For a better understanding of the differential impact of multilevel conditions on the achieved and ideal quantity and quality of social relations, we believe that it is important to distinguish between different types of loneliness. To that end, we supplement the cognitive approach with the interactionist approach to loneliness (Weiss, 1973) which emphasizes that loneliness is the outcome of the interplay between individual and structural factors, i.e., micro and macro conditions and that different factors lead to different types of loneliness. Emotional loneliness results from the absence of a close intimate attachment such as a spouse, whereas social loneliness occurs in the absence of meaningful friendships and a lack of sense of community (Weiss, 1973; Hawkley & Cacioppo, 2010; Dahlberg & McKee, 2014; Cacioppo & Cacioppo, 2018). A third type of loneliness that is gaining prominence is existential loneliness, which can be distinguished from social and emotional loneliness (van Tilburg, 2021). Existential loneliness can be described as a negative and painful feeling, yet an inevitable part of life and a characteristic of human beings (Álvarez et al., 2023).

Finally, for the empirical quantification of the impacts on different types of loneliness it is imperative to use measures that can distinguish between social and emotional loneliness. Besides being criticized for eliciting socially desirable answers (Lau & Gruen, 1992; Schoenmakers, 2020; Barreto et al., 2022), direct questions using the word "lonely" such as in "Do you feel lonely" cannot do that. One loneliness scale that can differentiate between social and emotional loneliness is the de Jong Gierveld Loneliness Scale (De Jong Gierveld & Kamphuis, 1985; De Jong Gierveld & van Tilburg, 2006), another is the Social and Emotional Loneliness Scale for Adults (SELSA) (DiTommaso & Spinner, 1993).

15.5 Conclusion

Our book set out to acknowledge and grasp loneliness as a socially embedded issue influenced by larger societal factors, with the ambition to be a catalyst for a deeper understanding of loneliness and for more innovative approaches to mitigate this pervasive phenomenon. How did we transform our understanding of loneliness with this state-of-the art volume?

Conceptually, loneliness provided us with unique lenses to assess the extent to which the various socioeconomic and political contexts in European countries grant citizens the meso- and macro-level conditions that foster social integration and enable individuals to be and feel part of their communities and societies. In doing so, the concept of loneliness became an epistemological tool that framed our inquiry and allowed us to examine the role of macro social factors, challenge existing assumptions about its psychological nature, and generate new knowledge.

Theoretically, we are currently on the path to enhanced integration of the various perspectives that have been put forward in science so far. By integrating theories across multiple levels, our book provides a comprehensive framework that enriches our understanding and encourages further investigation into the social dimensions of loneliness. Mapping micro, meso and macro level influences and highlighting theoretical models showing the interplay between societal influences and personal experiences of loneliness sheds light on the complexities of this multifaceted issue and underscores the importance of a sociological approach in addressing loneliness. In the end, much like suicide in the influential work of Durkheim, loneliness, even though a profound individual experience, is a *social fact*, a collective phenomenon that exists externally to individuals and cannot be reduced to psychology alone. Its social nature is evident in the way it is shaped by social structures and cultural norms around relationships and societal expectations of connection that exist beyond individuals; the (coercive) power that exerts on individuals regardless of their will, as people cannot decide not to experience loneliness in societies that value connection; patterns of loneliness across populations that reflect social circumstances; and in its social origin as it is influenced by major social transformations like urbanization, technological change, and shifting family structures.

Methodologically, a key issue surrounding the measurement of different types of loneliness has an important bearing on our current understanding of loneliness. Another key issue revolves around the potential lack of measurement invariance across groups, especially when direct questions are used, which compromises the generalizability and comparisons between social groups. Our book provides avenues for tackling these types of challenges that are still present in loneliness research. From a *policy* perspective, our book highlighted how, despite an evolving policy landscape with a clear direction towards comprehensive and multifaceted approaches to address loneliness in later life, challenges remain in designing effective interventions and in ensuring their implementation across diverse contexts. More work is needed to understand how the meso- and macro-level translate into meso- and macro-level strategies that are essential to increasing the impact of loneliness interventions.

Our book was written during (yet again) turbulent times marked by technological change and the rise of AI, pressures generated by migration in various European societies, uncertainty around the social consequences of climate change, fears related to an ongoing war in Europe, and signs of weakening democracies in some European countries, while the lessons of the pandemic have not yet had time to set in. This specific context provides an even greater argument to continue to focus our loneliness research on macro frameworks that impact people's lives and the subjective experience of loneliness.

Competing Interests The authors have no conflicts of interest to declare that are relevant to the content of this chapter.

References

Abrams, Z. (2025, March 12). *Using generic AI chatbots for mental health support: A dangerous trend. American Psychological Association Services Inc.* https://www.apaservices.org/practice/business/technology/artificial-intelligence-chatbots-therapists

Allen, K.-A., Kern, M. L., Crawford, J., Cowling, M., Vo, D., & Waters, L. (2024). The SEARCH for AI-informed wellbeing education: A conceptual framework. In *Applications of generative AI* (pp. 277–291). Springer. https://doi.org/10.1007/978-3-031-46238-2_14

Álvarez, M. G., Haugan, G., Larsson, H., Saarelainen, S. M., Duppen, D., & Dezutter, J. (2023). Mapping existential loneliness: A scoping review on existential loneliness/isolation conceptualizations and operationalizations. *Journal of Humanistic Psychology*, 00221678231193780. https://doi.org/10.1177/00221678231193780

Auliya, S. F., Kudina, O., Ding, A. Y., & Van de Poel, I. (2024). AI versus AI for democracy: Exploring the potential of adversarial machine learning to enhance privacy and deliberative decision-making in elections. *AI and Ethics*, 1–13. https://doi.org/10.1007/s43681-024-00588-2

Ayalon, L. (2025). Climate change and the risk of loneliness. In M. Aartsen, I. Precupetu, & B. Suanet (Eds.), *Macro social influences on loneliness in later life. Towards a better understanding of the loneliness paradox in later life*. Springer.

Barbosa Neves, B., Waycott, J., & Maddox, A. (2023). When technologies are not enough: The challenges of digital interventions to address loneliness in later life. *Sociological Research Online, 28*(1), 150–170. https://doi.org/10.1177/13607804211029298

Barreto, M., Doyle, D. M., & Qualter, P. (2024). Changing the narrative: Loneliness as a social justice issue. *Political Psychology, 45*(S1), 157–181. https://doi.org/10.1111/pops.12965

Barreto, M., van Breen, J., Victor, C., Hammond, C., Eccles, A., Richins, M. T., & Qualter, P. (2022). Exploring the nature and variation of the stigma associated with loneliness. *Journal of Social and Personal Relationships, 39*(9), 2658–2679. https://doi.org/10.1177/02654075221103780

Berridge, C., Zhou, Y., Robillard, J. M., & Kaye, J. (2023). Companion robots to mitigate loneliness among older adults: Perceptions of benefit and possible deception. *Frontiers in Psychology, 14*, 1106633. https://doi.org/10.3389/fpsyg.2023.1106633

Bierwiaczonek, K., Kunst, J. R., & Pich, O. (2024). The role of loneliness in the rise of populism and conspiracy theories. *Political Psychology, 45*(1), 123–140. https://doi.org/10.1111/pops.12966

Borjas, G. J. (2000). Ethnic enclaves and assimilation. *Swedish Economic Policy Review, 7*(2), 89–122.

Boucher, E. M., Harake, N. R., Ward, H. E., Stoeckl, S. E., Vargas, J., Minkel, J., et al. (2021). Artificially intelligent chatbots in digital mental health interventions: A review. *Expert Review of Medical Devices, 18*(sup1), 37–49. https://doi.org/10.1080/17434440.2021.2013200

Bronfenbrenner, U. (1995). Developmental ecology through space and time: A future perspective. In P. Moen, G. H. Elder Jr., & K. Lüscher (Eds.), *Examining lives in context: Perspectives on the ecology of human development* (pp. 619–647). American Psychological Association. https://doi.org/10.1037/10176-018

Cacioppo, J. T., & Cacioppo, S. (2018). Loneliness in the modern age: An evolutionary theory of loneliness (ETL). *Advances in Experimental Social Psychology, 59*, 127–197. https://doi.org/10.1016/bs.aesp.2018.03.003

Chiarenza, A., Dauvrin, M., Chiesa, V., Baatout, S., & Verrept, H. (2019). Supporting access to healthcare for refugees and migrants in European countries under particular migratory pressure. *BMC Health Services Research, 19*, 513. https://doi.org/10.1186/s12913-019-4353-1

Cinelli, M., Morales, G. D. F., Galeazzi, A., Quattrociocchi, W., & Starnini, M. (2021). The echo chamber effect on social media. *Proceedings of the National Academy of Sciences, 118*(9), e2023301118. https://doi.org/10.1073/pnas.2023301118

Ciobanu, R. O., Fokkema, T., & Nedelcu, M. (2017). Ageing as a migrant: Vulnerabilities, agency and policy implications. *Journal of Ethnic and Migration Studies, 43*(2), 164–181. https://doi.org/10.1080/1369183X.2016.1238903

Colantone, I., & Stanig, P. (2018). The trade origins of economic nationalism: Import competition and voting behavior in Western Europe. *American Journal of Political Science, 62*(4), 936–953. https://doi.org/10.1111/ajps.12358

Crowe, C., Liu, L., Bagnarol, N., & Fried, L. (2024). Loneliness prevention and the role of the public health system. *Perspectives in Public Health, 144*(1), 31–38.

Dahlberg, L., & McKee, K. J. (2014). Correlates of social and emotional loneliness in older people: Evidence from an English community study. *Aging & Mental Health, 18*(4), 504–514. https://doi.org/10.1080/13607863.2013.856863

De Freitas, J., Uğuralp, A. K., Uğuralp, Z., & Puntoni, S. (2024). AI companions reduce loneliness. *arXiv preprint arXiv*:2407.19096.

de Jong-Gierveld, J., & Kamphuis, F. (1985). The development of a Rasch-type loneliness scale. *Applied Psychological Measurement, 9*(3), 289–299. https://doi.org/10.1177/014662168500900307

de Jong-Gierveld, J., & van Tilburg, T. G. (2006). A 6-item scale for overall, emotional, and social loneliness: Confirmatory tests on survey data. *Research on Aging, 28*(5), 582–598. https://doi.org/10.1177/0164027506289723

DiTommaso, E., & Spinner, B. (1993). The development and initial validation of the social and emotional loneliness scale for adults (SELSA). *Personality and Individual Differences, 14*(1), 127–134. https://doi.org/10.1016/0191-8869(93)90182-390182-3)

Dwyer, P., & Papadimitriou, D. (2007). The social security rights of older international migrants in the European Union. *Journal of Ethnic and Migration Studies, 33*(8), 1301–1319. https://doi.org/10.1080/13691830600927773

Esaiasson, P., & Sohlberg, J. (2024). Social order in Sweden's politicized and vulnerable neighborhoods: The perspective of residents. *European Journal of Political Research*. Advance online publication. https://doi.org/10.1111/1475-6765.12723

Fokkema, T., & Ciobanu, R. O. (2021). Older migrants and loneliness: Scanning the field and looking forward. *European Journal of Ageing, 18*(3), 291–297. https://doi.org/10.1007/s10433-021-00646-2

Fokkema, T., & Naderi, R. (2013). Differences in late-life loneliness: A comparison between Turkish and native-born older adults in Germany. *European Journal of Ageing, 10*, 289–300. https://doi.org/10.1007/s10433-013-0267-7

Gest, J., Reny, T., & Mayer, J. (2018). Roots of the radical right: Nostalgic deprivation in the United States and Britain. *Comparative Political Studies, 51*(13), 1694–1719. https://doi.org/10.1177/0010414017720705

Gheнța, M., & Matei, A. (2025). Policy recommendations to address loneliness in later life. In M. Aartsen, I. Precupetu, & B. Suanet (Eds.), *Macro social influences on loneliness in later life: Towards a better understanding of the loneliness paradox in later life*. Springer.

Gidron, N., & Hall, P. A. (2017). The politics of social status: Economic and cultural roots of the populist right. *The British Journal of Sociology, 68*(S1), 57–84. https://doi.org/10.1111/1468-4446.12319

Gidron, N., & Hall, P. A. (2020). Populism as a problem of social integration. *Comparative Political Studies, 53*(7), 1027–1059. https://doi.org/10.1177/0010414019879947

Han, K. J. (2016). Income inequality and voting for radical right-wing parties. *Electoral Studies, 42*, 54–64. https://doi.org/10.1016/j.electstud.2016.02.001

Hansen, E. B. (2013). Older immigrants' use of public home care and residential care. *European Journal of Ageing, 11*(1), 41–53. https://doi.org/10.1007/s10433-013-0289-1

Hansen, T., Johansen, R., Straiton, M., Stene-Larsen, K., Tornes, R., & Reneflot, A. (2025). Digital bridges to social connection: A systematic review of digital interventions for loneliness and social isolation. Available at SSRN 5199280.

Hansen, T., Nes, R. B., Hynek, K., Nilsen, T. S., Reneflot, A., Stene-Larsen, K., Tornes, R. A., & Bidonde, J. (2024). Tackling social disconnection: An umbrella review of RCT-based interventions targeting social isolation and loneliness. *BMC Public Health, 24*(1), 1917.

Hawkley, L. C., & Cacioppo, J. T. (2010). Loneliness matters: A theoretical and empirical review of consequences and mechanisms. *Annals of Behavioral Medicine, 40*(2), 218–227.

Huxhold, O., Suanet, B., & Wetzel, M. (2022). Perceived social exclusion and loneliness: Two distinct but related phenomena. *Sociological Science, 9*, 430–453. https://doi.org/10.15195/v9.a17

Joshi, M., Finney, N., & Hale, J. M. (2024a). Loneliness and social isolation of ethnic minority/immigrant older adults: A scoping review. *Ageing & Society*. Advance online publication. https://doi.org/10.1017/S0144686X24000205

Joshi, M., Finney, N., & Hale, J. M. (2024b). Loneliness and social isolation of ethnic minority/immigrant older adults: A scoping review. *Ageing & Society*, 1–31. https://doi.org/10.1017/S0144686X24000205

Kim, M., Lee, S., Kim, S., Heo, J. I., Lee, S., Shin, Y. B., et al. (2025). Therapeutic potential of social Chatbots in alleviating loneliness and social anxiety: Quasi-experimental mixed methods study. *Journal of Medical Internet Research, 27*, e65589.

Klaesson, J., & Öner, Ö. (2021). Ethnic enclaves and segregation—self-employment and employment patterns among forced migrants. *Small Business Economics, 56*(3), 985–1006. https://doi.org/10.1007/s11187-019-00313-y

Klasen, L. J., Bünning, M., Kelle, N., Tesch-Römer, C., & Huxhold, O. (2025). The influence of societal crises on social integration and loneliness. In M. Aartsen, I. Precupetu, & B. Suanet (Eds.), *Macro social influences on loneliness in later life. Towards a better understanding of the loneliness paradox in later life*. Springer.

Klok, J., van Tilburg, T. G., Suanet, B., Fokkema, T., & Huisman, M. (2017). National and transnational belonging among Turkish and Moroccan older migrants in The Netherlands: Protective against loneliness? *European Journal of Ageing, 14*, 341–351. https://doi.org/10.1007/s10433-017-0420-9

Langenkamp, A. (2021a). Enhancing, suppressing or something in between—loneliness and five forms of political participation across Europe. *European Societies, 23*(3), 311–332. https://doi.org/10.1080/14616696.2021.1916554

Langenkamp, A. (2021b). Lonely hearts, empty booths? The relationship between loneliness, reported voting behavior and voting as civic duty. *Social Science Quarterly, 102*(4), 1239–1254. https://doi.org/10.1111/ssqu.12946

Langenkamp, A., & Bienstman, S. (2022). Populism and layers of social belonging: Support of populist parties in Europe. *Political Psychology, 43*(5), 931–949. https://doi.org/10.1111/pops.12827

Lasgaard, M. (2022). Are loneliness interventions effective in reducing loneliness? A meta-analytic review of 128 studies. *European Journal of Public Health, 32*. https://doi.org/10.1093/eurpub/ckac129.266

Lau, S., & Gruen, G. E. (1992). The social stigma of loneliness: Effect of target person's and perceiver's sex. *Personality and Social Psychology Bulletin, 18*(2), 182–189.

Lee, S. (2025). Understanding late-life loneliness: Micro and meso-level determinants. In M. Aartsen, I. Precupetu, & B. Suanet (Eds.), *Macro social influences on loneliness in later life. Towards a better understanding of the loneliness paradox in later life*. Springer.

Li, L., Carrino, L., Reinhard, E., & Avendano, M. (2024). Has the UK campaign to end loneliness reduced loneliness and improved mental health in older age? A difference-in-differences design. *The American Journal of Geriatric Psychiatry, 32*(3), 358–372. https://doi.org/10.1016/j.jagp.2023.10.007

Lykes, V. A., & Kemmelmeier, M. (2014). What predicts loneliness? Cultural difference between individualistic and collectivistic societies in Europe. *Journal of Cross-Cultural Psychology, 45(3), 468–490.*

Maples, B., Cerit, M., Vishwanath, A., & Pea, R. (2024). Loneliness and suicide mitigation for students using GPT-3-enabled chatbots. *Mental Health Research, 3*(4). https://doi.org/10.1038/s44184-023-00047-6

Morrish, N., Choudhury, S., & Medina-Lara, A. (2023). What works in interventions targeting loneliness: A systematic review of intervention characteristics. *BMC Public Health, 23*(1), 2214.

Mudde, C., & Kaltwasser, R. C. (2018). Studying populism in comparative perspective: Reflections on the contemporary and future research agenda. *Comparative Political Studies, 51*(13), 1667–1693. https://doi.org/10.1177/0010414018789490

Norman, A. (1985). *Triple jeopardy: Growing old in a second homeland.* Centre for Policy on Ageing.

Norris, P., & Inglehart, R. (2019). *Cultural backlash: Trump, Brexit, and authoritarian populism.* Cambridge University Press. https://doi.org/10.1017/9781108595841

Nyqvist, F., McHugh Power, J., & Coll-Planas, L. (2025). Theorizing loneliness in later life - micro, meso and macro perspectives. In M. Aartsen, I. Precupetu, & B. Suanet (Eds.), *Macro social influences on loneliness in later life. Towards a better understanding of the loneliness paradox in later life. Springer.*

Pani, B., Crawford, J., & Allen, K. A. (2024). Can generative artificial intelligence Foster belongingness, social support, and reduce loneliness? A conceptual analysis. In Z. Lyu (Ed.), *Applications of generative AI.* Springer. https://doi.org/10.1007/978-3-031-46238-2_13

Perlman, D., & Peplau, L. A. (1981). Toward a social psychology of loneliness. In S. Duck & R. Gilmour (Eds.), *Personal relationships in disorder* (pp. 31–56). Academic Press.

Petersen, M. B., Osmundsen, M., & Areceneux, K. (2023). The "Need for Chaos" and motivations to share hostile political rumors. *American Political Science Review, 117*(4), 1486–1505. https://doi.org/10.1017/S0003055422001447

Pew Research Center. (2022). *Populists in Europe—especially those on the right—have increased their vote shares in recent elections.*

Precupetu, I., Pop, C., & Aartsen, M. (2025). Macro-level influences on loneliness in later life. An fsQCA analysis. In M. Aartsen, I. Precupetu, & B. Suanet (Eds.), *Macro social influences on loneliness in later life. Towards a better understanding of the loneliness paradox in later life.* Springer.

Rapolienė, G., & Aartsen, M. (2022). Lonely societies: Low trust societies? Further explanations for national variations in loneliness among older Europeans. *European Journal of Ageing, 19*(3), 485–494. https://doi.org/10.1007/s10433-021-00649-z

Reinhardt, G. Y., Vidovic, D., & Hammerton, C. (2021). Understanding loneliness: A systematic review of the impact of social prescribing initiatives on loneliness. *Perspectives in Public Health, 141*(4), 204–213.

Rietdijk, N. (2021). Radicalizing populism and the making of an Echo chamber: The case of the Italian anti-vaccination movement. *Krisis Journal for Contemporary Philosophy, 41*(1), 114–134. https://doi.org/10.21827/krisis.41.1.37163

Rooduijn, M., Bonikowski, B., & Parlevliet, J. (2021). Populist and nativist attitudes: Does ingroup-outgroup thinking spill over across domains? *European Union Politics, 22*(2), 248–265. https://doi.org/10.1177/1465116521992876

Schoenmakers, E. (2020). Why and how to talk about loneliness. *Journal of Social Intervention: Theory and Practice, 29*(4), 4–18. https://doi.org/10.18352/jsi.646

Seifert, A. (2025). Information and communication technologies and the risk to loneliness. In M. Aartsen, I. Precupetu, & B. Suanet (Eds.), *Macro social influences on loneliness in later life. Towards a better understanding of the loneliness paradox in later life*. Springer.

Sha, S., Loveys, K., Qualter, P., Shi, H., Krpan, D., & Galizzi, M. (2024). Efficacy of relational agents for loneliness across age groups: A systematic review and meta-analysis. *BMC Public Health, 24*(1), 1802. https://doi.org/10.1186/s12889-024-19153-x

Skjuve, M., Følstad, A., Fostervold, K. I., & Brandtzaeg, P. B. (2021). My chatbot companion-a study of human-chatbot relationships. *International Journal of Human-Computer Studies, 149*, 102601. https://doi.org/10.1016/j.ijhcs.2021.102601

Smith, K., Weinschenk, A., & Panagopoulos, C. (2023). On pins and needles: Anxiety, politics and the 2020 U.S. presidential election. *Journal of Elections, Public Opinion and Parties, 34*(3), 409–426. https://doi.org/10.1080/17457289.2023.2189258

Song, X., Xu, B., & Zhao, Z. (2022). Can people experience romantic love for artificial intelligence? An empirical study of intelligent assistants. *Information & Management, 59*(2), 103595. https://doi.org/10.1016/j.im.2021.103595

Steptoe, A., Shankar, A., Demakakos, P., & Wardle, J. (2013). Social isolation, loneliness, and all-cause mortality in older men and women. *Proceedings of the National Academy of Sciences, 110*(15), 5797–5801.

Stoetzer, L. F., Giesecke, J., & Klüver, H. (2021). How does income inequality affect the support for populist parties? *Journal of European Public Policy, 30*(1), 1–20. https://doi.org/10.1080/13501763.2021.1981981

Stone, P. (2020). A broader, more inclusive definition of AI. *Journal of Artificial General Intelligence, 11(2), 63–65.* https://doi.org/10.2478/jagi-2020-0003

Suanet, B., & Aartsen, M. (2025). Linking life course theory to multi-level explanations of loneliness: Towards a sociology of loneliness. In M. Aartsen, I. Precupetu, & B. Suanet (Eds.), *Macro social influences on loneliness in later life: Towards a better understanding of the loneliness paradox in later life*. Springer.

Suanet, B., & Pavlidis, G. (2025). And, you know: There's such a thing as society: Towards a clarification of the 'loneliness paradox' by a macrofication of loneliness studies. In M. Aartsen, I. Precupetu, & B. Suanet (Eds.), *Macro social influences on loneliness in later life: Towards a better understanding of the loneliness paradox in later life*. Springer.

Ten Kate, R. L. F., Bilecen, B., & Steverink, N. (2020). A closer look at loneliness: Why do first-generation migrants feel more lonely than their native Dutch counterparts? *The Gerontologist, 60*(2), 291–301. https://doi.org/10.1093/geront/gnz192

Tufa, L. (2025). The social infrastructure of loneliness. A scoping review of societal influences and their implications. In M. Aartsen, I. Precupetu, & B. Suanet (Eds.), *Macro social influences on loneliness in later life: Towards a better understanding of the loneliness paradox in later life*. Springer.

Van Regenmprtel, S., Tiilikainen, E., Ristolainen, H., Burholt, V., & Dahlberg, L. (2025). Social exclusion perspective on loneliness in later life. In M. Aartsen, I. Precupetu, & B. Suanet (Eds.), *Macro social influences on loneliness in later life: Towards a better understanding of the loneliness paradox in later life*. Springer.

van Tilburg, T. G. (2021). Social, emotional, and existential loneliness: A test of the multidimensional concept. *The Gerontologist, 61*(7), e335–e344. https://doi.org/10.1093/geront/gnaa082

van Tilburg, T. G. (2025). Unravelling the socio-cultural influence on loneliness. In M. Aartsen, I. Precupetu, & B. Suanet (Eds.), *Macro social influences on loneliness in later life. Towards a better understanding of the loneliness paradox in later life*. Springer.

van Tilburg, T. G., & Fokkema, T. (2021). Stronger feelings of loneliness among Moroccan and Turkish older adults in The Netherlands: In search for an explanation. *European Journal of Ageing, 18*(3), 311–322. https://doi.org/10.1007/s10433-020-00562-x

Vasile, M., & Aartsen, M. (2025). Loneliness prevalence in different age groups in Europe. In M. Aartsen, I. Precupetu, & B. Suanet (Eds.), *Macro social influences on loneliness in later life: Towards a better understanding of the loneliness paradox in later life*. Springer.

Vidovic, D., Reinhardt, G. Y., & Hammerton, C. (2021). Can social prescribing foster individual and community Well-being? A systematic review of the evidence. *International Journal of Environmental Research and Public Health, 18*(10), 5276. https://doi.org/10.3390/ijerph18105276

Wang, P. (2019). On defining artificial intelligence. *Journal of Artificial General Intelligence, 10*(2), 1–37.

Weiss, R. S. (1973). *Loneliness: The experience of emotional and social isolation*. MIT Press.

Wu, Z., & Penning, M. J. (2015). Immigration and loneliness in later life. *Ageing & Society, 35*(1), 64–95. https://doi.org/10.1017/S0144686X13000470

Xie, T., & Pentina, I. (2022). Attachment theory as a framework to understand relationships with social chatbots: A case study of Replika. *Proceedings of the 55th Hawaii international conference on system sciences*, 2046-2055. DOI: https://doi.org/10.24251/hicss.2022.258.

Yang, K., & Victor, C. (2011). Age and loneliness in 25 European nations. *Ageing & Society, 31*(8), 1368–1388. https://doi.org/10.1017/S0144686X1000139X

Marja Aartsen , PhD, is currently research professor and social gerontologist at NOVA – Norwegian Social Research at OsloMet. She is specialized in longitudinal research on social relations, social exclusion, loneliness, and cognitive functioning in the second half of life. She is interested in social issues related to aging in place and active or successful ageing. Resent research projects and collaborations include gendered pathways to exclusion from social relations (GENPATH), reducing old-age social exclusion (ROSENET) and a multidimensional approach to social exclusion and its health consequences (AMASE). She was editor of the European Journal of Ageing from 2017 until summer 2022.

Bianca Suanet , PhD, is a sociologist, specializing in loneliness, social relations, and care use among older adults, especially in relation to the impact of societal and policy changes. She was formerly Professor of Ageing and Social Change at the Linköping University in Sweden and Associate Professor in Sociology and Head of the Social Functioning Group of the Longitudinal Aging Study Amsterdam at the Vrije Universiteit Amsterdam in the Netherlands. Currently, her research projects encompass studies on the relationship between macro-level factors and loneliness, and optimizing interventions against loneliness based on scientific evidence for older migrants.

Thomas Hansen , PhD, is a research professor at the Norwegian Institute of Public Health, specializing in subjective well-being, loneliness, and aging. His research also covers childlessness, volunteering, and caregiving. He is currently involved in developing a national strategy on loneliness, leading two government-commissioned systematic reviews on the effectiveness of interventions—one broad and one focused on digital approaches. He is also leading a related project, commissioned by the Ministry of Health, mapping mental health and loneliness among older adults.

Iuliana Precupetu , PhD, is a senior researcher at the Research Institute for Quality of Life, Romanian Academy, and the Research Institute of the University of Bucharest. She is a sociologist specializing in quality of life, health inequalities and social exclusion in later life. Her current interests include the relationship between social exclusion in older age and mental health, as well as the application of life course methods to quality of life research. Most recently, she coordinated the AMASE research project - A multidimensional approach to social exclusion in later life – health consequences for ageing populations.

Open Access This chapter is licensed under the terms of the Creative Commons Attribution 4.0 International License (http://creativecommons.org/licenses/by/4.0/), which permits use, sharing, adaptation, distribution and reproduction in any medium or format, as long as you give appropriate credit to the original author(s) and the source, provide a link to the Creative Commons license and indicate if changes were made.

The images or other third party material in this chapter are included in the chapter's Creative Commons license, unless indicated otherwise in a credit line to the material. If material is not included in the chapter's Creative Commons license and your intended use is not permitted by statutory regulation or exceeds the permitted use, you will need to obtain permission directly from the copyright holder.

The manufacturer's authorised representative in the EU is Springer Nature Customer Service Centre GmbH, Europaplatz 3, 69115 Heidelberg, Germany. If you have any concerns regarding our products, please contact ProductSafety@springernature.com

Printed and bound by CPI Group (UK) Ltd, Croydon, CR0 4YY

30/09/2026

02225570-0013